P9-BYC-423

Delmar's HANDBOOK OF Essential Skills and Procedures for Chairside Dental Assisting

Donna J. Phinney, CDA, BA, MEd
Spokane Community College
Judy H. Halstead, CDA, BA
Spokane Community College

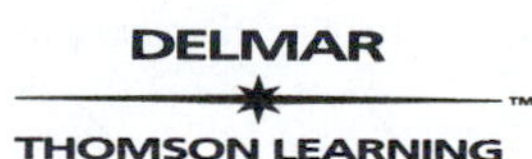

Australia Canada Mexico Singapore Spain United Kingdom United States

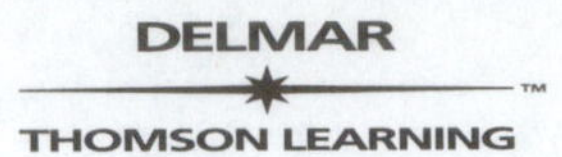

Delmar's Handbook of Essential Skills and Procedures for Chairside Dental Assisting
Donna J. Phinney, Judy H. Halstead

Business Unit Director:
William Brottmiller

Acquisitions Editor:
Marie Linvill

Editorial Assistant:
Jennifer Frisbee

Executive Marketing Manager:
Dawn F. Gerrain

Project Editor:
Maureen M. E. Grealish

Production Coordinator:
Nina Lontrato

Art/Design Coordinator
Connie Lundberg-Watkins

Cover Design:
Connie Lundberg-Watkins

COPYRIGHT © 2002 by Delmar, a division of Thomson Learning, Inc. Thomson Learning™ is a trademark used herein under license

Printed in the United States of America
1 2 3 4 5 XXX 05 04 03 02 01

For more information, contact Delmar,
3 Columbia Circle, PO Box 15015,
Albany, NY 12212-0515.

Or find us on the World Wide Web at
http://www.delmar.com

ALL RIGHTS RESERVED. No part of this work covered by the copyright hereon may be reproduced or used in any form or by any means—graphic, electronic, or mechanical, including photocopying, recording, taping, Web distribution or information storage and retrieval systems—without written permission of the publisher.

For permission to use material from this text or product, contact us by
Tel (800) 730-2214
Fax (800) 730-2215
www.thomsonrights.com

Library of Congress Cataloging-in-Publication Data

Phinney, Donna J.
Delmar's handbook of essential skills and procedures for chairside dental assisting / Donna J. Phinney, Judy H. Halstead.
p. cm.
Includes index.
ISBN 0-7668-3457-3 (alk. paper)
1. Dental assistants—Handbooks, manuals, etc. 2. Dentistry—Handbooks, manuals, etc. 3. Dental technicians—Handbooks, manuals, etc. I. Title: Handbook of essential skills and procedures for chairside dental assisting. II. Halstead, Judy H. III. Title.
RK60.5.P483 2001
617.6'0233—dc21

2001037291

NOTICE TO THE READER

Publisher does not warrant or guarantee any of the products described herein or perform any independent analysis in connection with any of the product information contained herein. Publisher does not assume, and expressly disclaims, any obligation to obtain and include information other than that provided to it by the manufacturer.

The reader is expressly warned to consider and adopt all safety precautions that might be indicated by the activities herein and to avoid all potential hazards. By following the instructions contained herein, the reader willingly assumes all risks in connection with such instructions.

The Publisher makes no representation or warranties of any kind including, but not limited to, the warranties of fitness for a particular purpose or merchantability, nor are any such representations implied with respect to the material set forth herein, and the publisher takes no responsibility with respect to such material. The publisher shall not be liable for any special, consequential, or exemplary damages resulting, in whole or part, from the readers' use of, or reliance upon, this material.

CONTENTS

PREFACE

This book is designed as a learning tool for dental assistants who have no previous professional education or are in a short-term training program. It is also ideal as an office handbook for new dental assisting staff. The book is a resized and reformatted approach of the main dental assisting textbook, *Delmar's Dental Assisting, A Comprehensive Approach.* Rather than the comprehensive coverage of the main text, this handbook focuses on the essential clinical dental assisting skills without going into depth in the background information. The text is divided into four primary sections. The first section, "Introduction to Dental Assisting and Basic Dental Sciences" (Chapters 1–5), provides information about the profession of dental assisting, along with oral health, head and neck anatomy, tooth anatomy and supporting structures, and dental charting. The second section, "Preclinical Dental Skills" (Chapters 6–8), covers infection control and management of hazardous materials. This section also covers preparing the patient, reviewing health history, and reading vital signs. The third section, "Clinical Dental Procedures" (Chapters 9–21), covers chairside assisting skills, dental instruments and tray systems, dental radiography, topical and local anesthesia, dental cements and laboratory materials, and the dental specialties. The final section, "Advanced Functions" (Chapters 22–24), covers coronal polish, cavity liners, varnish and cement bases, pit and fissure sealants, bleaching techniques, dental dam, matrix and wedge techniques, retraction cord, and temporary restorations.

The chapters include the following pedagogical features:

- Chapter objectives
- Key terms
- In-text icons indicating handwashing, gloves, mask and protective eyewear, basic setup, and expanded function
- Step-by-step procedures
- Detailed information on dental assisting competencies
- Icons at the beginning of procedures to indicate which function, instruments, and protective equipment are needed
- Equipment and supplies lists prior to procedures
- Boxed information containing tips and summaries

SECTION I

Introduction to Dental Assisting and Basic Dental Sciences

1 Dental Assisting—The Profession

2 Oral Health

3 Head and Neck Anatomy

4 Tooth Anatomy and Supporting Structures

5 Dental Charting

CHAPTER 1

Dental Assisting—The Profession

CDA

OBJECTIVES

The student should strive to meet the following objectives and demonstrate an understanding of the facts and principles presented in this chapter:

1. Explain what DDS and DMD stand for.
2. Identify the eight specialties of dentistry.
3. Describe generally what career skills are performed by dental hygienists, dental assistants, and dental laboratory technicians.
4. List the education required for and the professional organizations that represent each profession.
5. Define the Dental Practice Act and what it encompasses.
6. Identify who oversees the Dental Practice Act and how licenses for the dental field are obtained.
7. Define expanded functions.
8. Identify due care and give examples of malpractice.
9. Identify the responsibilities of the dental team with regard to dental records.
10. Define ethics.

KEY TERMS

American Dental Assistants Association (ADAA) (p. 10)

American Dental Association (ADA) (p. 8)

American Dental Hygienists Association (ADHA) (p. 9)

American Dental Laboratory Technicians Association (ADLTA) (p. 12)

certified dental assistant (CDA) (p. 9)

Dental Assisting National Board, Inc. (DANB) (p. 9)

dental jurisprudence (p. 12)

Dental Practice Act (p. 12)

dental public health (p. 7)

Doctrine of Respondeat Superior (p. 13)

Dr. C. Edmund Kells (p. 8)

due care (p. 13)

endodontics (p. 7)

ethics (p. 12)

expanded functions (p. 12)

expert witnesses (p. 14)

forensic dentistry (p. 7)

Juliette Southard (p. 10)

malpractice (p. 14)

negligence (p. 14)

oral and maxillofacial surgery (p. 7)

oral pathology (p. 7)

orthodontics (p. 7)

pediatric dentistry (p. 7)

periodontics (p. 7)

prosthodontics (p. 7)

statutes (p. 12)

The Career of Dental Assisting

Dental assisting is an allied health profession that offers many exciting opportunities. Today's dental assistant can choose employment in a solo or partnership dental practice, a group practice, dental specialty practice, or from many other opportunities. The dental assistant can work as a chairside assistant, dental receptionist, clinical coordinator, or dental practice manager assistant. The opportunities are numerous because the modern dentist employs an average of four dental auxiliaries.

The dental assistant's salary and benefits vary according to the specific position, the responsibilities within the position, the location of the practice, and the skill level of the dental assistant.

Employment for the Dental Assistant

Whether graduating from an accredited program, secondary, or postsecondary dental assisting program, it is advisable to evaluate the opportunities available.

Solo Practices

The majority of dentists practice in solo offices. The majority of dental assistants are employed in solo practices. Each practice is as different as the dental team employed in that practice.

Partnership Practices

Many dentists work in a partnership practice where two dentists work together and share the responsibilities. In a partnership practice, a dental assistant may work for the dentists jointly or for only one of the dentists. Often the hours available to patients will be extended and therefore the need will arise for dental assistants to work different shifts. This may be an option for a dental assistant who needs to work evenings or has a varying schedule.

Group Practice

Another type of dental office is the group practice. In a group practice, any number of dentists (both general and specialty) may share a building and still remain independent. Because there is usually interaction between each staff in a group practice, a dental assistant who likes to work with a larger number of individuals may be attracted to employment in a group practice.

Dental Specialty Practice

A number of dental practices are specialty practices. If a dental assistant likes to assist primarily in oral and maxillofacial surgery, endodontics, periodontics, orthodontics, prosthodontics, pathology, pediatric dentistry, or dental public health, specialty practices provide this option. However, few employment opportunities are available in the areas of pathology and dental public health.

Other Employment Choices

Dental assistants may secure employment in government clinics that care for patients who are eligible to receive dental treatment at a reduced rate. Often federal or state grants fund programs to meet the specific needs of people who cannot afford dental care. Usually the guidelines of the programs change or have to be renewed annually. A dental assistant is an employee hired by the overseer of the grant. This dental assistant may receive great satisfaction treating patients in this type of employment.

School Clinics and Laboratories. Dental schools and dental assisting schools also employ dental assistants to work in the clinic with students, to teach, and/or to be administrators of the program.

Veterans' Hospitals. Veterans' hospitals hire dental assistants to help the dentists on staff in the clinics. Employment in the area must be obtained through the civil service office.

Dental Supply Companies. Dental supply companies hire dental assistants as sales representatives of equipment and supplies. Normally, a dental assistant in this position does not utilize his or her chairside skills, but becomes knowledgeable about the products and travels to various dental offices, giving product knowledge and ordering supplies.

Insurance Companies. Dental assistants are also hired by insurance companies to process dental insurance claims. Having knowledge and background in dental terminology and procedures is an asset in understanding procedures and processing dental insurance claims.

Upon learning the skills necessary to become a dental assistant, the employment opportunities are plentiful. The career of dental assisting is a very rewarding one, both professionally and personally. The work environment is pleasant and usually does not require overnight or evening shifts. The goal of dental offices is to provide the best care possible for the patients. The patients are in turn appreciative of the dental assistants who care for their needs. Most days, dental assistants go home feeling good about having the skills and knowledge to provide quality dental care to the patients. Today's dental assistants are lifelong learners. They continue to improve their dental assisting skills and knowledge through continuing education to stay knowledgeable about new techniques and materials.

The Dental Team

Dentists

The requirements to become a dentist include an undergraduate education and graduate education from a dental school approved by the American Dental Association (ADA) Commission on Dental Accreditation. Currently, two to four years of undergraduate study and four years of dental school preparation (five at Harvard) are required to earn a dental degree. Depending upon the school, a Doctor of Dental Surgery (DDS) or Doctor of Medical Dentistry (DMD) degree is conferred.

Training to become a dental specialist requires two or more years of post-graduate dental education. To become licensed to practice, all dentists must take and pass both written and clinical examinations for the state(s) in which they wish to practice. All dental team members are required to follow the dental practice rules and regulations (statutes) promulgated by their respective state dental practice acts enforced by the state dental board. These statutes are designed to protect the health, safety, and welfare of the public. The dental practice act in each state specifies those acts that can legally be performed by licensed or otherwise credentialed dental professionals in that state. The dentist, whether owner of the practice or an employee of the practice, is legally responsible for supervising dental team members.

Specialties of Dentistry. A dentist who practices all phases of dentistry is referred to as a general dentist or general practitioner. Occasionally, when the treatment required exceeds the scope of his or her training, the general dentist refers cases to a dental specialist. The ADA recognizes the following eight dental specialties:

1. **Dental public health** is the specialty concerned with the prevention of dental disease. The public health dentist works with the community to promote dental health.
2. **Endodontics** is concerned with the pathology and morphology of the dental pulp and surrounding tissues due to injury and disease. If a patient is referred for a root canal, he or she would see an endodontist.
3. **Oral pathology** is the specialty concerned with the diagnosis and nature of the diseases that affect the oral cavity. A patient who has a lesion unknown to the general dentist may be referred to the oral pathologist for further diagnosis and treatment.
4. **Oral and maxillofacial surgery** is concerned with the diagnosis and surgical treatment of the oral and maxillofacial region due to injury, disease, or defects. A patient having third molars (wisdom teeth) removed may be referred to an oral and maxillofacial surgeon.
5. **Orthodontics** is concerned with diagnosis, supervision, guidance, and correction of the malocclusion of the dentofacial structures. Braces for straightening teeth are placed by the orthodontist.
6. **Pediatric dentistry** is concerned with prevention of oral disease and the diagnosis and treatment of oral care in children, from birth through adolescence. Other patients requiring special care due to emotional, mental, or physical problems are referred to the pediatric dentist.
7. **Periodontics** is the specialty concerned with the diagnosis and treatment of the diseases of the supporting and surrounding tissues of the tooth. The periodontist is also concerned with the prevention of periodontal disease. If a patient has plaque and calculus buildup and has lost some of the bone around the tooth due to periodontal disease, he or she would be referred to the periodontist for further evaluation and treatment.
8. **Prosthodontics** is concerned with the diagnosis, restoration, and maintenance of oral functions. This specialty is also concerned with the replacement of missing teeth through artificial means.

Another area that requires additional training but is not regarded as a specialty of dentistry is **forensic dentistry**. This is a relatively new area that deals with a wide range of services, such as identification of bite marks on the body and/or identification of an individual through tooth restorations and morphology utilizing dental records.

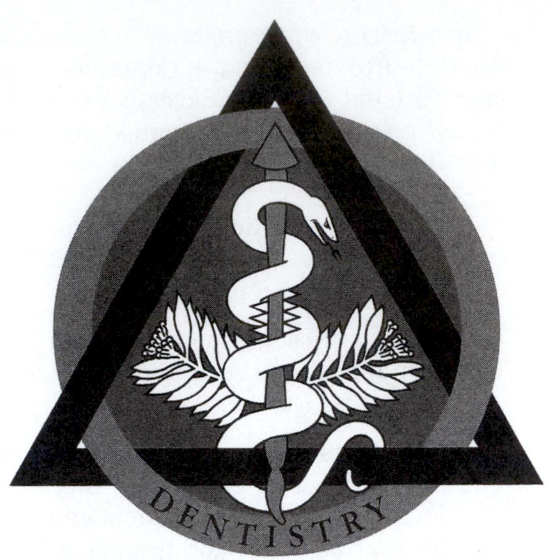

FIGURE 1–1 Logo for Dentistry.

The specialist works with the general dentist to provide the optimum oral health and patient care. During and once the specialty treatment is completed, the patient continues regular visits with his or her general dentist.

American Dental Association. In 1859, twenty-five delegates gathered in Niagara Falls, New York, and organized the **American Dental Association (ADA)** (Figure 1–1). The association was small at first, but after grouping all local associations according to states and then all states having representation to the national organization, the membership began to increase. Each state now has its own organization with bylaws approved by the ADA, and each local (regional) organization has ADA-approved bylaws that are sent to each state organization. For instance, Texas is represented by the Texas State Dental Association to the ADA, and the Texas State Dental Association comprises individual local dental associations. The official publication of the ADA is the *Journal of the American Dental Association (JADA).* The ADA also has a website, ADAONLINE (*http://www.ada.org*), which provides a link to the ADA for dental professionals and dental customers.

Dental Hygienists

Early in the 1900s in Bridgeport, Connecticut, several dentists, along with a leader, Dr. Alfred Civilon Fones, stated that they would not be able to be surgeons and to give preventive treatments. It was suggested that women be trained to clean teeth because "they have smaller and more gentle hands." At that time, it was uncommon for women to work outside the home. A dental assistant, Irene Morgan, was the first to be trained by Dr. Fones in dental hygiene. Dr. Fones developed a school in 1913, and it survives today as the Fones School of Dental Hygiene, University of Bridgeport. Graduates of either two- or four-year dental hygiene schools receive the title registered dental hygienist (RDH) after passing both written and clinical tests in the states in which they practice, and they are granted licenses. Dental hygienists specialize in providing dental prophylaxis, including the removal of plaque, stains, and calculus from the teeth, along with patient education. Many state practice acts allow licensed hygienists to apply tooth sealants; to expose, process, and mount dental radiographs; and to chart the conditions in the oral cavity. Some of the states allow hygienists to place restorative materials, to remove sutures, and to administer local anesthetics. The **American Dental Hygienists' Association (ADHA)** represents dental hygienists.

Dental Assistants

Prior to the early twentieth century, dentists hired men and boys to assist them in their dental practices. **Dr. C. Edmund Kells**, who practiced in New Orleans, hired a female to replace a male assistant in 1885. He wanted this "lady assistant" to be "quick, quiet, gentle, and attentive." A number of dentists were unsure about a female in the dental office, but the public accepted it quickly. It now allowed a woman to go to a dental office without being accompanied by her husband or maiden aunt. Due to the popularity of "Ladies in Attendance," dentists advertised the fact that they had hired female dental assistants by displaying signs in their windows.

Today, the educationally qualified dental assistant graduates from an institution accredited by the American Dental Association Commission on Dental Accreditation. Training is approximately one academic year in length and includes didactic, laboratory, and clinical content. Each state has a dental practice act that governs which duties dental assistants can perform. This varies from performing invasive procedures, such as placing retraction cord and dental dams, to noninvasive procedures, such as patient education. Dental assistants enable dentists to care for many more patients and to produce much more dentistry than they could alone. In the office, the person working directly with the dentist during patient procedures is the dental assistant.

Certified Dental Assistants. A 104-hour course was developed in 1947 to give credentials to assistants who passed the written and clinical examination. The **Dental Assisting National Board, Inc. (DANB)**, provides a pathway for competent, qualified dental assistants to obtain credentials. By passing a comprehensive written examination from DANB, the dental assistant can use the title of **certified dental assistant (CDA)**.

Dental Receptionists/Dental Practice Management Assistants. The *dental receptionist* position is becoming a more specialized area of dental assisting with the use of computers and computerized insurance claims. The dental receptionist or practice management assistant attends seminars to upgrade skills in the front office, computer technology, marketing, and accounting.

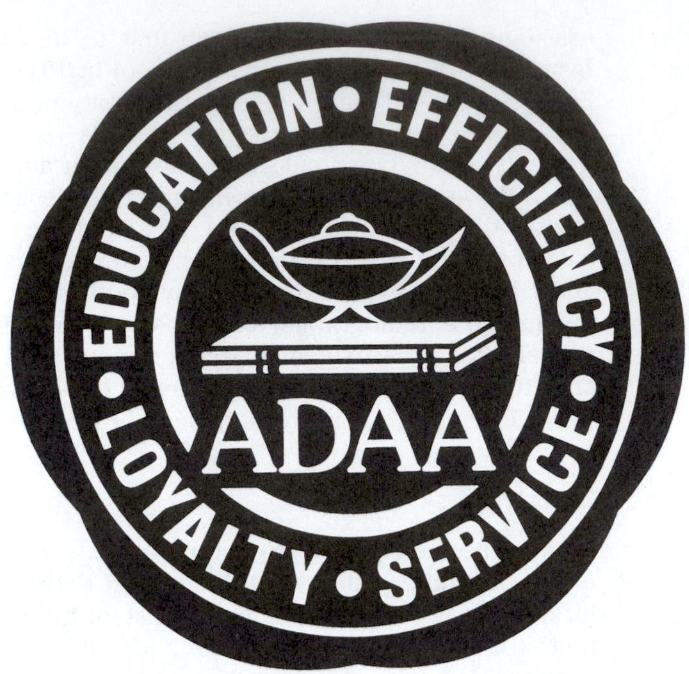

FIGURE 1–2 Logo for American Dental Assistants. (*Courtesy of American Dental Assistants Association; Chicago, IL.*)

American Dental Assistants Association. The **American Dental Assistants Association (ADAA)** was founded in 1924 by **Juliette Southard**, who was also its first president (Figures 1–2 and 1–3). The ADAA was founded on four principles: education, efficiency, loyalty, and service. Membership in the ADAA offers the dental assistant participation in national affairs of concern to the profession of dental assisting, opportunities in continuing education, professional liability insurance, and interaction with other professionals in the dental field. Another benefit of membership in ADAA is a subscription to *The Dental Assistant/Journal of the American Dental Assistants Association;* members may also access the ADAA's website at *http://dentalassistant.org* or through email at adaa1@aol.com.

Dental Laboratory Technicians

The dental laboratory technician may not work in the dental office with the other members of the team but is an essential member of the team. Some dental laboratory technicians are employed by the dentist; others work in privately owned dental laboratories.

Originally, dentists performed their own laboratory procedures; however, they eventually became too busy to complete the laboratory work and hired trained technicians to perform these skills. Today, whether the technicians are

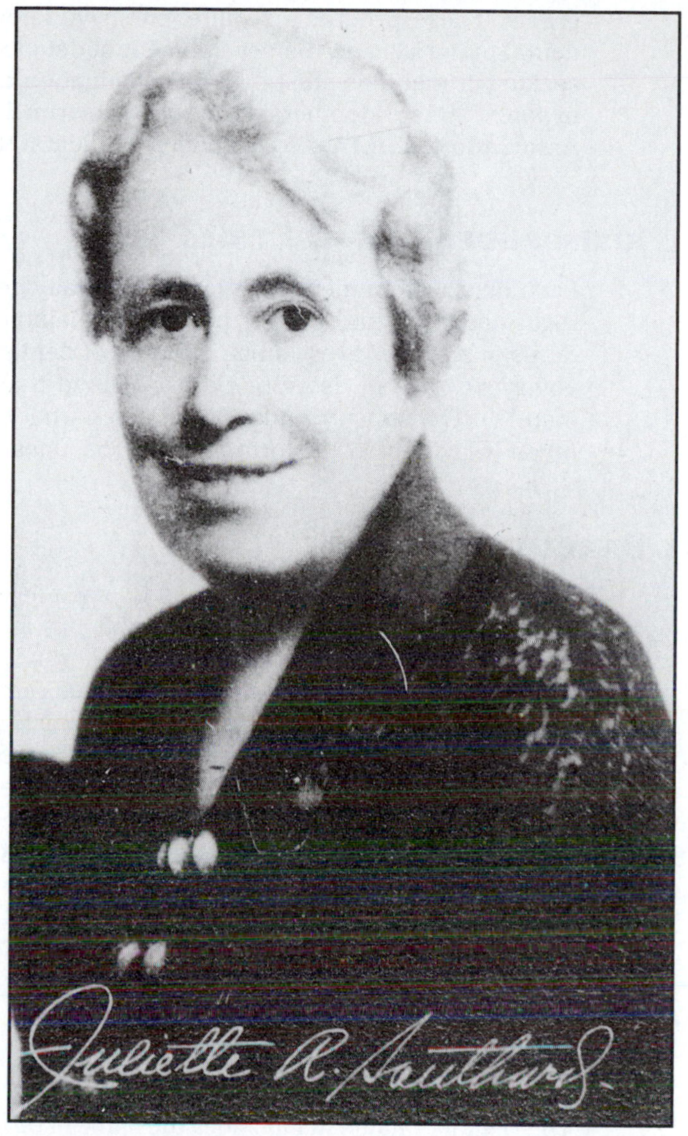

FIGURE 1–3 Juliette Southard, founder and first president of the American Dental Assistants Association. (*Courtesy of the American Dental Assistants Association, Chicago, IL*)

in the dental office or outside in a commercial dental laboratory, they provide such extra oral services as fabricating gold and porcelain restorations and partial and full dentures.

In most states, a dental laboratory technician is not required to have formal training and may be trained on the job. A large number of technicians have graduated from two-year ADA-accredited dental laboratory technician programs. These programs require extensive knowledge in dental anatomy and dental materials and the development of detailed mechanical skills. Individuals seeking credentials must pass an examination to become certified dental technicians (CDTs). Membership in the **American Dental Laboratory Technicians Association (ADLTA)** is also offered to dental technicians.

Dental Jurisprudence and Ethics

Each dental team member is faced with daily decisions that require judgments regarding legal and ethical principles. Maintaining professional ethical standards at all times is essential. The area of **dental jurisprudence**, the law(s) that governs dentistry, is more clearly defined than dental **ethics**, or moral judgment(s). The consequences of not doing what should be done can be imposed on an individual in the form of sanctions, fines, or imprisonment.

Dental Practice Act

In each state, **statutes** are enacted by each legislative body to make rules and regulations. The state board of dentistry is an administrative agency in each state that enforces these statutes and rules in regard to performance of specific functions. Each state has a **Dental Practice Act** that describes the legal restrictions and controls on the dentist, the hygienist, and, in some states, dental assistants. The Dental Practice Act describes the dental team members as licensed or nonlicensed and lists what are allowed or disallowed duties for each, including the **expanded functions** (delegated functions that require increased responsibility and skill) that may be performed by each dental team member. Even if the job classification or title is unused in the state Dental Practice Act, any employee working in a dental office is covered in the law. The Dental Practice Act of each state sets forth guidelines for eligibility for licensing and identifies the grounds by which this license can be suspended or repealed.

State Board of Dentistry

The Dental Practice Act includes the name of the administrative board that supervises the act, such as The State Board of Dental Examiners or Dental Quality Assurance Board, or Dental Board, of the state. This board has the responsibility of enforcing adherence to the Dental Practice Act of that specific state. The members of this board are appointed by the governor of that state, usually from a list of recommendations from the state dental association. The membership usually has one lay member from the state, and the rest of the board members are normally licensed dentists. Another function of this board is to examine applicants for dental licenses and to grant licenses if the criteria are met. Some state boards may also have a dental hygienist.

Licensed to Practice. A license is granted to a dentist who has met all minimum requirements. The license is to protect the public from unqualified individuals providing dental treatment. Each state requires that the dental hygienist become licensed as well. Some of the states require dental assistants to become licensed to perform specific dental tasks.

The factors for revoking, suspending, or denying a renewal of a license vary from state to state. Most states take action if the licensed person has a felony conviction and/or misdemeanors of drug addiction, moral corruptness, incompetence, or mental/physical disability that may cause harm to patients under his or her dental care.

Expanded Functions. Expanded functions are specific advanced tasks that require increased skill and responsibility. These functions are delegated by the dentist according to the Dental Practice Act within the state. Some states require additional education, certification, or registration to perform these functions. Like all functions the dental assistant performs, the expanded functions fall under the **Doctrine of Respondent Superior**. Translated from the Latin, this means "Let the master answer." So, if wrongdoing took place under the guidelines of employment, the dentist is liable for the negligent act. However, this does not mean that the dental assistant is not held responsible or cannot be sued. It merely means that a suit can be filed against either the employee or the dentist, or both.

The expanded functions are most often specified in the Dental Practice Act according to how they are to be delegated. They may be stipulated for general supervision, which means that the procedure authorized in the Dental Practice Act can be performed legally on a patient of record by the dental assistant under the general supervision of the dentist. If it is specified to be delegated under direct supervision, the dentist must be in the treatment facility to authorize this function and he or she must evaluate the performance of this procedure.

Certification, Licensure, and Registration. Dental assistants can become nationally certified by the Dental Assisting National Board, Inc. (DANB). Some states require dental assistants to be certified, licensed, or registered to perform specific functions in the dental office. The first state to grant licensure to dental assistants was Minnesota. Certification from DANB is granted after education or work requirements have been met, and a written test covering chairside, radiology, and infection control has been passed. Continuing education is required to maintain current certification from DANB, and many states require continuing education to maintain registration or licensure.

The Dentist, the Dental Assistant, and the Law

The dental assistant must thoroughly understand the law to protect the patient, the dentist, and the profession. Dental health care continues to change, and the dental assistant must understand how these changes are impacted by the law.

Standard of Care

The dentist and the dental team members have the responsibility to perform due care in treating all patients. **Due care** is what any reasonable and prudent dental care professional in the same circumstances would do. The dental professional must provide sufficient care, within his or her scope of training, in all dental procedures, not excluding prescribing, dispensing, or administering drugs.

Malpractice

Malpractice is failure to use due care in dental treatment, which is considered negligence. **Negligence** is the failure to exercise the standard of care that a reasonable person would exercise in similar circumstances. Negligence is the primary cause of malpractice suits. Negligence occurs when an individual suffers injury because of another person's failure to live up to the normal standard of care. Malpractice is professional negligence. There are four elements of negligence (sometimes called the four "Ds"): duty, derelict, direct cause, and damage. Dental professionals are held to a high standard of care by virtue of their knowledge, intelligence, and skills. It is their duty to provide high performance and not to be derelict (careless) in their skills. If they directly cause injury due to deviation from the normal standard of care and damage or harm occurs, they are negligent. At times, in a court of law, **expert witnesses** may testify with regard to the standard of care that is to be expected.

Dental Records

The dentist and dental team members must maintain accurate, up-to-date patient records. In litigation, the accuracy of the dental record directly relates to the credibility of the professionals. All treatment and charges must be reflected in patients' dental records. Charts must be written in ink and be legible and all necessary corrections should be made by drawing a line through the initial content and then making the correction, initialing it, and dating the new data.

Ethics

Ethics is defined in terms of what is right or wrong, or moral judgment of these two. In dentistry, it is defined by a code as The American Dental Association Principles of Ethics. Unlike the law, which rarely changes, ethics constantly change and evolve just as personal values and morals change and evolve.

The Dental Assistant and Jurisprudence

As the dental profession continues to advance, the dental assistant will have more decisions to make with regard to ethics and jurisprudence. Thus, it is necessary for the dental assistant to keep abreast of statutory changes and to make relevant decisions that reflect these changes. The dental assistant must always strive to practice work standards within the law, to manage patients in a professional manner, to maintain a high standard of care, to obtain prior written consent, to preserve patient confidentiality, to maintain legible accurate records, and to refrain from judging others who may possess differing belief systems.

CHAPTER 2

Oral Health

OBJECTIVES

The student should strive to meet the following objectives and demonstrate an understanding of the facts and principles presented in this chapter:

1. Describe how plaque forms and affects the teeth.
2. Demonstrate the Bass toothbrushing techniques.
3. Identify types of dental floss and demonstrate flossing technique.
4. Describe fluoride and its use in dentistry.
5. List and explain the forms of fluoride. Describe how to prepare a patient and demonstrate fluoride application.

KEY TERMS

caries (p. 17)
demineralization (p. 16)
plaque (p. 16)

Introduction

An important role of the dental assistant is preventive dentistry. Dentistry is about preventing oral disease, such as dental decay, and caring for periodontal disease. It is important to educate the public on how to prevent disease. The dental assistant must be knowledgeable about the many products available to aid patients in maintaining their teeth and gums. The dental assistant must be a good listener and be able to evaluate the needs of patients. Dental assistants must also know how to motivate patients to be effective in their oral hygiene care. Fluoride has been proven to be effective in reducing dental caries. The dental assistant needs to have background knowledge of fluoride to educate patients in its usage and benefits. A final area of oral health and prevention is nutrition. Many patients will not be knowledgeable about the kinds of foods to aid them in cleansing their teeth or which foods perpetuate decay. The dental assistant, after discussions with the patient, can identify nutritional concerns and further assist the patient in choosing foods that will benefit his or her oral health.

Preventive Dentistry

The goal of preventive dentistry is that each individual maintain optimal oral health. To be effective in preventive dentistry, the dental assistant must first care for his or her teeth properly and practice good nutrition.

- Brush and floss daily to remove plaque and bacteria.
- Disclose periodically to evaluate the effectiveness of brushing and flossing.
- Follow a fluoride program while the teeth are developing to allow them to be strong and decay resistant. The fluoride program includes office applications and home treatments.
- Follow a good nutrition and exercise program to maintain overall health. Good nutrition over a lifetime allows strong teeth and bones to develop and be maintained.
- Schedule regular dental visits for a thorough examination, oral prophylaxis, and necessary dental treatment.

Plaque Formation

Dental **plaque** is a sticky mass that contains bacteria and grows in colonies on the teeth. Most people have missed areas while brushing their teeth and noted that a soft, white, sticky mass forms. This is plaque and other soft deposits. The bacteria in plaque is fed by the sugar in foods. The bacteria-rich plaque converts the sugar into acid. In time, the acid attacks the tooth and eventually causes **demineralization,** where the minerals, calcium, and phosphate are lost from the enamel surface. Patients who have had orthodontic appliances may have demineralization on the tooth surface where the brackets were located. When the brackets are removed, demineralization appears as a whitish area on the tooth. It developed because plaque was not removed routinely around the brackets. If plaque continues to attack the tooth, it will cause decay, or **caries**. Once dental decay has begun, the area should be restored by a dentist.

Patient Motivation

Preventing dental disease is ultimately the responsibility of the patient. However, dental auxiliaries spend a great deal of time educating and motivating patients to care for their teeth and oral cavities. The first aspect of patient motivation is for the dental assistant to assess oral hygiene and listen to the patient. Listening to the patient provides insight into the patient's attitude toward oral hygiene and allows the assistant to get a better idea how to motivate and communicate with the patient. It will be best to work with the patients to help them recognize their dental problems, problem solve together to develop solutions, and then provide motivation and aid them in setting oral hygiene goals.

Each patient should be treated as an individual, taking into consideration the patient's age, oral hygiene knowledge, skills, attitude, and any special considerations. Different age groups have characteristics that are normally identifiable; however, these characteristics are not absolute.

Home Care

The patient has the ultimate responsibility of caring for his or her oral health. The dental assistant can suggest ideas to make this task simple. The dental assistant's goals should closely parallel the ideas that stimulated the patient's desire to meet these goals. These ideas, of course, will be different for each patient. If what the patient has been doing is working and he or she is not developing periodontal disease or dental decay, then acknowledge that he or she is doing a good job and encourage him or her to keep it up.

Oral Hygiene Aids

A number of oral hygiene aids are available today for patient use. It is important to keep in mind that the more simple the task, the more chance of getting it accomplished. Adding a large number of steps makes it more difficult to accomplish the task daily. Suggestions for the proper aid comes from the dental team members. The dental assistant should keep abreast of the aids on the market and know how they can help specific patients.

Disclosing Agents. Most individuals are visual in their approach to life. Being able to see plaque makes it easier for the dental assistant to show what it is and how and when it should be removed. Disclosing agents have been

PROCEDURE

2-1 Applying Disclosing Agent for Plaque Identification

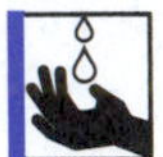 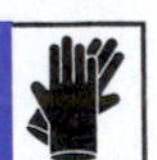 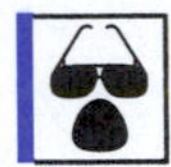 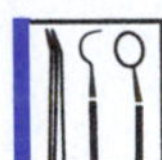

The procedure is performed by the dental assistant or dental hygienist. During the hygiene appointment, disclosing would be done to identify plaque and its location for the patient and operator. In some offices, a record of plaque location is charted and referred to during future appointments. Means of removing the plaque then are discussed and demonstrated.

EQUIPMENT AND SUPPLIES

- Basic setup: mouth mirror, explorer, and cotton pliers
- Saliva ejector, evacuator tip (HVE), and air/water syringe tip
- Cotton rolls, cotton tip applicator, and gauze sponges
- Petroleum jelly (lubricant)
- Disclosing agent (liquid or tablet) and dappen dish
- Plaque chart and red pencil

PROCEDURE STEPS

1. The operator examines the oral cavity and reviews the health history.
2. The operator applies the petroleum jelly (lubricant) to the patient's lips (some dentists may want the petroleum jelly on any tooth-colored restorations to prevent staining).
3. The operator applies the liquid using the dappen dish and a cotton tip applicator. Each attainable surface of the teeth should be stained with the disclosing solution.
4. If using the disclosing tablets, the operator instructs the patient to chew the tablets and then swish his or her saliva around for fifteen seconds.
5. The remaining solution is rinsed and evacuated from the area.
6. The patient uses a hand mirror to see the plaque and the operator uses a mouth mirror and an air/water syringe to identify and chart the plaque.
7. The operator demonstrates to the patient proper methods of brushing and flossing to remove plaque.

available for a number of years and are used as a motivating factor in oral hygiene. The agent is a temporary coloration (normally red) that makes plaque visible. The disclosing agent comes in a tablet that can be chewed, a solution that the dental assistant can paint on the teeth, or a drop that can be placed on the tongue (Procedure 2–1).

Toothbrushing

Most patients use toothbrushes; however, many have never been shown proper techniques and the methods recommended today. The patient should be shown that the toothbrush only cleans three of the five surfaces of the tooth. The proximal (between the teeth) tooth surfaces normally are not accessible with a toothbrush. Patients have a variety of toothbrushes to select from today. Dental assistants need to stay informed of the current choices available so that they can answer the patients' questions appropriately. Manual toothbrushes are powered by the human hand. Automatic toothbrushes are powered by electricity or batteries. The toothbrush itself does the moving while merely held by the individual. Automatic toothbrushes normally are supplied with recharging units.

Brushing Techniques for the Manual Toothbrush

There are several toothbrushing techniques that can be used to obtain proper oral hygiene. Any technique should allow for all the surfaces of all the teeth to be cleaned. Brushing does not clean the interproximal areas. Some patients will be successful in noting the amount of time spent on brushing by using a timer. Normally, two to three minutes is recommended to clean the facial, lingual, occlusal, and incisal surfaces of all the teeth. A pattern should be developed by the patient to ensure that no area is missed. Some patients like the counting system where five to ten strokes are made in each area. Starting at the same point each time when brushing is a good idea. The area could be the maxillary (upper) right facial surface (cheek and lip side), then continue around the entire surface to the maxillary left. From that position, the lingual side (tongue side) of the arch can be cleaned from the left to the right. The mandibular (lower) teeth can be cleaned in the same manner starting from the right, continuing to the left, and then cleaning the lingual side from the left to the right. It does not matter what the pattern is; it only matters that no teeth are left uncleaned. The heel or the toe of the toothbrush can be used effectively on the more narrow anterior areas. There are five commonly used brushing techniques: Bass or modified Bass, Charters, Modified Stillman, Rolling Stroke, and the Modified Scrub. The Bass or modified Bass is the most popular in the dental community.

Bass or Modified Bass Brushing Technique. The Bass technique is named for Dr. C. Bass, a dentist who was an early advocate of preventive dentistry. The Bass brushing technique is used to remove plaque next to and directly beneath the gingival margin (Procedure 2–2).

Flossing

Dental flossing (Procedure 2–3) is the second essential element of a good oral hygiene program and should be performed daily. Dental floss has been shown to be the most effective way to remove bacterial plaque and other debris from otherwise inaccessible areas, the proximal surfaces of the teeth.

PROCEDURE

2-2 Bass or Modified Bass Brushing Technique

The procedure is explained to the patient to teach a toothbrushing technique.

EQUIPMENT AND SUPPLIES

- Toothbrush

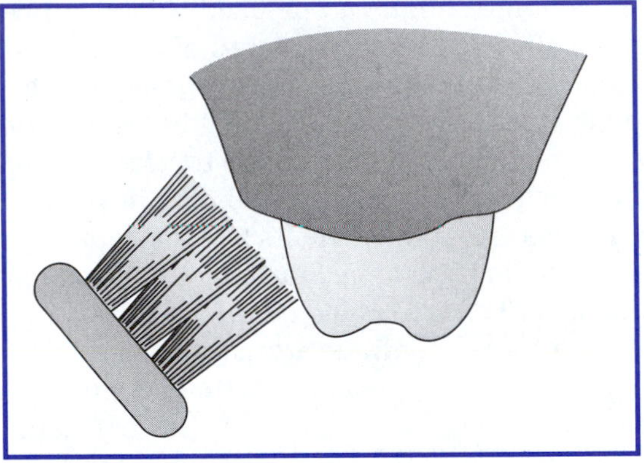

FIGURE 2–1 The initial position of the toothbrush when using the Bass technique.

PROCEDURE STEPS

Bass

1. Grasp the brush and place it so that the bristles are at a 45-degree angle, with the tips of the bristles directed straight into the gingival sulcus (Figure 2–1).
2. Using the tips of the bristles, vibrate back and forth with short, light strokes for a count of ten, allowing the tips of the bristle to enter the sulcus and cover the gingival margin.
3. Lift the brush and continue into the next area or group of teeth until all areas have been cleaned.
4. Use the toe bristles of the brush to clean the lingual (tongue) anterior area in the arch.

Modified Bass

1. Follow all the steps of the Bass technique.
2. After the vibratory motion has been completed in each area, sweep the bristles over the crown of the tooth, toward the chewing surface of the tooth.

Oral Hygiene for Special Needs Patients

Dental assistants may be called upon to become creative to meet the oral hygiene needs of patients who have special needs. Patients who are mentally or physically compromised are often fed soft foods that lack the cleaning effects of normal foods. Devices can be developed to clean these patients' teeth. The dental assistant may need to show the caregiver how to clean the patient's teeth routinely. For example, putty can be wrapped over the handle of a toothbrush to allow the patient to grasp it more easily, or the handle may be extended with a tongue depressor or ruler so that the patient can reach his or her oral cavity. Keep the focus on the desired outcome and establish methods to meet these goals. A moist washcloth can be used to wipe the surfaces of the teeth, if necessary.

PROCEDURE

2-3 Dental Flossing Technique

The procedure is explained to the patient to teach a dental flossing technique.

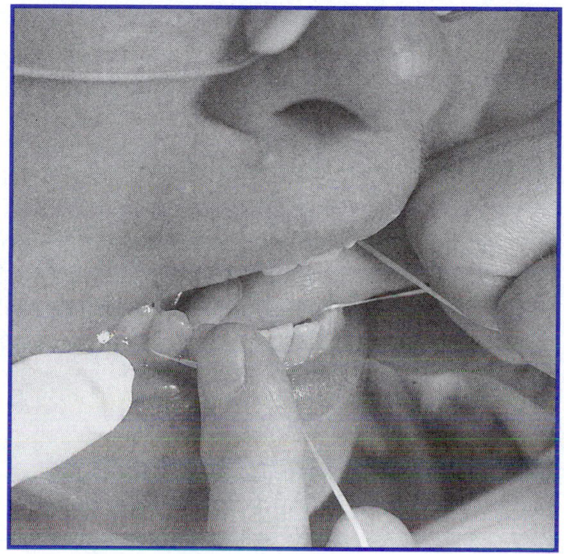

FIGURE 2–2 Placing the dental floss around the tooth, wrapped into the sulcus.

EQUIPMENT AND SUPPLIES

- Dental floss

PROCEDURE STEPS

1. Obtain the appropriate dental floss and dispense 18 inches in length.
2. Wrap the ends of the floss around the middle or ring finger as anchors.
3. Grasp the floss between the thumb and index finger of each hand, allowing ½ to 1 inch to remain between the two hands.
4. For the maxillary teeth, pass the floss over the two thumbs or a thumb and finger, and direct the floss upward. For the mandibular teeth, pass the floss over the two index fingers and guide it downward.
5. Direct the floss to pass gently between the teeth, using a sawing motion. Try not to snap the floss through the contacts because it may damage the interdental papilla (gingival tissue between teeth).
6. Curve the floss in a C-shape to wrap it around the tooth and allow access into the sulcus area (Figure 2–2). When a resistance is felt, it indicates that the bottom of the gingival sulcus has been reached.
7. Move the floss gently up and down the surface of the tooth to remove the plaque.
8. Lift slightly and wrap the floss in the opposite direction in a C-shape over the adjacent tooth.
9. Move the floss gently up and down the surface of this tooth prior to removing it from the area.
10. Rotate the floss on the fingers to allow for a fresh section to be used each time and continue to clean between every tooth. It is best to proceed in a systematic method to ensure that no area is missed.
11. Use the dental floss around the distal surface of the most posterior tooth by wrapping it in a tight C-shape and moving it gently up and down with a firm pressure. Do the most posterior teeth in all four quadrants in the same manner.

FLUORIDE

Introduction to Fluoride

The use of fluoride in dentistry is based on the knowledge that when the fluoride content of the teeth is increased to the "optimum level," there is significant reduction in dental caries. Once, fluoride was thought to be beneficial only during tooth development years, but through further research fluoride has been proven to have remineralization properties.

Effects of Fluoride

Fluoride is a natural substance needed for the development of healthy teeth and bones. It is absorbed almost entirely through the blood stream from the gastrointestinal tract. Fluorides also are absorbed through the lungs, as in industrial settings where people have occupational exposure to fluorine.

Once fluoride is absorbed by the body and deposited in the bones and teeth, the remaining fluoride is excreted. The developing child requires more fluoride than a forty-year-old person and so the body adjusts the amount and excretes the excess fluoride.

Fluoride in Dental Plaque

Fluoride in dental plaque has been found to have a favorable effect. The amount of fluoride in the plaque is relative to the amount of fluoride exposure. Fluoride in the plaque is bound within bacteria. This condition causes an **antibacterial effect** that inhibits the production of acids responsible for dental decay.

Forms of Fluorides Used in Dentistry

Fluorides are available for dental health care needs in two forms: **systemic fluoride** and **topical fluoride.** The fluoride compounds used in dentistry are **sodium fluoride, stannous fluoride,** and **acidulated phosphate fluoride.**

Systemic Fluoride. Systemic fluoride is ingested and then circulated through the body to the developing teeth. Sources of systemic fluoride include fluoridated water, foods with fluoride, fluoride tablets, and drops.

Topical Fluoride

Topical fluoride is another method to make the tooth more resistant to demineralization and also to assist in the remineralization of decalcified areas. Because topical fluoride only penetrates the outer layer of the enamel, it is most effective if the tooth is cleaned prior to application. The cleaning can be accomplished by toothbrushing or a rubber-cup polish.

Topical fluoride is available for direct application in a variety of forms, such as gels, rinses, foams, and liquids (Procedure 2–4). Polishing paste and dentifrice that are applied to the teeth also contain fluoride.

P R O C E D U R E

2-4 Fluoride Application

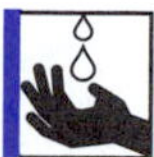
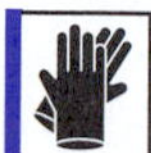
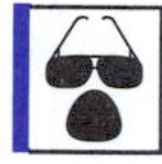
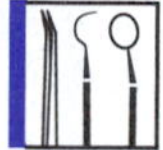
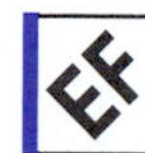

This procedure is performed by the dental assistant after the rubber-cup polish has been completed. In some states, the application of fluoride may be an expanded function.

EQUIPMENT AND SUPPLIES

- Basic setup: mouth mirror, explorer, and cotton pliers
- Saliva ejector, evacuator tip (HVE), air-water syringe tip
- Cotton rolls, gauze sponges
- Fluoride solution
- Appropriately sized trays
- Timer (for one or four minutes)

PROCEDURE STEPS *(Follow aseptic procedures)*

1. Seat the patient in an upright position, review health history, and confirm that he or she has not had allergic reactions to fluorides.
2. Explain the procedure to the patient. Inform the patient to try not to swallow the fluoride and show him or her how to use the saliva ejector.
3. Explain that for the fluoride to be most effective, he or she should not eat, drink, or rinse for thirty minutes after the fluoride treatment.
4. Select the trays and try them in the patient's mouth to ensure coverage of all the exposed teeth.
5. Place the fluoride gel or foam in the tray. The tray should be about one-third full.
6. Dry all the teeth with the air syringe. To keep the teeth dry while reaching for the tray, keep your finger in the patient's mouth and tell him or her to keep it open.
7. Place the tray over the dried teeth. The maxillary and mandibular arches can be done at the same time or individually (Figure 2–3).

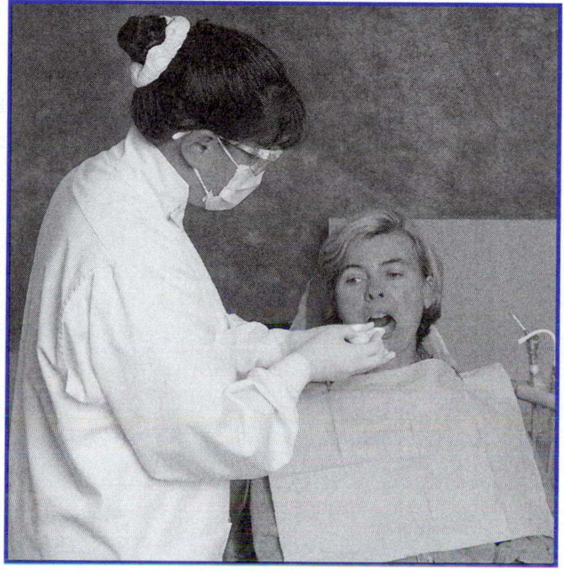

FIGURE 2–3 Dental assistant placing a loaded fluoride tray into the patient's mouth.

8. Move the trays up and down to dispense the fluoride solution around the teeth.
9. Place the saliva ejector between the arches and have the patient close gently.
10. Set the timer for the designated amount of time.
11. When the timer goes off, remove the saliva ejector and the trays from the patient's mouth.
12. Quickly evacuate the mouth with the saliva ejector or the evacuator (HVE) completely to remove any excess fluoride.
13. Remind the patient not to eat, drink, or rinse for thirty minutes.
14. Make the chart entry, including the date, the fluoride solution applied, and any reactions.

Dual benefit of chewing fluoride tablets.

If fluoride tablets are chewed before being swallowed, the teeth benefit both from topical and systemic fluoride applications.

Fluoride Rinses

Fluoride rinses are supplied in a liquid that is a higher concentration and, because it is easy to swallow, the patient must be reminded *not to swallow after rinsing.*

After the patient's teeth have been cleaned with a toothbrush or a rubber-cup polish, administer the fluoride rinse. Follow the instructions for the individual rinse. Usually, the patient is directed to take half the dosage and then swish for a specific time (one minute). The patient then empties this amount and repeats with the second portion for the same amount of time.

Because of the taste of the fluoride, patients do not always look forward to the fluoride treatments. The dental assistant can be the motivating factor for the patient's attitude. Children under six years should not use the fluoride rinses or mouthwashes because they may accidentally swallow them.

CHAPTER 3

Head and Neck Anatomy

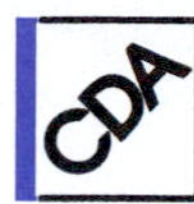

OBJECTIVES

The student should strive to meet the following objectives and demonstrate an understanding of the facts and principles presented in this chapter:

1. Identify the bones of the cranium and the face. Identify the landmarks on the maxilla and the mandible.
2. List and identify the muscles of mastication.
3. List and identify the nerves of the maxilla and the mandible.
4. Identify the arteries and veins of the head and the neck.

KEY TERMS

alveolar process (p. 29)
buccal branch (p. 32)
common carotid (p. 33)
ethmoid bone (p. 28)
external pterygoid muscles (p. 31)
frena (p. 26)
inferior alveolar branch (p. 32)
internal pterygoid muscles (p. 31)
lacrimal bones (p. 29)
lingual branch (p. 32)
masseter muscles (p. 31)
oral vestibule (p. 26)
parotid glands (p. 26)
sphenoid bone (p. 28)
temporal muscles (p. 31)
uvula (p. 26)
Wharton's duct (p. 27)
zygomatic bones (p. 29)

INTRODUCTION

This chapter provides information on the anatomy of the head and neck. The dental assistant must be able to describe the anatomy, including the locations of the structures and their functions. Identifying the anatomy of the head and face in normal, healthy tissues enables the dental assistant to recognize dental abnormalities.

Landmarks of the Oral Cavity

Understanding the landmarks of the oral cavity aids the dental assistant when taking radiographs, placing topical anesthetic, recognizing healthy tissue, and recording information or medical history on a patient's chart.

The landmarks of the oral cavity include the following: vestibule, vestibule fornix, labial mucosa, buccal mucosa, parotid papilla, Stensen's duct, linea alba, alveolar mucosa, gingiva, labial frenum, and the buccal frenum.

Inside the mouth, a pocket is formed by the soft tissue of the cheeks and the gingiva. This is the **oral vestibule.** The tissue that lines the inner surface of the lips and cheeks is called **mucosa.** The mucosa is named according to location. The inner surface of the lips is called the **labial mucosa,** and the inner surface of the cheeks is the **buccal mucosa.** Mucosa also covers the alveolar bone that supports the teeth. It is called the **alveolar mucosa.** Alveolar mucosa is loosely attached and is highly vascular, giving the mucosa a reddish color. Moving from the alveolar mucosa toward the teeth is the **gingiva.** The gingiva is firmly attached and usually pale pink or brownish pink, depending on pigmentation.

When the lips are retracted, **frena** become visible. Frena (plural form of frenum) are raised lines of mucosal tissue that extend from the alveolar mucosa through the vestibule to the labial and buccal mucosa.

The Palate Area of the Oral Cavity

On the inside of the maxillary teeth is the **palate,** or the "roof of the mouth." The palate is divided into hard and soft sections. The hard palate, the anterior portion, is a bony plate covered with pink to brownish-pink keratinized tissue. The soft palate, the posterior portion, covers muscle tissue and is darker pink or yellowish. Occasionally, in the middle of the palate a lump or prominence of bone (exostosis) may be found. This excess bone is called a **torus** (plural is tori), or a torus palatinus. The **uvula** is a projection that extends off the back of the soft palate.

The Salivary Glands

There are three major pairs of **salivary glands** that supply the oral cavity: the parotid glands, submandibular glands, and sublingual glands (Figure 3–1). These glands secret saliva to assist in chewing, swallowing, lubrication, and digestion. The largest of the salivary glands are the **parotid glands,** which lie

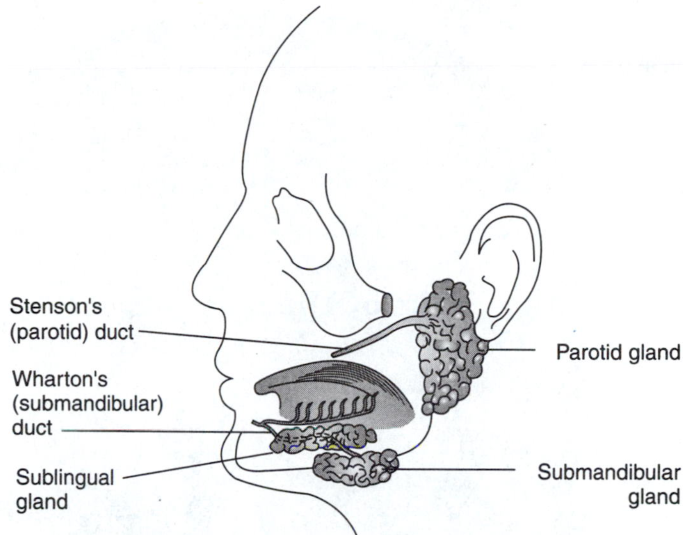

FIGURE 3–1 Salivary glands and ducts.

just below and in front of the ear. The parotid glands empty into the mouth through the **parotid duct** (also known as the Stensen's duct). The **submandibular glands** are approximately the size of a walnut and lie on the inside of the mandible in the posterior area. They empty the saliva into the mouth through the **Wharton's duct.** The third set of glands are the **sublingual.** These are the smallest of the glands and are located on the floor of the mouth. These glands empty directly into the mouth.

BONES OF THE HEAD

The skull is divided into two sections: the **cranium** and the **face.** The cranium covers and protects the brain and is comprised of eight bones (Figure 3–2). The face consists of fourteen bones, including the maxilla and the mandible (Figure 3–3).

Bones of the Cranium

The **frontal bone** forms the forehead, the main portion of the roof of the eye socket (orbit), and part of the nasal cavity. On the skull just behind the frontal bone are the two parietal bones, right and left halves joining at the midline. The **parietal bones** form most of the roof of the skull and the upper half of the sides. Below each parietal bone, forming the lower sides and the base of the skull, are the **temporal bones.** Each temporal bone contains the following landmarks: the external auditory meatus, the mastoid process, the glenoid fossa, and the styloid process. The **external auditory meatus** is the opening for the ear. The **mastoid process** is the bony projection found on the bottom border of

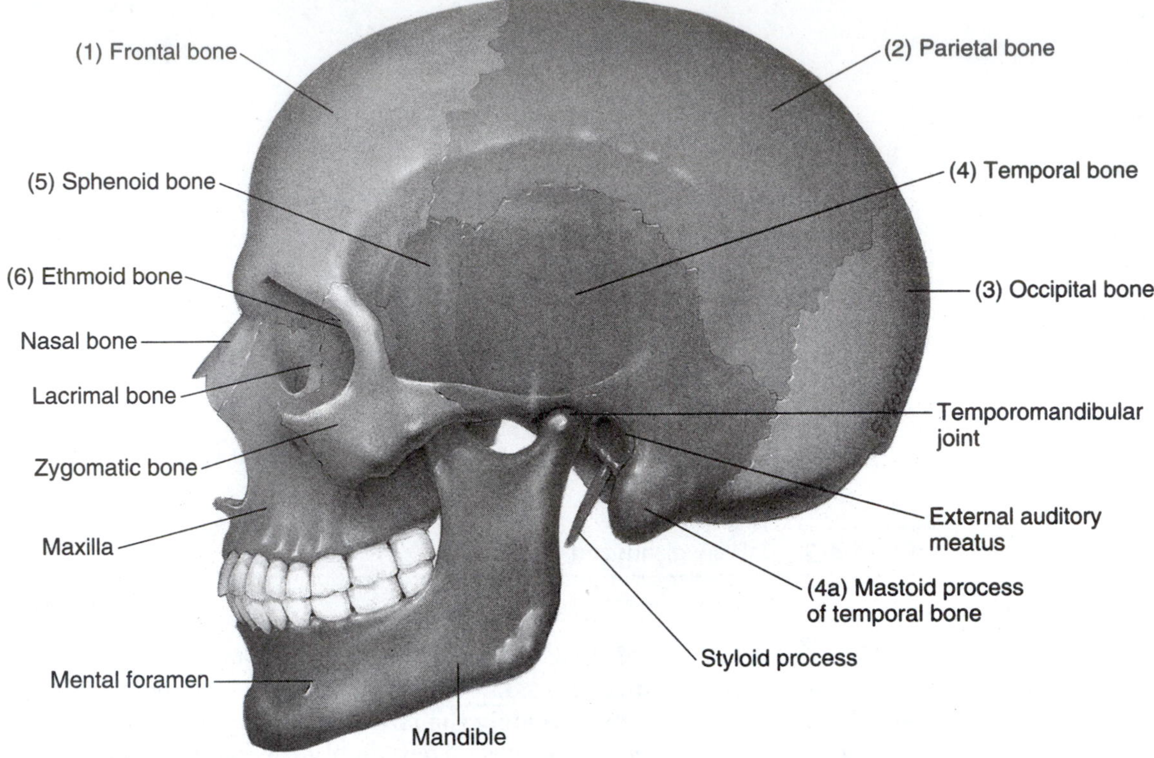

FIGURE 3–2 Lateral aspect of the cranium.

the temporal bone. A pit or depression found anterior to the mastoid process is the **glenoid fossa,** the location where the mandible articulates with the skull. The **styloid process** is a sharp projection on the under-surface of the temporal bone between the glenoid fossa and the mastoid process. The **occipital bone** forms the back and base of the skull. The occipital bone contains a large opening, the foramen magnum, through which the spinal cord passes. The **sphenoid bone** is a wedge-shaped bone that goes across the skull anterior to the temporal bones. It is one continuous bone, shaped like a bat with its wings spread out. The wings of the sphenoid bone are called the **pterygoid** process. The sphenoid bone forms the anterior base of the skull behind the orbit and contains the **sphenoid sinuses.** The **ethmoid bone** forms part of the nose, the orbits, and the floor of the cranium. This bone is thin and spongy or honeycombed in appearance. It contains the **ethmoid sinuses**.

Bones of the Face

The **nasal bones** form the bridge of the nose. The **vomer bone** is a single bone on the inside of the nasal cavity. It forms the posterior and the bottom of the

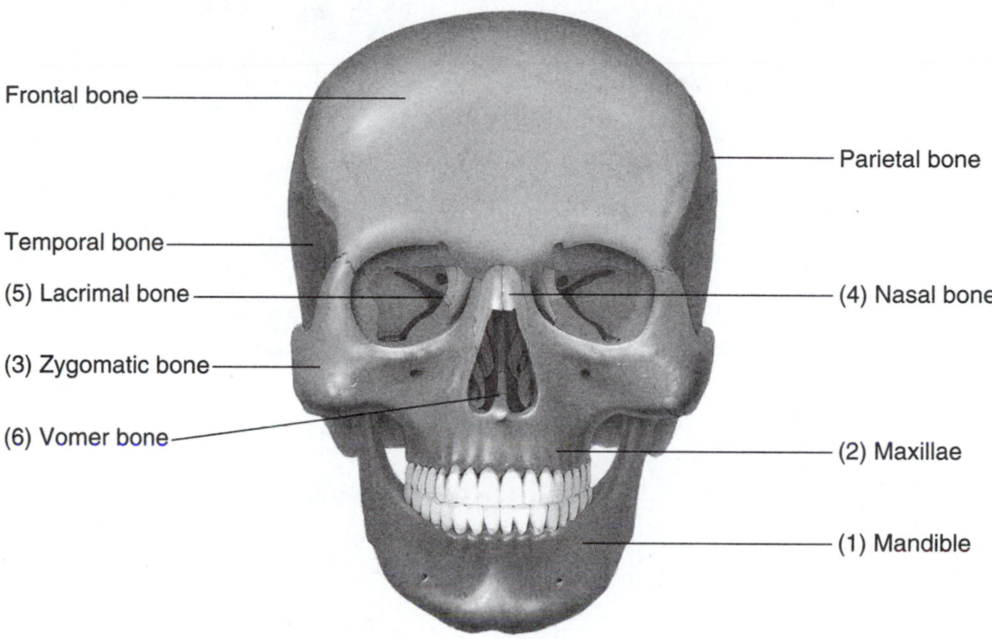

FIGURE 3–3 Bones of the face.

nasal septum (the nasal septum is a cartilage structure that divides the nasal cavities). On the outside of the nasal cavities are scroll-like bones called inferior nasal conchae. Each concha consists of thin, cancellous bone. The **lacrimal bones** are small and very delicate. They are anterior to the ethmoid bone, making part of the orbit (the corner of the eye). The tear ducts pass through the lacrimal bones. The **zygomatic bones** form the cheeks.

Maxilla. The maxilla is the largest of the facial bones and is composed of two sections of bone joined at the median suture. The maxilla extends from the floor of each orbit and the floor and exterior walls of the nasal cavity to form the roof the mouth. The maxilla is formed by *four processes* (outgrowths of bone). The *frontal* and the *zygomatic processes* meet the frontal and the zygomatic bones. The **alveolar process** forms the bone that supports the maxillary teeth, and the *palatine process* is the main portion of the hard palate.

Mandible. The **mandible** is the only movable bone of the face (Figure 3–4). The mandible consists of a horseshoe-shaped body that is horizontal, with two vertical extensions called **rami** (plural form of ramus). At the top of the rami are two projections. The posterior projection is the **condyle** or **condyloid process,** and the anterior projection is the **coronoid process.** The condyle articulates with the temporal bone to form the **temporomandibular joint (TMJ).**

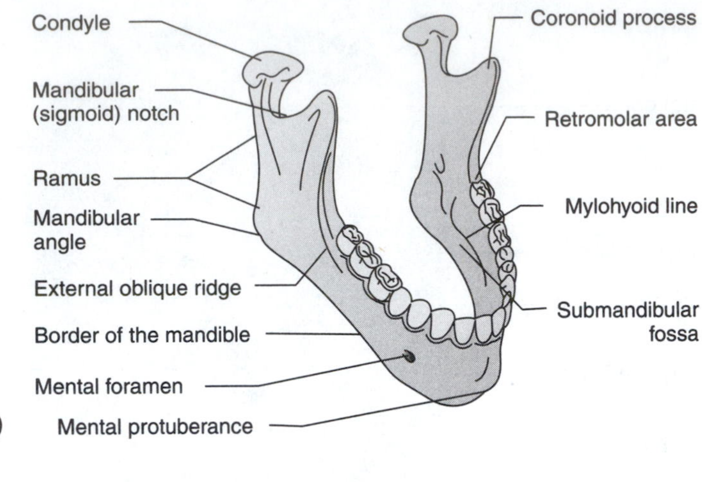

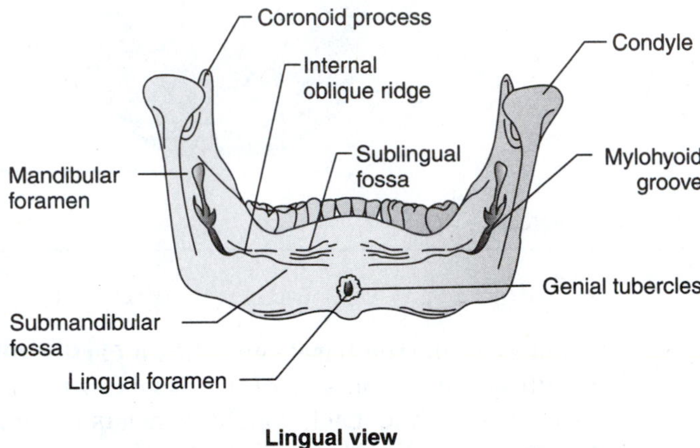

FIGURE 3–4 (A) External surface of the mandible. (B) Internal (lingual) view of the mandible.

Temporomandibular Joint (TMJ)

Once the bones of the cranium and the face have been identified, it is easy to locate the temporomandibular joint (TMJ). The joint is named for the two bones that form the union: the temporal and the mandible bones.

The temporomandibular joint is supported by ligaments and the muscles of mastication control the movements. The left and right TMJs function in unison and move in two ways: hinge (swinging) motion and gliding movement.

Muscles of Mastication

Muscles expand and contract to make movement possible and each muscle has an **origin** (fixed point) and **insertion** (movable point).

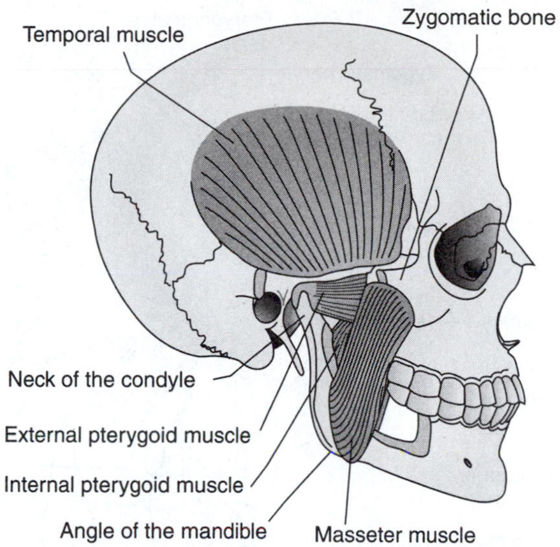

FIGURE 3–5 Muscles of mastication. Lateral view of the internal pterygoid muscle and the external pterygoid muscle. The temporal muscle and the masseter muscle.

There are four pairs of muscles of mastication, known as the **temporal muscles**, **masseter muscles**, **internal pterygoid muscles**, and **external pterygoid muscles**. These muscles provide movement for the mandible as they protrude, retract, elevate, and provide lateral movements (Figure 3–5). Nerves to the muscles of mastication originate from the mandibular division of the trigeminal labor.

Nerves of the Head and Neck

Four cranial nerves innervate the face and oral cavity: **trigeminal, facial, glossopharyngeal,** and **hypoglossal.** The largest cranial nerve and the most important to dental auxiliaries is the trigeminal nerve, because this cranial nerve innervates the maxilla and the mandible. The trigeminal nerve divides at the semi-lunar (gasserian) ganglion into three branches: the ophthalmic nerve, maxillary nerve, and mandibular nerve.

The Maxillary Branch of the Trigeminal Nerve

Maxillary Nerve Branch. The maxillary nerve branch (Figure 3–6) is a sensory nerve that innervates the nose, cheeks, palate, gingiva, maxillary teeth, maxillary sinus, tonsils, nasophynarynx, and other facial structures.

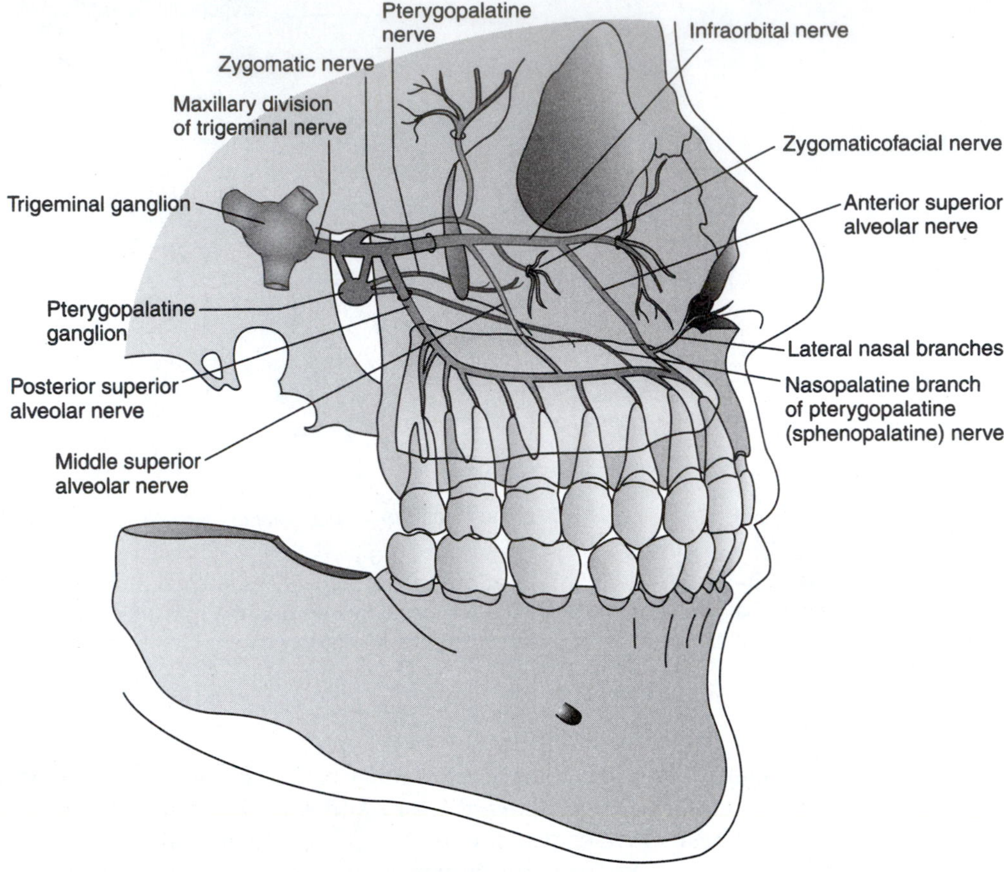

FIGURE 3–6 Nerves of the maxillary arch.

The Mandibular Branch of the Trigeminal Nerve

The **mandibular nerve branch** is the largest division. The three branches of the mandibular nerve are the buccal branch, the lingual branch, and the inferior alveolar branch. The mandibular nerve innervates the mucosa, gingiva, the floor of the mouth, the tongue, the chin, the lower lip area, and the teeth.

Circulation to the Head and Neck

The arteries and veins of the face and oral cavity are located near each other. They supply blood and nutrients to the area and drain unoxygenated blood and waste products from the area.

Arteries of the Face and Oral Cavity

The **common carotid** supplies blood to most of the head and neck. As the common carotid ascends up the neck, it divides into the internal and external carotid arteries. The internal carotid artery supplies blood to the brain and eyes, while the external carotid artery supplies blood to the face and oral cavity and has numerous branches.

Veins of the Face and Oral Cavity

Some of the veins of the face and oral cavity are located with corresponding arteries and have similar names. There are many variations of venous drainage, but ultimately the blood from the face and oral cavity drains into either the external jugular vein or internal jugular vein.

C H A P T E R 4

Tooth Anatomy and Supporting Structures

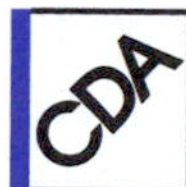

OBJECTIVES

The student should strive to meet the following objectives and demonstrate an understanding of the facts and principles presented in this chapter:

1. Identify the substances of enamel, dentin, cementum, and pulp and their distinguishing marks.
2. Identify the components of the periodontium and the considerations of the alveolar bone.
3. Describe the structures of the gingiva and the oral mucosa.
4. Identify the dental arches and quadrants using the correct terminology.
5. List the primary and permanent teeth by name and location.
6. Identify the different divisions of the tooth.
7. Identify the surfaces of each tooth and their locations.

KEY TERMS

alveolus (p. 37)
apical foramen (p. 45)
bifurcated (p. 45)
buccal (p. 45)
cementum (p. 36)
cingulum (p. 45)
cusp of Carabelli (p. 45)
cusps (p. 41)
dentin (p. 36)
dentition (p. 38)
developmental groove (p. 45)
distal (p. 42)
enamel (p. 36)
facial (p. 43)
fissure (p. 45)
fossa (p. 45)
furcation (p. 45)
gingiva (p. 38)
incisal edge (p. 41)
lingual (p. 43)
lobes (p. 45)
mamelons (p. 45)
mandibular arch (p. 38)
marginal ridge (p. 45)
maxillary arch (p. 38)
mesial (p. 42)
midline (p. 38)
oblique ridge (p. 46)
occlusal (p. 45)
periodontium (p. 36)
pit (p. 46)
posterior (p. 41)
pulp (p. 36)
ridge (p. 46)
succedaneous (p. 42)
supplemental groove (p. 46)
transverse ridge (p. 46)
triangular ridge (p. 47)
trifurcated (p. 47)

TOOTH STRUCTURE

Each tooth is comprised of four primary structures (Figure 4–1). The **enamel** is the structure that covers the outside of the crown of the tooth. It is the hardest living tissue in the body. Enamel can be very brittle if not supported by dentin and a vital pulp. **Dentin** makes up the bulk of the tooth structure but is not normally visible. It surrounds the pulp cavity and lies under the enamel, within the anatomical crown and under the cementum within the root. The **cementum** is the third structure and covers the dentin on the root portion of the tooth. At the center of the tooth, within the **pulp** cavity, is the pulp tissue. It is made up of the nerves and blood vessels that provide nutrients to the tooth. The pulp cavity is made up of a pulp chamber with pulp horns and pulp canal(s). The **pulp canal**(s) is (are) located in the root(s) of the teeth. The **pulp chamber** is a large portion of the pulp, which is located in the crown of the tooth. The **pulp horns,** pointed elongations of the pulp, extend toward the incisal or occlusal portion of the tooth.

COMPONENTS OF THE PERIODONTIUM

The **periodontium** consists of portions of the tooth structure, supporting hard and soft dental tissues, and the alveolar bone.

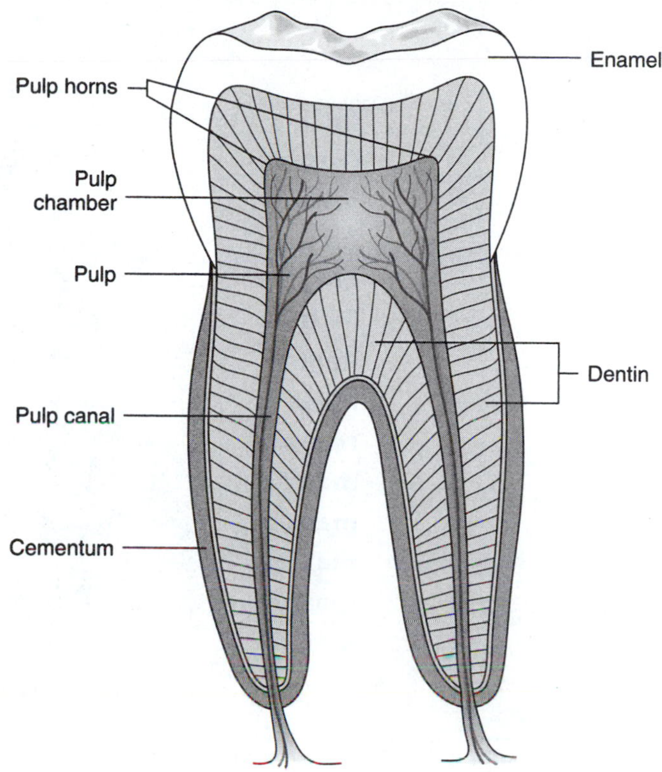

FIGURE 4–1 Tissues of the tooth.

Cementum

Surrounding the root of the tooth, attaching it to the alveolar bone by anchoring the periodontal ligaments, is the cementum (Figure 4–2).

Alveolar Bone

The bone that surrounds the root of the tooth, the socket, is the **alveolus**.

Periodontal Ligament

The **periodontal ligament,** like all connective tissue, is formed by fibroblast cells and secures the tooth into the socket by a number of organized fiber groups.

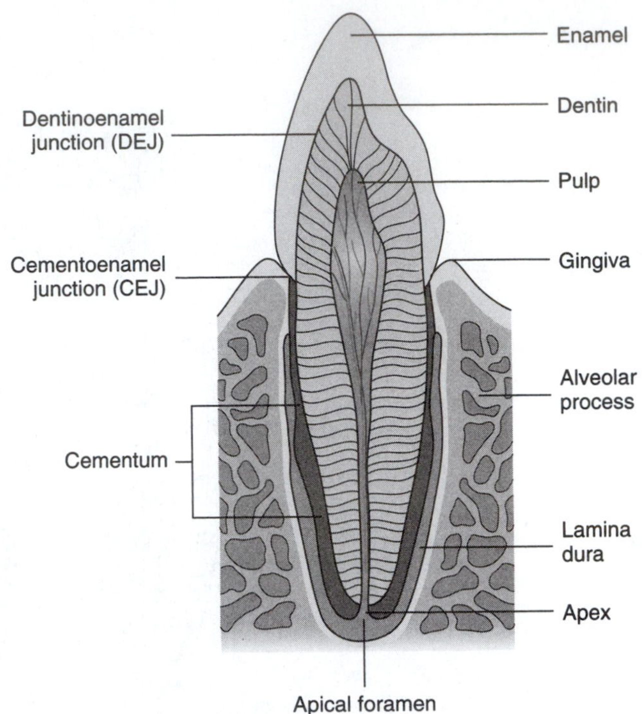

FIGURE 4–2 Tooth and surrounding tissues.

Gingiva

The **gingiva**, composed of a mucosa that surrounds the necks of the teeth and covers the alveolar processes, is commonly referred to as the **gums.** (The plural of gingiva is gingivae.) The gingival tissue surrounds the teeth and, in a healthy state, is firm and tightly adapted to the tooth.

Dental Arches

The **dentition** (natural teeth in position) are arranged in two arches. The upper arch is the **maxillary arch**, because the teeth are set in the maxilla bone. The lower teeth are located in the mandible bone, therefore located in the **mandibular arch**.

Dental Quadrants

Each of the dental arches is divided in two halves by an imaginary line called the **midline** (median line), which creates two sections called **quadrants.** Thus, there are four quadrants, containing eight permanent teeth each. The arrange-

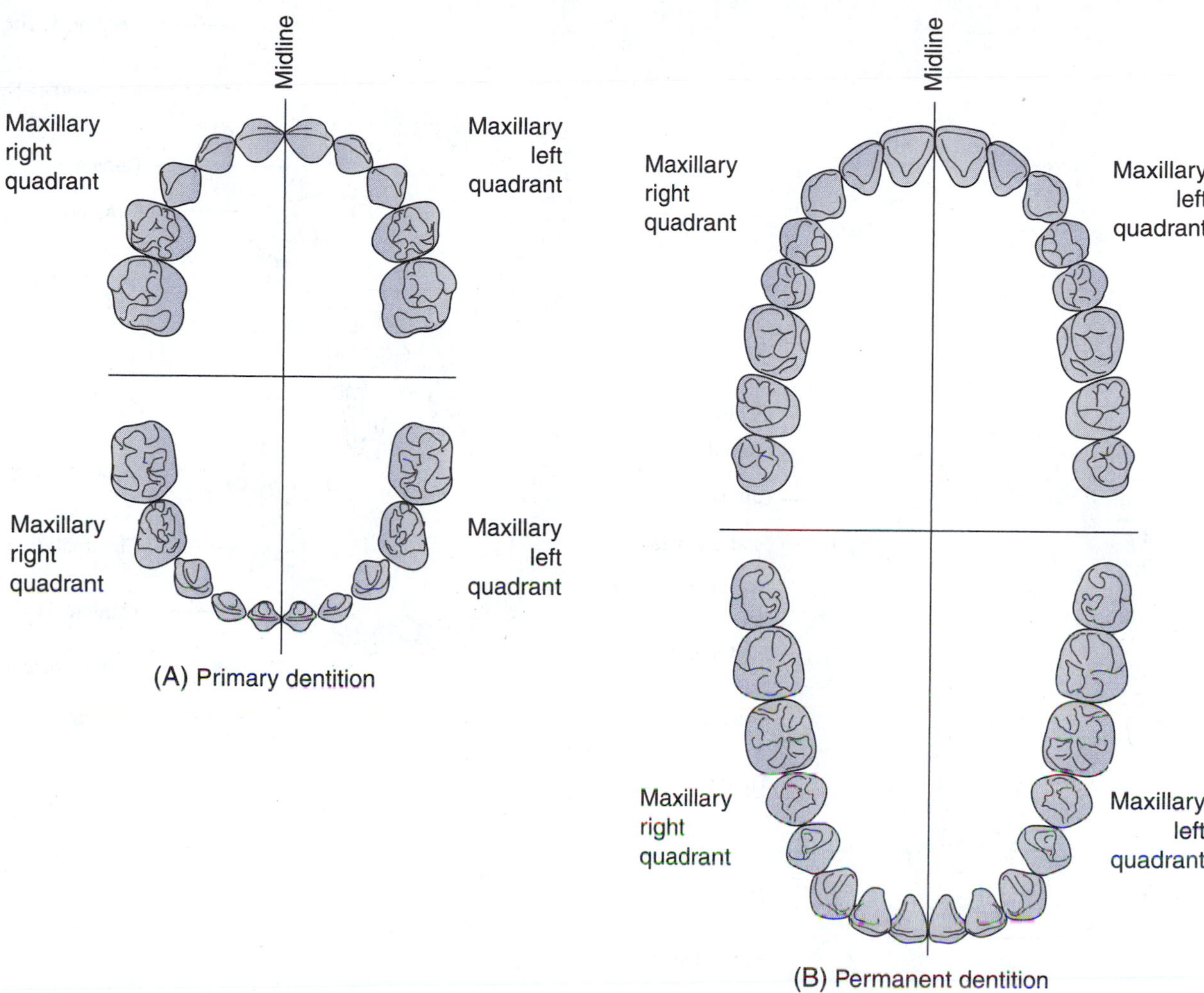

FIGURE 4–3 Dental arches of (A) primary (deciduous) dentition and (B) permanent dentition divided into quadrants with the midline identified.

ment of the teeth is identical in each quadrant, and each quadrant is named according to its location in the oral cavity (Figure 4–3).

The quadrants are labeled according to the patient's right or left.

Types of Teeth and Their Functions

Primary Teeth

The primary (**deciduous**) teeth in each quadrant have names similar to the permanent teeth. The deciduous dentition has twenty teeth total: ten in each arch and five in each quadrant. The following teeth are found in each quadrant.

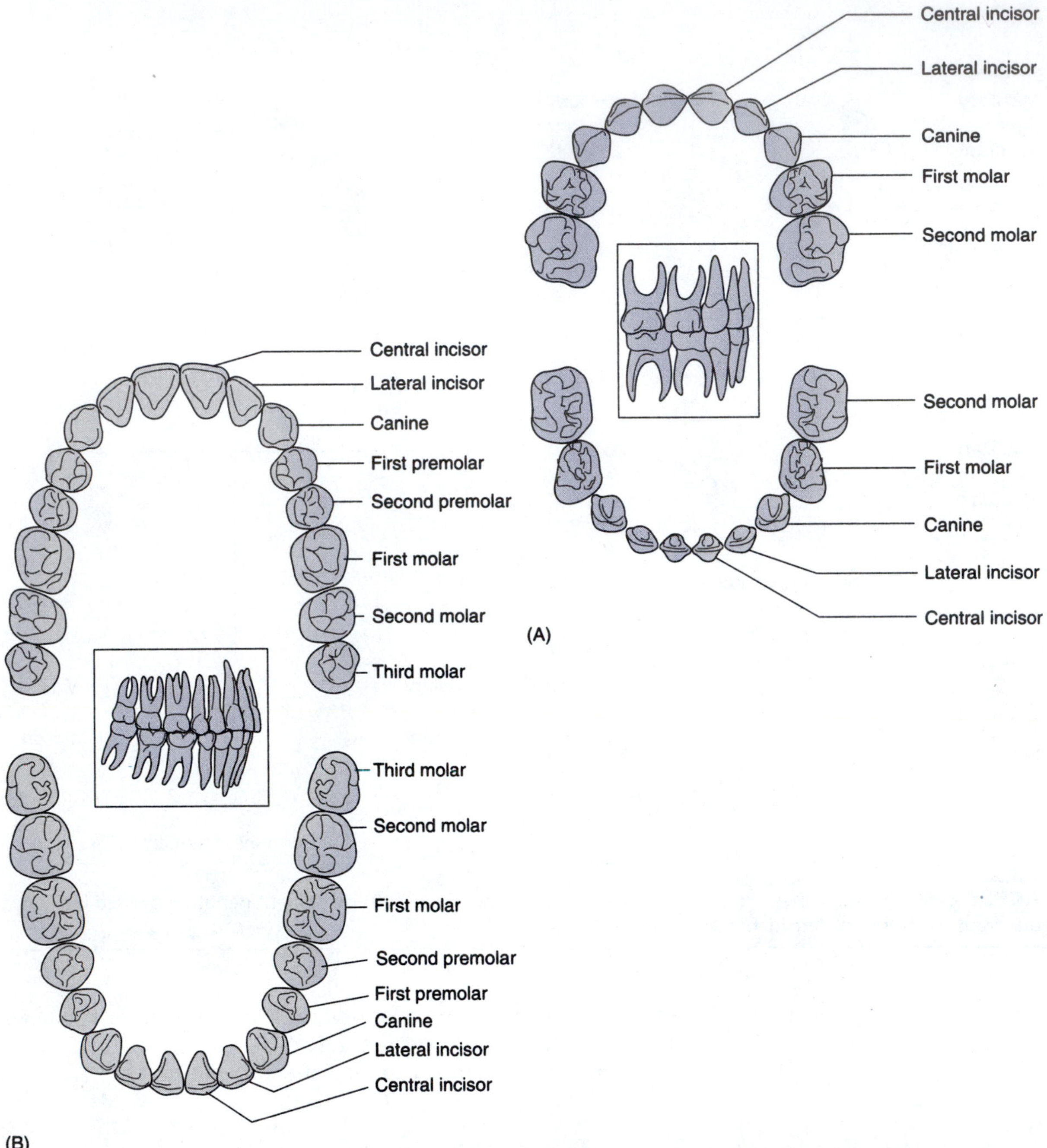

FIGURE 4–4 (A) The deciduous dentition identifying each tooth by name. (B) The permanent dentition identifying each tooth by name.

Starting from the midline, the first tooth is called the **central incisor** and is used to cut or bite the ingested food. The second tooth from the midline, the **lateral incisor,** is also used for cutting. The third tooth from the midline is the **canine** (cuspid). This tooth is slightly more bulky in size and aids in tearing food. The next two teeth are molars and are named the first molar, which is the one closest to the midline, and the second molar. **Molars** are used to grind food (Figure 4–4).

Permanent Teeth

Permanent teeth are arranged similarly to the deciduous teeth. Adults have thirty-two permanent teeth: sixteen in each arch and eight in each quadrant. Each quadrant has the permanent central incisor, the lateral incisor, and the canine (cuspid), as did the deciduous quadrant. Directly after the canine (cuspid) in the permanent dentition are the first and second **premolars** (Figure 4–4).

The premolars are often called **bicuspids** because they usually have two (bi) **cusps** (pointed or rounded mounds on the crown of the tooth). However, two of the eight bicuspids may have three cusps; therefore, the term is technically incorrect. It is important to be aware of the different names commonly used for the same teeth (for example, canines or cuspids and premolars or bicuspids).

The premolars are used to pulverize food. They break the food down into smaller sizes to ready them for the chewing and grinding process, which is done by the molars.

Behind the premolars, the permanent dentition has the first, second, and third molars. The first molars are closest to the midline and the third molars, farthest from the midline, are commonly termed the "wisdom teeth."

The teeth in either arch that are toward the front of the mouth from cuspid to cuspid are the anterior teeth, commonly referred to as the anterior sextant. The central incisors, lateral incisors, and canines (cuspids) are termed anterior teeth for both the deciduous and permanent dentition. Anterior teeth have single roots and a cutting or tearing edge called the **incisal edge**.

The teeth in either arch that are located in the back of the mouth are termed **posterior** teeth. The molars are posterior teeth in the deciduous dentition, and the premolars (bicuspids) and molars are posterior teeth in the permanent dentition. Posterior teeth normally have more than one root and multiple cusps for pulverizing and chewing.

Eruption Schedule

Humans have two dentitions. The primary dentition (deciduous teeth) begins eruption (proceeds into the oral cavity) around six months of age. All twenty teeth are normally erupted by the age of three years (Table 4–1). The period when both primary teeth and permanent teeth are in the dentition is called the mixed dentition period. This period lasts from approximately six to twelve

TABLE 4-1 ERUPTION AND EXFOLIATION DATES FOR PRIMARY TEETH

Tooth	Eruption Date	Exfoliation Date	Maxillary Order
Central incisor	6–10 months	6–7 years	#1
Lateral incisor	9–12 months	7–8 years	#2
Canine	16–22 months	10–12 years	#4
First molar	12–18 months	9–11 years	#3
Second molar	24–32 months	10–12 years	#5
			Mandibular Order
Central incisor	6–10 months	6–7 years	#1
Lateral incisor	7–10 months	7–8 years	#2
Canine	16–22 months	9–12 years	#4
First molar	12–18 months	9–11 years	#3
Second molar	20–32 months	10–12 years	#5

years of age. After the age of twelve, most of the primary teeth have exfoliated (shed from the oral cavity). The permanent dentition begins to erupt from about six years of age until around seventeen to twenty-one years of age (Table 4–2).

The permanent teeth that replace the primary teeth are called **succedaneous** teeth. This refers to succeeding deciduous teeth. Therefore, because there are twenty primary teeth, there are also twenty succedaneous teeth. The only permanent teeth that are not succedaneous teeth are the molars, because the premolars replace the primary molars.

Surfaces of the Teeth

All teeth have five surfaces on the crown portion. Each surface, or side, has a specific name (Figure 4–5).

Anterior Teeth

- **Mesial**—The surface *toward* the midline.
- **Distal**—The surface *away* from the midline.
- **Labial**—The "outside" surface, which is toward the lips.

TABLE 4-2 ERUPTION DATES FOR PERMANENT TEETH

Tooth	Eruption Date	Order of Eruption (Maxillary)
Central incisor	7–8 years	#2
Lateral incisor	8–9 years	#3
Canine	11–12 years	#6
First premolar	10–11 years	#4
Second premolar	11–12 years	#5
First molar	6–7 years	#1
Second molar	12–13 years	#7
Third molar	17–21 years	#8
		Order of Eruption (Mandibular)
Central incisor	6–7 years	#2
Lateral incisor	7–8 years	#3
Cuspid	9–10 years	#4
First premolar	10–11 years	#5
Second premolar	11–12 years	#6
First molar	6–7 years	#1
Second molar	11–13 years	#7
Third molar	17–21 years	#8

- **Lingual**—The "inside" surface, which is toward the tongue. On the maxillary arch, the lingual side may be referred to as the **palatal** surface.
- **Incisal edge**—The biting or cutting edge.

Facial Surface

The term **facial** may be used for either the labial surface of the anterior teeth or the buccal surface of the posterior teeth.

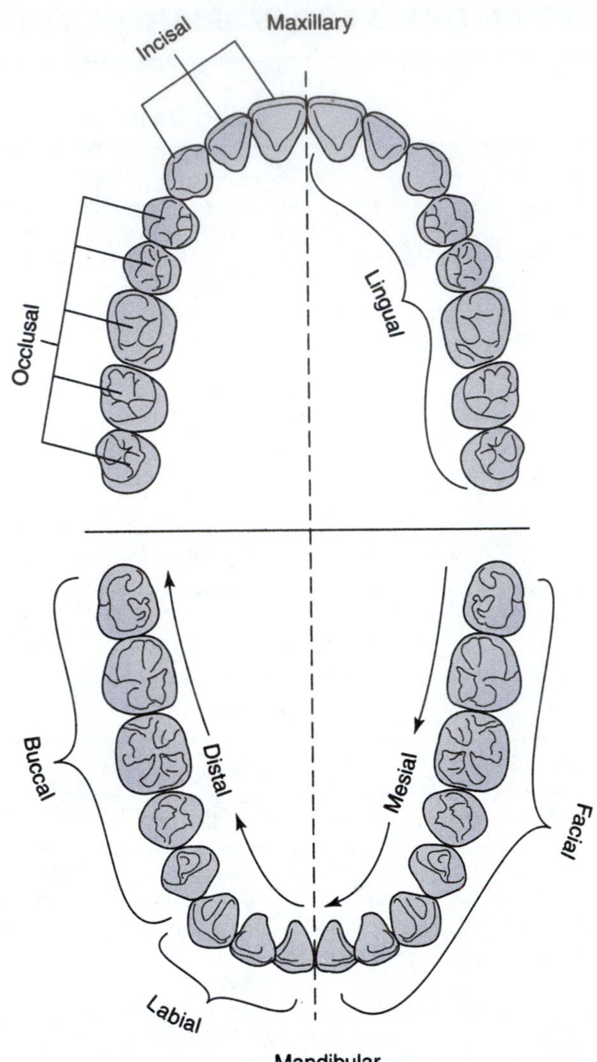

FIGURE 4–5 The surfaces of the teeth identified on the dental arches.

Posterior Teeth

- **Mesial**—The surface *toward* the midline.
- **Distal**—The surface *away* from the midline.
- **Lingual**—The "inside" surface, which is toward the tongue.

- **Buccal**—The "outside" surface, which is toward the cheek.
- **Occlusal**—The pulverizing or chewing surface.

Anatomical Structures

It is important to be able to identify the landmarks on each individual tooth. Each area's name should be used when identifying the anatomical structures.

- **Apex**—At or near the end of the root (Figure 4–6).
- **Apical foramen**—An opening in the end of the tooth through which nerves and blood vessels enter. There may be more than one opening at the end of the root.
- **Bifurcated**—When there are two roots on one tooth, they are said to be bifurcated, or branched in two (bi means two and furca means fork) (Figure 4–6).
- **Buccal groove**—A linear depression forming a groove that extends from the middle of the buccal surface to the occlusal surface of the tooth (Figure 4–6).
- **Cingulum**—A convex or bulging area on the lingual surface of the anterior teeth, near the gingiva.
- **Cusp**—A pointed or rounded mound on the crown of the tooth.
- **Cusp of Carabelli**—A fifth cusp located on the mesial lingual surface of most maxillary first molars.
- **Developmental groove**—A groove formed by the uniting of lobes during development of the crown of the tooth.
- **Fissure**—A developmental groove that has an imperfect union where the lobes come together. Decay often initiates in the fissure.
- **Fossa**—A shallow rounded or angular depression.
- **Furcation**—The dividing point of a multi-rooted tooth.
- **Lobes**—The separate divisions that come together to form a tooth. Often in the molars, the lobes become cusps.
- **Mamelons**—Three bulges on the incisal edge of the newly erupted central incisor. Mamelons normally disappear from normal wear.
- **Marginal ridges**—Elevated area of enamel that forms the mesial and distal borders of the lingual surface of the anterior teeth and the mesial and distal borders of the occlusal surface of the posterior teeth (Figure 4–7).

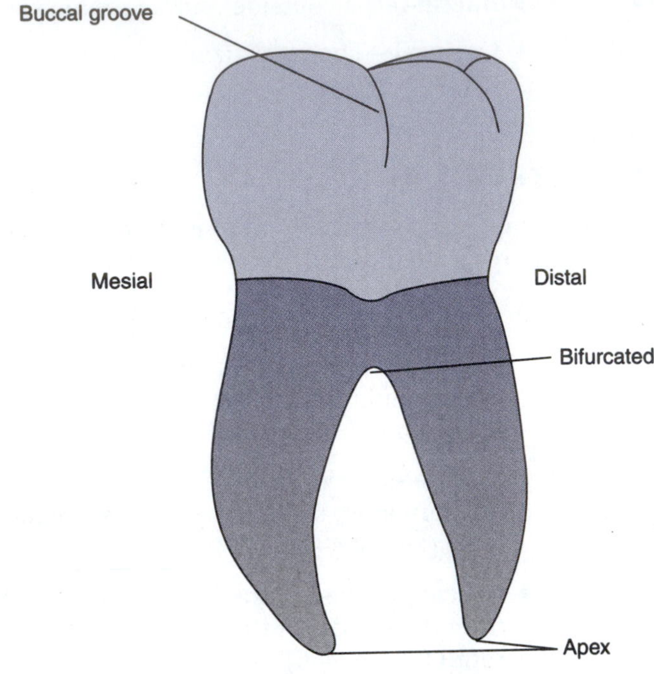

FIGURE 4–6 Mandibular molar with the buccal groove bifurcated and apex identified.

- **Oblique ridge**—Elevated area of enamel that extends obliquely across the occlusal of the tooth. On the maxillary first molars, the oblique ridge extends from the disto-buccal cusp to the mesio-lingual cusp.
- **Pit**—The place where the grooves come together or the fissures cross. Decay often begins in the pit.
- **Ridge**—A linear elevation of enamel found on the tooth.
- **Supplemental groove**—Shallow, linear groove that radiates from the developmental groove. It often gives the tooth surface a wrinkled appearance. These grooves do not denote any major divisions of the tooth.
- **Transverse ridge**—The union of two triangular ridges that produces a single ridge of elevation across the occlusal surface of a posterior tooth.

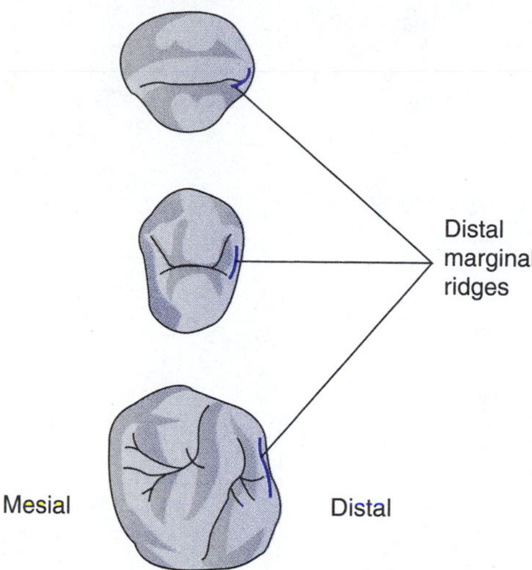

FIGURE 4–7 The marginal ridges of the maxillary central, premolar, and molar.

- **Triangular ridge**—A ridge or an elevation that descends from the cusp and widens as it runs down to the middle area of the occlusal surface.
- **Trifurcated**—Where there are three roots (*tri* means "three") coming from the main trunk of the tooth.

CHAPTER 5

Dental Charting

OBJECTIVES

The student should strive to meet the following objectives and demonstrate an understanding of the facts and principles presented in this chapter:

1. Explain why charting is necessary in dental practices.
2. Identify charts that use symbols to represent conditions present in the oral cavity.
3. List and explain the systems used for charting the permanent and deciduous dentitions.
4. Define G.V. Black's six classifications of cavity preparations.
5. List common abbreviations used to identify simple, compound, and complex cavities.
6. Describe basic terminology used in dental charting.
7. Explain color indicators and identify charting symbols.

KEY TERMS

abscess (p. 55)
bridge (p. 55)
crown (p. 55)
denture (p. 55)
drifting (p. 55)
Fédération Dentaire Internationale (FDI) system for numbering (p. 51)
incipient (p. 55)
mobility (p. 56)
overhang (p. 56)
Palmer System for numbering (p. 53)
periodontal pocket (p. 56)
restoration (p. 56)
root canal (p. 56)
sealant (p. 56)
Universal/National System for numbering (p. 50)

INTRODUCTION

Recording the conditions present in the patient's oral cavity on a dental chart using symbols, numbers, and colors is a shorthand technique called charting. Numerous symbols and various charts are used. The dental assistant needs to learn the doctor's preferred system in order to ensure that accurate charting is accomplished. Charting is part of the patient's legal record that is maintained in the office. As with all legal and medical records, each patient's chart should be complete and correct. The initial charting is recorded during the patient's first examination. The dentist dictates his or her findings to the dental assistant, who charts them on a tooth diagram. The doctor indicates the existing conditions, the dental services that have been completed, and the dental services that need to be completed. The patient's dental record (chart) is used for billing purposes, diagnosis, and consultation. Forensic dentistry also uses the patient's dental record to provide information and to identify individuals involved in homicides, abuse, fires, auto accidents, or other tragedies.

DENTAL CHARTS

There are several types of dental charts. Each chart has an area designed for dental charting and an area in which to record treatment. The most commonly used chart is one with diagrams of the teeth that may show an anatomic or a geometric representation of the teeth. Most charts show both the permanent and the primary dentition. The anatomical chart shows the crown of the tooth, the crown and a small portion of the root, or the crown and the complete root. The geometric chart shows the teeth as circles. Each circle represents one tooth and is sectioned into five areas indicating the corresponding surfaces of the tooth.

NUMBERING SYSTEMS

Dental offices have several numbering systems available for their use, and the dentists indicate the preferred systems to be used in their offices. All patient records in one office are documented according to one numbering system to prevent confusion.

Universal/National System for Numbering

The **Universal/National System for numbering** is currently the most commonly used in the United States (Figure 5–1). Each permanent tooth has its own number, starting from the maxillary right third molar as #1 and moving in a clockwise direction to the maxillary left third molar as #16. The mandibular left third molar is #17, and the mandibular right third molar is #32. Therefore, #1 and #32 occlude together and #16 and #17 occlude together. It is the *patient's* right side where tooth #1 and #32 are located; thus, they are not reversed during charting. The primary teeth are each given a letter or a "d" with a number.

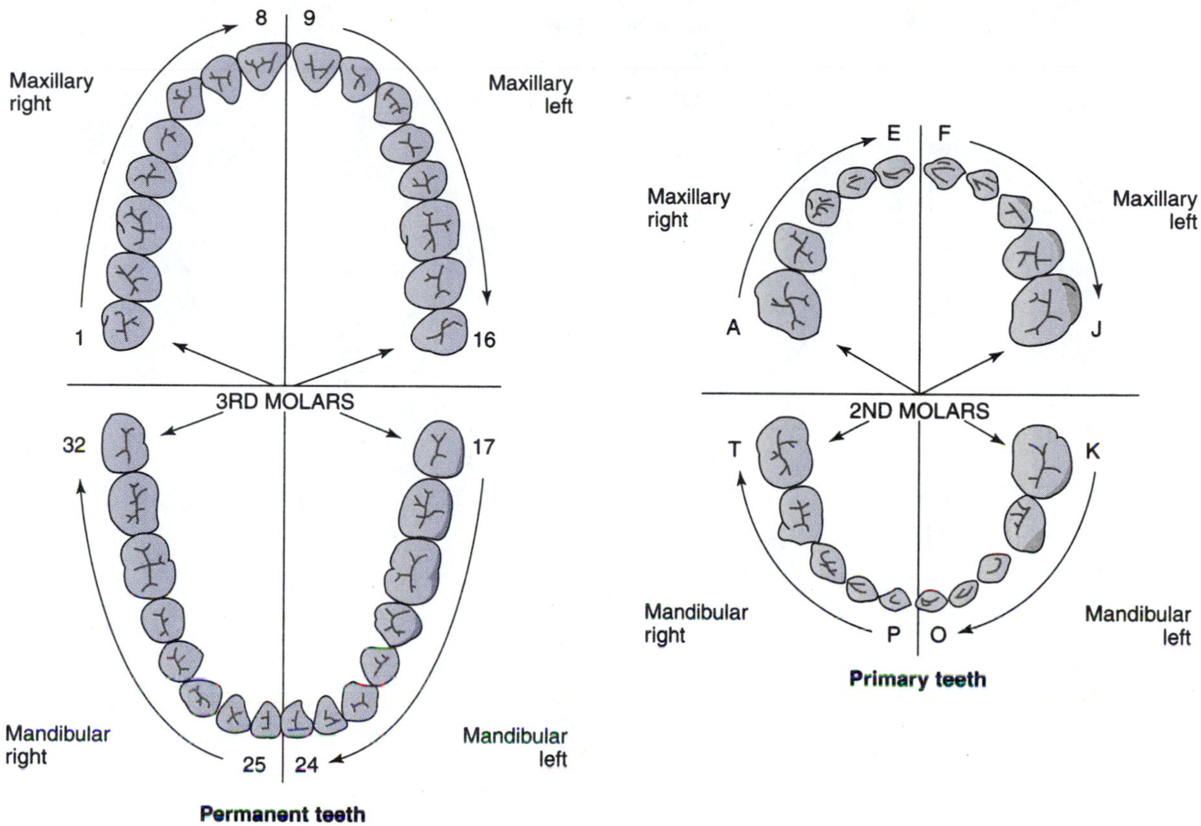

FIGURE 5–1 Permanent and primary dentition showing the Universal/National numbering and lettering system.

The maxillary right deciduous second molar is lettered "A" or "d-1," and this continues across the maxillary arch, with the maxillary left second deciduous molar as "J" or "d-10." The mandibular left second deciduous molar is "K" or "d-11," and this continues across the mandibular arch, with the mandibular right second deciduous molar lettered as "T" or "d-20." Most standardized charts in the United States are printed with diagrams of the primary and permanent teeth using the Universal System for numbering.

Fédération Dentaire Internationale (FDI) System for Numbering

The **Fédération Dentaire Internationale (FDI) system for numbering** can be adapted easily to the computer and is widely used in most other countries (Figure 5–2). In this system, each quadrant is assigned a number. The oral cavity is assigned two digits. If two 00s are noted, the entire oral cavity is designated.

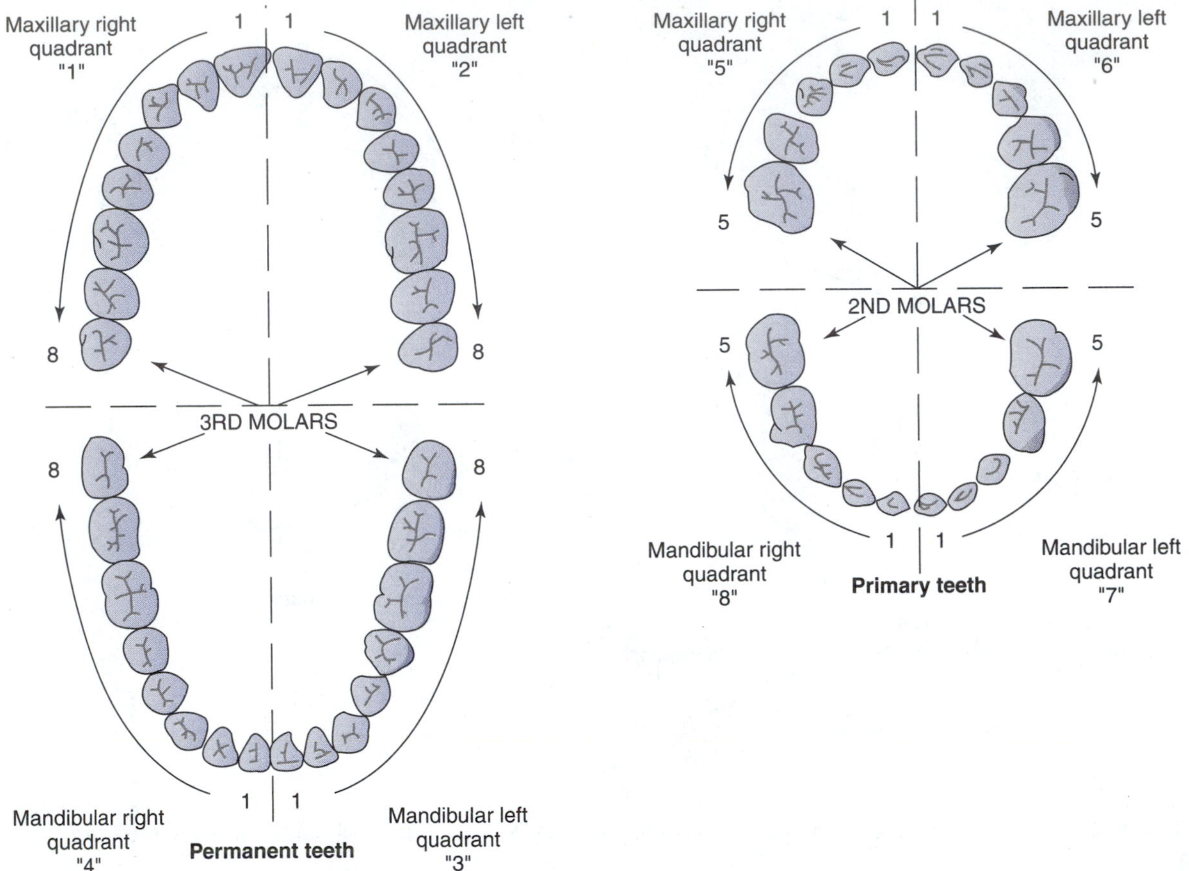

FIGURE 5–2 Permanent and primary dentition showing the International Standards Organization (ISO) TC 106 Designation System/Fédération Dentaire Internationale system.

If 01 is used, it designates the entire maxillary arch; 02 designates the entire mandibular arch. For example, a full denture on the upper (maxillary) arch is noted as denture 01.

The permanent dentition is assigned 1 for the upper right quadrant, 2 for the upper left quadrant, 3 for the lower left quadrant, and 4 for the lower right quadrant. The deciduous dentition is assigned 5 through 8 for the corresponding quadrants. Each quadrant is numbered from 1 to 8, at the midline, starting with the centrals and ending with the molars. The primary teeth are numbered from 1 to 5 in the same manner. When the FDI system is used, the quadrant number is recorded first. For example, the maxillary right lateral incisor is numbered 12 in the permanent dentition and the maxillary right lateral incisor in the deciduous dentition is 52.

Palmer System for Numbering

The **Palmer System for numbering** and lettering the teeth is used in some dental offices. The permanent teeth are numbered 1 through 8 in each quadrant: The centrals are 1 and the third molars are 8. For each number, a quadrant bracket is used to denote which quadrant it is referring to. For example, the maxillary right first bicuspid is charted as 4⅃. The deciduous teeth are identified in a similar manner except that the teeth are lettered "A" through "E" for each quadrant. "A" represents the central incisors and "E" represents the primary second molars. Again, the quadrant bracket is used to denote which quadrant it is referring to. For example, the deciduous mandibular right central incisor is charted as A⅂.

CAVITY CLASSIFICATIONS

Five standard cavity classifications were developed by G.V. Black, and a sixth class was added later. These classifications are useful in recording the type of dental **caries** (cavity) on a patient's chart.

Class I

Class I caries are developmental cavities in the pit and fissures of teeth. They are located in:

- The occlusal surfaces of the posterior teeth (premolars and molars)
- The buccal or lingual pits on the molars
- The lingual pit near the cingulum of the maxillary incisors

Class II

Class II caries form on the proximal (mesial or distal) surfaces on the posterior teeth (premolars and molars).

Class III

Class III caries form on the interproximal surface (mesial or distal) of anterior teeth (canines, lateral incisors, and central incisors).

Class IV

Class IV caries form on the interproximal surface (mesial or distal) of anterior teeth and include the incisal edge.

Class V

Class V caries form on the cervical third of the facial or lingual surfaces of the teeth. Often Class V caries form because the patient habitually sucks on sweets.

The dental assistant may note severe Class V carious lesions in one quadrant because the patient takes medications that cause drying of the oral tissues (xerostomia), chews gum, or ingests soft drinks over long periods. Class V caries are common in older patients with cervical recession.

Class VI

Class VI caries were not part of the original standard classification of cavities developed by G.V. Black. They were later identified to more clearly label cavities that involve the incisal or occlusal surface that has been worn away due to abrasion.

ABBREVIATIONS FOR TOOTH SURFACES

Terms such as simple, compound, and complex are used in cavity classification. A simple cavity involves only one tooth surface, a compound cavity involves two surfaces, and a complex cavity involves more than two surfaces.

When documenting the chart to record the surfaces of the teeth that need to be restored or that have been restored, the dental assistant abbreviates the notations. Each surface is abbreviated using the first letter of the surface, capitalized. For example, an abbreviated form of a mesial restoration on tooth #8 is #8 M. If two or more surfaces are restored, then a combined word is used. The *"al"* is normally dropped and *"o"* is substituted on the first word. For example, to identify the restoration that is on the distal and occlusal surfaces, the term is disto-occlusal restoration, pronounced "D-O." If three surfaces are combined, the same principle is applied to the second word as well. If the tooth has a mesial-occlusal-distal restoration, the correct term is mesio-occluso-distal or MOD restoration, pronounced "M-O-D." If a mesial surface of the tooth is restored with another surface, it is always used first. Occlusal and lingual normally fall in the last position.

Commonly Used Abbreviations

Some commonly used abbreviations for simple, compound, or complex cavities include the following:

- MOD Mesio-occluso-distal
- DO Disto-occlusal
- MO Mesio-occlusal
- MI Mesio-incisal
- DI Disto-incisal
- LI Linguo-incisal
- DL Disto-lingual

- MODBL Mesio-occluso-disto-bucco-lingual
- I Incisal
- M Mesial
- D Distal
- B Buccal

Basic Charting Terms

- **Abscess**—A localized area of infection.
- **Bridge**—A prosthetic device placed in the mouth where a tooth is missing, normally attached on each side and covering the space created by the missing tooth or teeth. The attaching sides are called **abutments** and the middle area is called the **pontic.** A **cantilever bridge** is attached only to one tooth. This is useful in an area that has little stress, such as a missing lateral. The abutment side could then be on the canine, which is a strong support. The **Maryland bridge** has wings on the pontic, attached to the lingual sides of the adjacent (abutment) teeth.
- **Crown**—Some crowns are cast in a laboratory and made to fit the patient's tooth exactly. They are made of several types or combinations of materials, such as gold, porcelain and gold, or porcelain. Crowns can be permanent or temporary, or made for the anterior or posterior. Preformed (temporary) crowns are manufactured in quantities. The dentist sizes and forms the crown to fit the tooth. These crowns are made from stainless steel or mylar plastic. All crowns are "fixed" or cemented into place in the patient's mouth and are not removable like partial and full dentures. Crowns cover the complete tooth, as in a full crown, or three-quarters of the tooth, as in a three-fourths crown.
- **Denture** (complete and partial)—A full denture replaces the complete arch of a patient's dentition. If all the natural teeth in one arch are missing, a full denture is needed. If some of the natural teeth are missing, a partial denture (artificial teeth mounted on a metal framework) is fabricated.
- **Drifting**—All teeth are supported by each other in the dentition. If a maxillary tooth is removed, the opposing mandibular tooth may drift, or **over-erupt,** into the space. Also, the teeth adjacent to the space created by the removed tooth can drift into the space.
- **Incipient**—Beginning decay that has not broken through the enamel. The doctor may choose to watch this area for further breakdown

rather than immediately restore this area. Incipient caries appear as a chalky area on the tooth. It is not yet decay, but the surface has begun to decalcify. Some doctors note this on the chart by placing the word "watch" on that area. Other doctors use a series of red dots, a symbol that represents an incipient area of decay.

- **Mobility**—When the tooth moves in the socket, normally due to periodontal disease or trauma. A numbering system is used to indicate how many millimeters the tooth moves and is recorded in Roman numerals, or from 0–4.
- **Overhang**—Excessive restorative material normally found interproximally near the gingiva.
- **Periodontal pocket**—The space in the gingival sulcus created by periodontal disease. It is measured using a periodontal probe marked in millimeters. A healthy sulcus depth is 1–3 millimeters; beyond this depth it is a periodontal pocket.
- **Restoration**—A material used to replace the missing tooth structure. Several different materials are used to make dental restorations, the most common of which include gold, amalgam, and composite.
- **Root canal**—When the pulp is removed and replaced with a filling material.
- **Sealant**—A resin (plastic) material used to cover or protect pits and fissures to prevent potential decay.

Charting Color Indications and Symbols

Colors and symbols are used in charting to indicate the existing condition of the patient's teeth and surrounding tissues and the restorative services required (Figure 5–3). There are some established symbols that allow for common references when interaction takes place between dental professionals.

Per industry standards red is used to represent the dentistry that needs to be done, and blue indicates that the work has been completed. (For the purposes of this textbook, light blue will be used to represent work that needs to be done, and dark blue will represent work that has already been completed.) Some of the symbols can be charted in either color. For instance, if a tooth is fractured but not causing any discomfort to the patient or not affecting the patient's appearance, the dentist may decide not to restore it. A notation is made on the chart that nothing is to be done at this time and it is charted in either color.

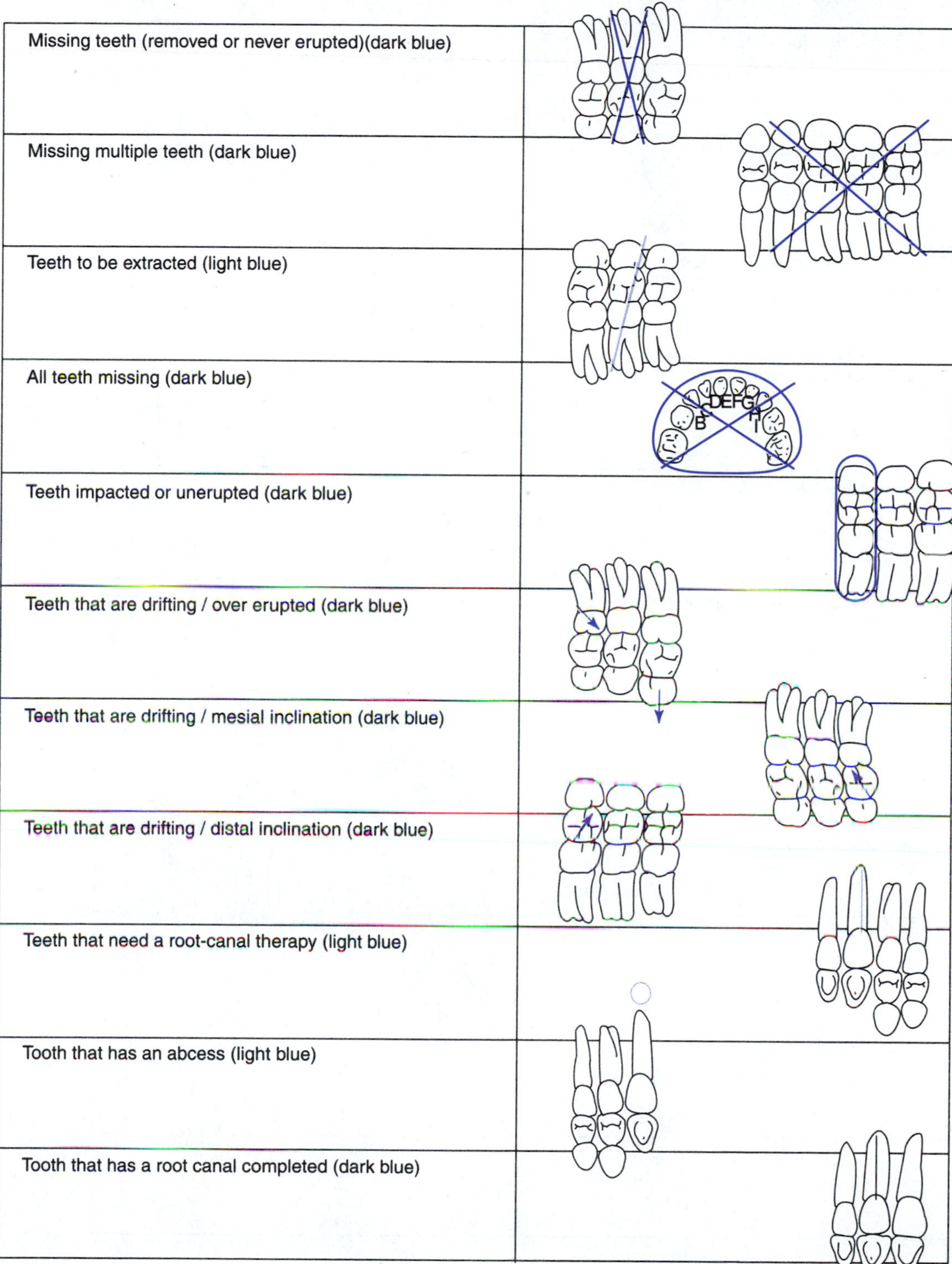

Charting symbol	
Missing teeth (removed or never erupted)(dark blue)	
Missing multiple teeth (dark blue)	
Teeth to be extracted (light blue)	
All teeth missing (dark blue)	
Teeth impacted or unerupted (dark blue)	
Teeth that are drifting / over erupted (dark blue)	
Teeth that are drifting / mesial inclination (dark blue)	
Teeth that are drifting / distal inclination (dark blue)	
Teeth that need a root-canal therapy (light blue)	
Tooth that has an abcess (light blue)	
Tooth that has a root canal completed (dark blue)	

FIGURE 5–3 Charting symbols.

(continued)

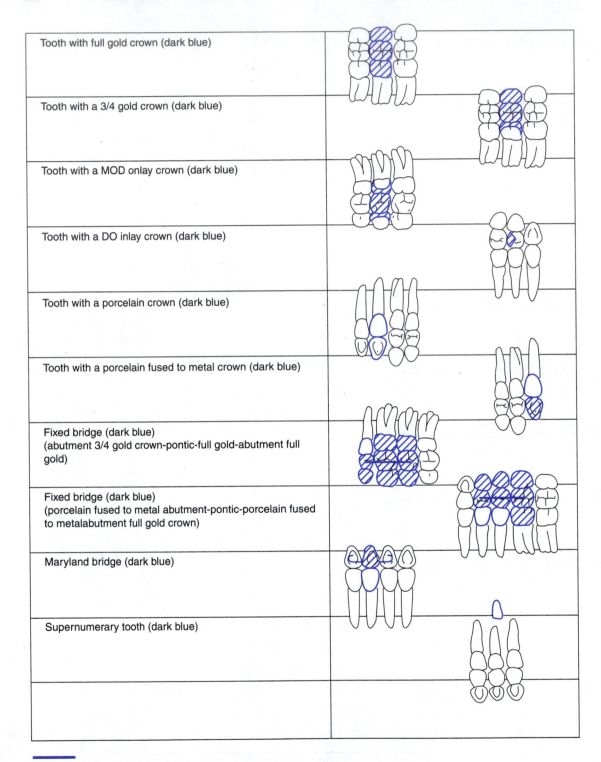

Tooth with full gold crown (dark blue)	
Tooth with a 3/4 gold crown (dark blue)	
Tooth with a MOD onlay crown (dark blue)	
Tooth with a DO inlay crown (dark blue)	
Tooth with a porcelain crown (dark blue)	
Tooth with a porcelain fused to metal crown (dark blue)	
Fixed bridge (dark blue) (abutment 3/4 gold crown-pontic-full gold-abutment full gold)	
Fixed bridge (dark blue) (porcelain fused to metal abutment-pontic-porcelain fused to metalabutment full gold crown)	
Maryland bridge (dark blue)	
Supernumerary tooth (dark blue)	

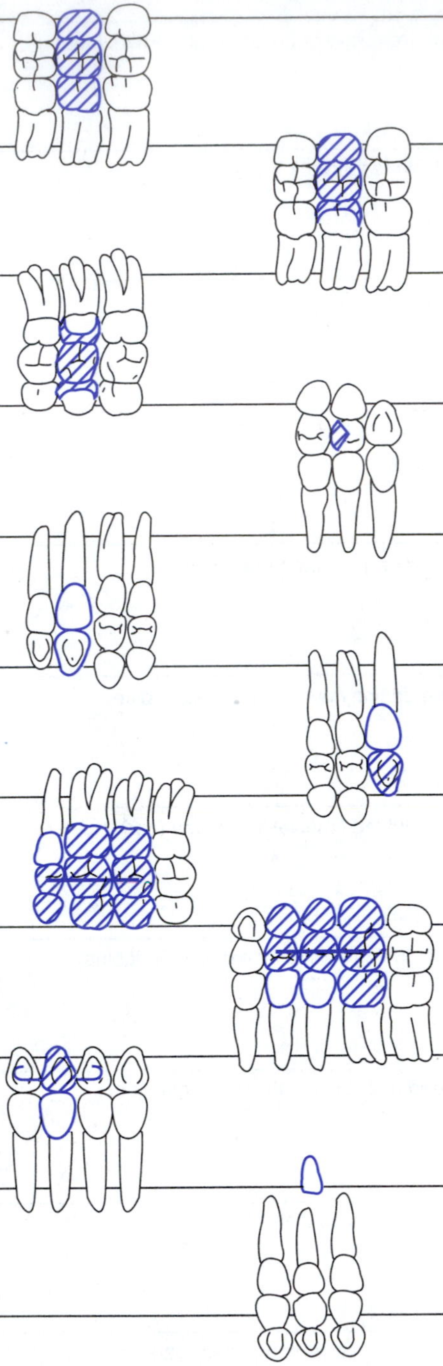

FIGURE 5–3 *(continued)*

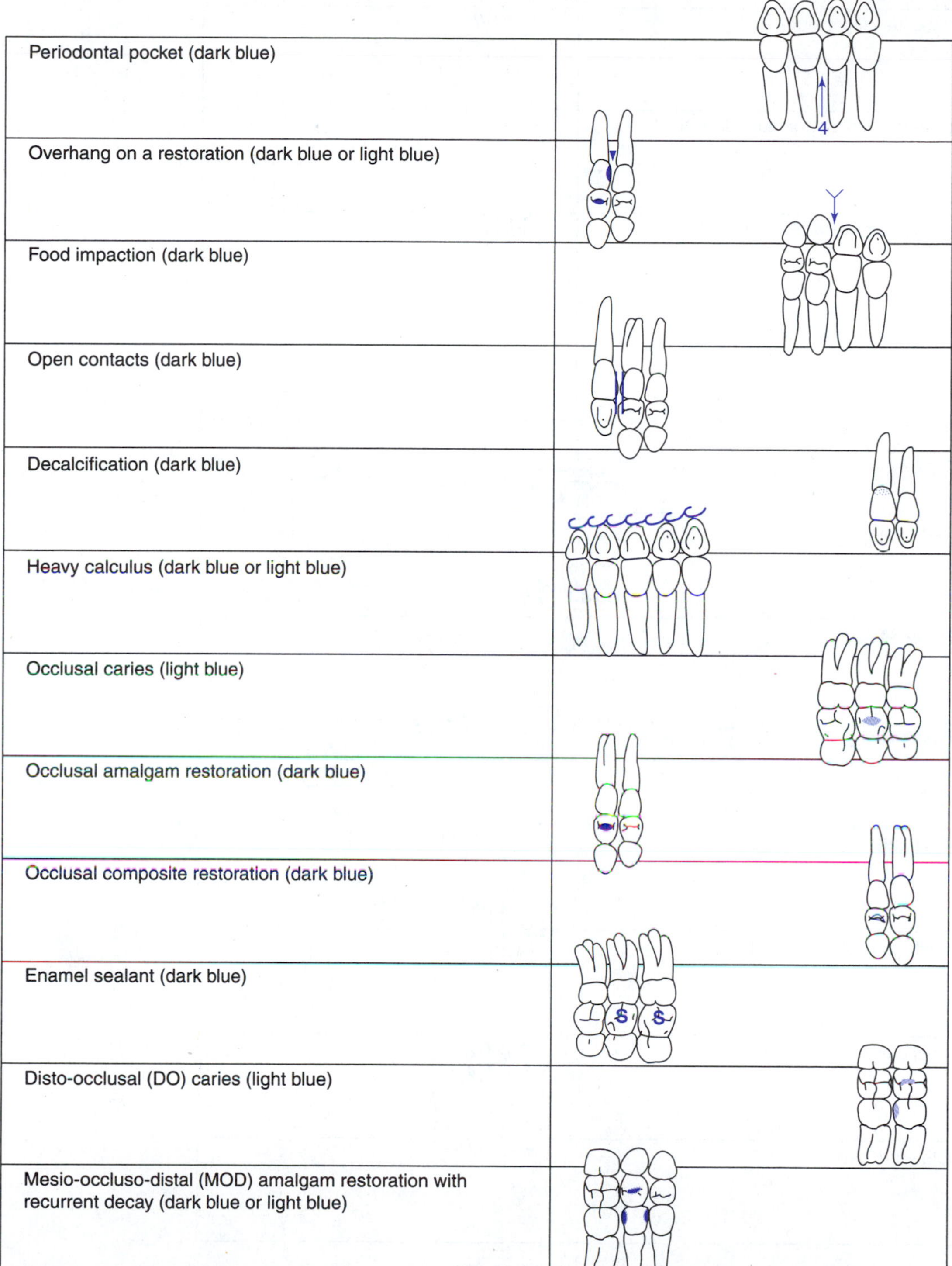

Periodontal pocket (dark blue)
Overhang on a restoration (dark blue or light blue)
Food impaction (dark blue)
Open contacts (dark blue)
Decalcification (dark blue)
Heavy calculus (dark blue or light blue)
Occlusal caries (light blue)
Occlusal amalgam restoration (dark blue)
Occlusal composite restoration (dark blue)
Enamel sealant (dark blue)
Disto-occlusal (DO) caries (light blue)
Mesio-occluso-distal (MOD) amalgam restoration with recurrent decay (dark blue or light blue)

FIGURE 5–3 *(continued)*

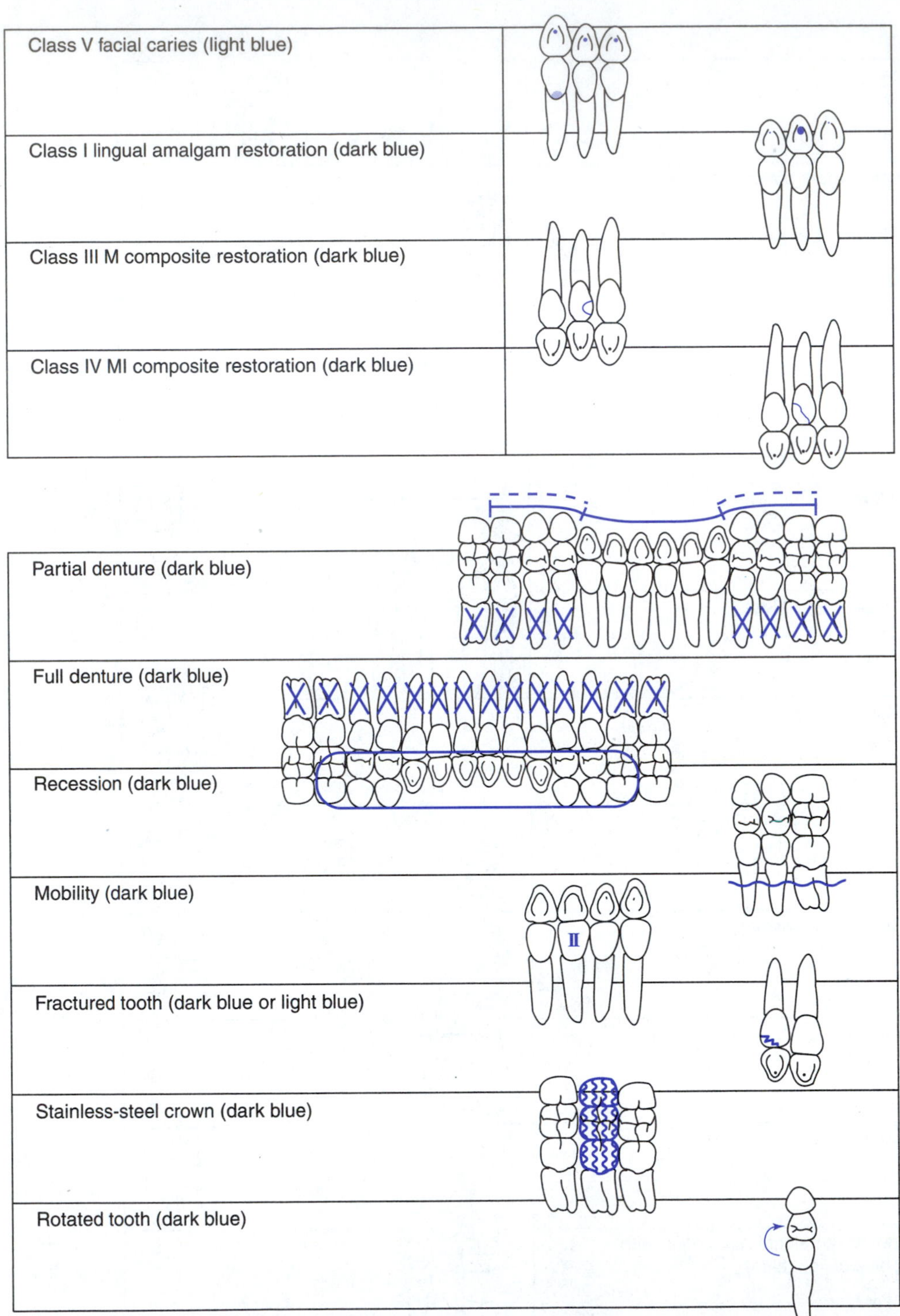

Class V facial caries (light blue)
Class I lingual amalgam restoration (dark blue)
Class III M composite restoration (dark blue)
Class IV MI composite restoration (dark blue)
Partial denture (dark blue)
Full denture (dark blue)
Recession (dark blue)
Mobility (dark blue)
II
Fractured tooth (dark blue or light blue)
Stainless-steel crown (dark blue)
Rotated tooth (dark blue)

FIGURE 5–3 *(continued)*

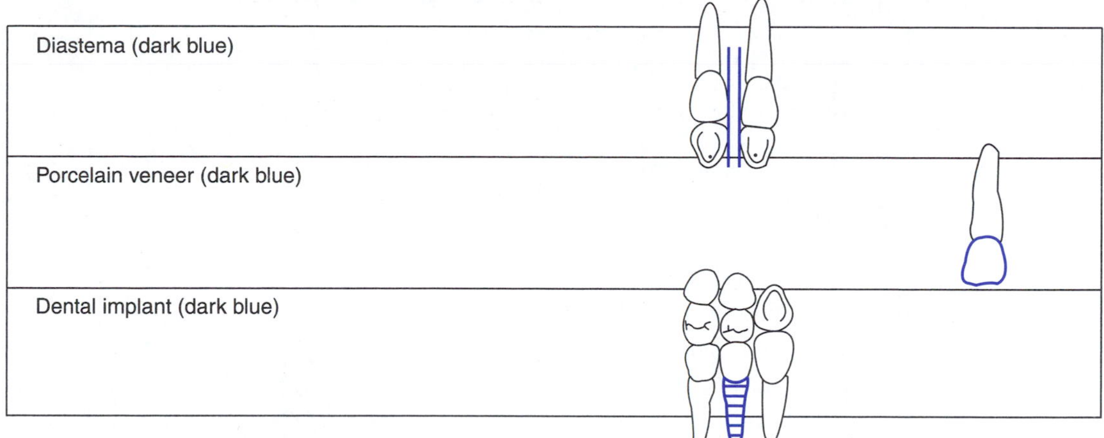

Diastema (dark blue)
Porcelain veneer (dark blue)
Dental implant (dark blue)

FIGURE 5–3 *(continued)*

Charting Example 1

(Charting Using the Anatomical Representation of the Teeth and the Universal System for Numbering) (Figure 5–4)

Tooth	#1	impacted
	#2	Class II DO amalgam restoration present
	#4	Class II MOD amalgam restoration present
	#6	Class III M composite restoration present
	#8	Class IV MI composite restoration present
	#9	Class III M decay (light blue)
	#13	Class II MOD amalgam restoration with recurrent decay (dark blue and light blue)
	#14	Class II MO amalgam restoration present,; food impaction between 13 & 14
	#16	has been removed
	#17	partially impacted and needs to be removed (light blue)
	#19	bridge present, abutment full gold crown
	#20	bridge present, pontic porcelain with gold
	#21	bridge present, abutment porcelain with gold
	#24	mobility of III, periodontal pocket on M and D of 4mm each, heavy calculus from mandibular left cuspid to mandibular right cuspid
	#25	periodontal pocket on IV and D of 3mm each
	#28	needs a full gold crown with a porcelain facing (light blue)
	#28	has a root canal completed
	#30	Class I O decay (light blue)
	#31	Class II MO amalgam restoration present
	#32	has been removed

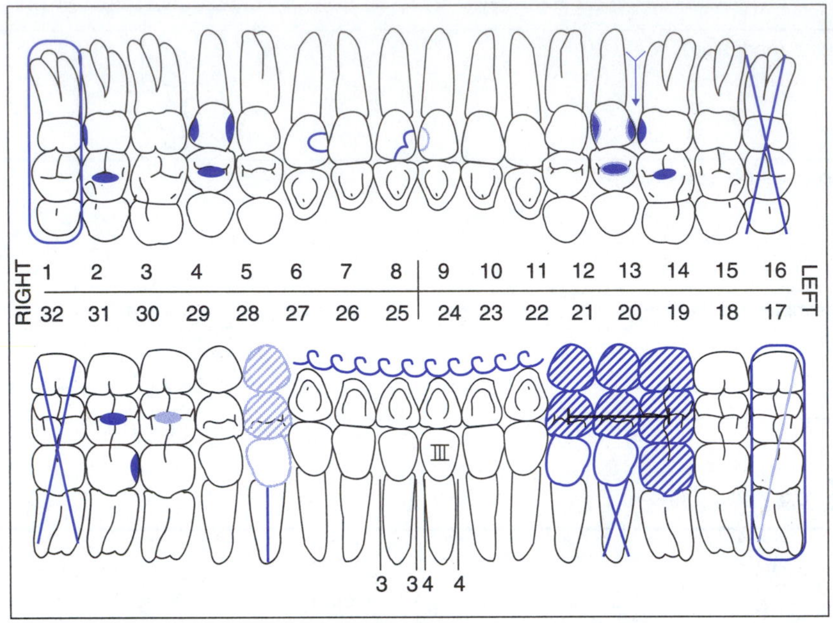

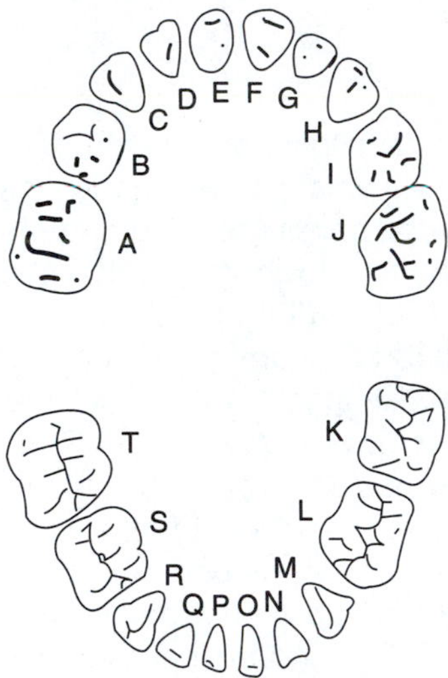

FIGURE 5–4 Charting using the anatomical teeth and the Universal numbering system.

Charting Example 2

(Charting Using the Geometric Representation of the Teeth and the International Standards Organization System for Tooth Identification) (Figure 5–5).

Tooth	#18	impacted
	#16	full porcelain with gold crown present
	#15	Class II MO amalgam restoration present
	#14	Class I O sealant present
	#12	Class III M composite present with recurrent decay (light blue)
	#11	Class I L composite present
	#24	bridge present, abutment full porcelain with gold
	#25	bridge present, pontic full porcelain with gold
	#26	bridge present, abutment full porcelain with gold
	#28	has been removed
	#38	has been removed
	#36	has a full gold crown
	#34	has an abscess and needs a root canal (light blue)
	#33	is missing and the deciduous tooth is retained
	#31	Class IV MI composite restoration present
	#42	has a fracture on the MI edge
	#45	Class II DO amalgam restoration with an overhang
	#47	has been removed
	#48	mesial inclination

Charting Example Review

1. Which tooth has a pit and fissure sealant?
2. Which primary tooth is present in the patient's mouth?
3. Which tooth needs endodontic therapy?

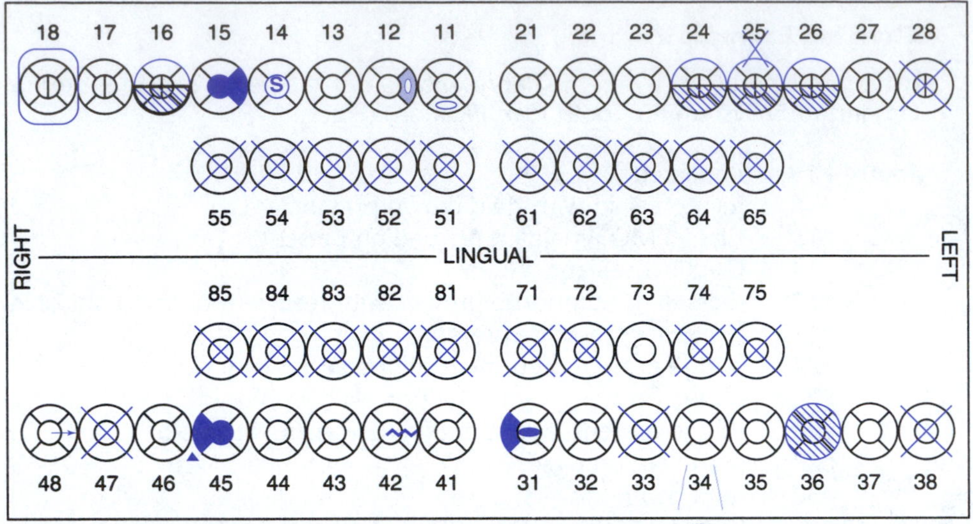

FIGURE 5–5 Charting using the geometric representation of the teeth and the International Standards Organization (ISO) TC 106 designation system for the teeth.

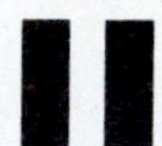

Preclinical Dental Skills

CHAPTER 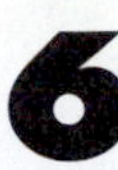

Infection Control/ Sterilization Procedures

CDA

OBJECTIVES

The student should strive to meet the following objectives and demonstrate an understanding of the facts and principles presented in this chapter:

1. Identify the regulations and training that govern infection control in the dental office.
2. Describe how pathogens travel from person to person in the dental office.
3. List the three primary routes of microbial transmission and the associated dental procedures that affect the dental assistant.
4. Demonstrate the principles of infection control, including medical history, handwashing, personal protective equipment, barriers, chemical disinfectants, ultrasonic cleaners, sterilizers, and instrument storage.
5. List various disinfectants and their applications in dentistry.
6. Demonstrate the usage of several types of sterilizers.
7. Identify and demonstrate the correct protocol for disinfecting, cleaning, and sterilizing instruments and surfaces prior to seating the patient, as well as at the end of the dental treatment, and in the dental laboratory.

KEY TERMS

antimicrobial (p. 74)
asepsis (p. 68)
aseptic technique (p. 68)
Bloodborne Pathogens Standard (p. 69)
contamination (p. 69)
direct contact (p. 73)
disinfect (p. 79)
Environmental Protection Agency (p. 80)
indirect contact (p. 73)
infection control (p. 73)
inhalation (p. 73)
instrument sterilizing system (p. 83)
Occupational Safety and Health Administration (OSHA) (p. 69)
other potentially infectious materials (OPIM) (p. 69)
pathogens (p. 68)
standard precautions (p. 68)
sterilization (p. 80)
universal precautions (p. 68)

Introduction

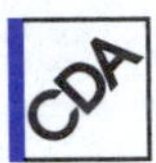

The dentist is responsible for ensuring that the process of infection control is adequate. Compliance with all regulations must be accomplished on a continuing basis; staff must be trained at the time of initial employment or when job tasks change (before the employee is placed in a position where occupational exposure may occur) and annually thereafter. The records must be maintained for the duration of employment plus thirty years, in accordance with federal regulations. Even though the dentist is ultimately responsible, often an employee is designated as the infection control and hazard waste coordinator. This person ensures that the office is in compliance with all regulations, reads updated information on infection control and hazard waste, and presents the information to the dental team for review. The infection control and hazard waste coordinator schedules staff training, oversees the entire process of infection control, and makes sure that procedures ensure complete **asepsis**. Asepsis means the creation of an environment free of **pathogens** (disease-causing microorganisms). It also includes the steps, or **aseptic technique**, used to provide this environment. Aseptic technique is necessary for all procedures in which there is a potential risk of introducing infection or disease into a human's body.

Rationales and Regulations

Rationale of Infection Control

All efforts are made to prevent infectious diseases from spreading. Routine practices eliminate mistakes from being made. **Universal precautions** mean that all patients are treated as if they are infectious. **Standard precautions** (universal precautions and body substance isolation techniques) are practiced prior to, during, and after each procedure in the dental office. Therefore, every precaution is taken to ensure that the chain of asepsis (aseptic procedures ensuring that no cross-contamination occurs) is not broken and that **contamination** does not occur.

Occupational Safety and Health Administration. The **Occupational Safety and Health Administration (OSHA)** is a regulating body that enforces the requirements that employers must protect their employees from exposure to blood and **other potentially infectious materials (OPIM)** when employees are at work. This agency is part of the United States Department of Labor. Its overall mission is to protect workers in the United States from physical, chemical, or infectious hazards while in the workplace. The OSHA **Bloodborne Pathogens Standard** became effective in 1992. This standard applies to any facility where employees can or have the potential to be exposed to body fluids, such as in hospitals, funeral homes, emergency medical services, medical and dental offices, and research laboratories.

Compliance with these standards is monitored through investigations of the facilities by OSHA compliance inspectors. If the facility fails to come into compliance, a citation resulting in a possible fine is issued. If the facility continues to refuse to comply, the fine increases and additional steps are taken to ensure that the conditions are corrected.

When Investigations of Dental Offices for Compliance Are Conducted

- After an employee or a patient complaint is made
- In any office having eleven or more employees, on a random basis
- By invitation of the office when an inspection is requested

Overview of the 1992 OSHA Bloodborne Pathogens Standard

Every facility must:

- Review the Bloodborne Pathogens Standard
- Prepare a written exposure control plan and means to protect and train employees
- Train all employees in a timely manner (initially, after a job task change, and annually thereafter)
- Provide employees with everything needed to meet standard regulations
- Provide personal protective equipment (PPE)
- Maintain and dispose of necessary PPE

- Establish standard operating procedures (SOP) in infection control
- Offer the hepatitis B vaccination series to all employees free of charge
- Establish a post-exposure plan, including medical evaluation and follow-up procedures (for example, occupational exposure needle stick)
- Provide communication on biohazards
- Establish standards for handling and disposing of hazardous waste
- Maintain records of training, hepatitis B vaccinations, and exposure incidents

Written Exposure Plan This plan documents the specific exposure determination for each employee and identifies a schedule of implementation (how and when the provisions of the standard will be implemented). This document must list how the situations surrounding an exposure will be evaluated and what measures will be taken to correct the situation (if necessary).

Exposure Determination To evaluate an employee's risk for an occupational exposure to bloodborne pathogens, an exposure determination is made. An occupational exposure is any reasonably anticipated eye, mucosa, skin, parenteral (cut, needlestick, puncture, or abrasions), or any contact with blood or saliva that may be a result of employment tasks. The determination is made based on three categories:

Step 1. All employees make a list of tasks they perform in each job classification and then identify under which category they fall. Any employee who may have any occupational exposure at any time is covered under the standard.

- **Category 1**—includes all tasks that involve exposure to blood, body fluids such as saliva, and body tissues. (This group includes the dentist, dental assistant, dental hygienist, and dental laboratory technician.)
- **Category 2**—includes all tasks that involve no exposure to blood, body fluids such as saliva, or body tissues, but occasionally may involve unplanned tasks from Category 1. (This group includes the receptionist, coordinating assistant, etc.)
- **Category 3**—includes all tasks that involve no exposure to blood, body fluids such as saliva, or body tissues. (This group includes the accountant, insurance assistant, etc.)

Step 2. The office must have a schedule for implementation. This schedule must designate how and when each provision of the standard will be implemented.

- How and when are the hepatitis B vaccinations being offered to employees?

- How and when is communication of hazards to employees being covered?
- How and when are the post-exposure evaluation and office follow-up procedures being accomplished?
- How and when is the recordkeeping being accomplished and updated?

Step 3. A manual and procedure plan must be written to cover methods of compliance for office PPE and safety issues. For example, the office must have written information covering all aspects of the following:

- Personal protective equipment
- Engineering controls
- Housekeeping controls
- Work practice controls

Step 4. A written policy on how exposure incidents are evaluated is required. Included in this area are the circumstances that surround the incident and how they can be corrected. What type of evaluation will be done by the office if an exposure incident occurs?

OSHA-Mandated Training of Employees in the Dental Office

All employers must ensure that employees (full time, part time, and temporary) who fall into Category 1 and/or 2, where tasks involve exposure to blood, body fluid such as saliva, and/or body tissues, have training. This training must be provided at no cost to the employee. The training must be given prior to placement in a position where bloodborne pathogens are a factor, to all new employees within ten days of employment, and to all employees reclassifying into different positions.

Mandated OSHA Training of Dental Employees

The following must be available to all dental employees:

- A copy of the Bloodborne Pathogens Standard and specific information regarding the meaning of the standard
- Information about bloodborne pathogens, both the epidemiology and symptoms of the diseases
- Information about the cross-contamination pathways of bloodborne pathogens
- A written copy or means for employees to obtain the employer's/office's written exposure control plan

- Information on the tasks, category placement of employee classifications, and how each is identified in relation to bloodborne pathogens and other potentially infectious materials (OPIM)
- Information regarding the hepatitis B vaccine
- Information about exposure reduction, including PPE; work practices; standard precautions, including universal precautions; and engineering practices
- Information about the selection, placement, use, removal, disinfection, sterilization, and disposal of PPE
- Information about what to do and whom to contact if an emergency involving blood or OPIM arises
- Information about the procedure to follow if an incident of blood exposure occurs, how to report the incident, and what type of medical follow-up is available at no cost to the employee
- Information about the post-exposure evaluation and follow-up the employer provides
- A copy of the OSHA Hazard Communication Standard
- Material Safety Data Sheets (MSDS) and information about labeling and hazardous waste
- Opportunity for employees to ask questions of the individual providing the training

The training cannot be provided by videos or interactive computer training programs alone. It must be provided by an individual who has the background necessary to answer questions and to supplement the training with in-office (on-site), specific information. The information must be communicated in a manner for all to understand. If an employee is unable to understand the content due to a language barrier or a disability, the employer must provide an interpreter or convey this information in a manner for the employee to understand completely.

A record of the date of the training session, employees present, and qualifications of the trainer must be maintained.

Cross-Contamination Pathways

Pathogens can travel from patients to dentists, dental assistants, dental hygienists, dental laboratory technicians, and other patients. Pathogens can also travel from dental personnel to patients. The transfer then can go to the families and friends of the dental personnel. This cycle must be broken through aseptic techniques.

Routes of Microbial Transmission

In dentistry, three primary routes transmit most microorganisms: direct contact, indirect contact, and inhalation/aerosol. Microorganisms may be missed because they appear as a mist or dry clear on the surfaces that are touched. The dental assistant is the primary provider of infection control practices. Using the correct barriers, PPE, treating all patients as if they are infectious, using proper disinfection, and sterilization break the cycle of infection and eliminate cross-contamination. The possible routes of microbial transmission are:

1. **Direct contact**: An individual has direct contact with a lesion or pathogenic microorganism while performing intraoral dental procedures.
2. **Indirect contact**: An individual contacts the pathogenic microorganism through another means, such as contaminated instruments, supplies, or equipment.
3. **Inhalation**/aerosol: An individual contacts the microorganism through inhalation. This normally happens when the high speed handpiece or the ultrasonic cavitron is used.

Infection Control in the Dental Office

A number of steps must be followed to accomplish the goal of **infection control**, or asepsis. The first step is for the dental assistant to maintain good health standards. Eating and sleeping properly facilitates staying healthy. Proper exercise, along with maintaining a positive mental attitude, provides the energy to attain individual goals for good overall health.

Immunizations

The dental assistant should have the immunizations necessary to fight off pathogens that are encountered due to the close proximity to patients during dental treatment. If the dental assistant has not had the hepatitis B series, the employer must provide the vaccine and is required to pay for the series.

Medical History

Taking the patient's medical history and updating it at each appointment is a good way to gather information but may not identify infectious diseases patients have. It is important to update this information both verbally and in writing. Patients are sometimes more willing to disclose information during conversation. The majority of individuals infected with HBV and HIV are **asymptomatic,** having no symptoms. Therefore, the medical history may give information to the healthcare worker, but it cannot be used alone to identify patients who place dental personnel at high risk. Incorporating universal precautions and practicing infection control standards with each and every patient are essential in infection control.

Handwashing

One of the most important ways to prevent the transfer of microorganisms from one person or object to another person is handwashing. Handwashing is the vigorous rubbing together of well-lathered soapy hands (ensuring friction on all surfaces), concluding with a thorough rinsing under a stream of warm water and proper drying (Procedure 6–1). Handwashing is both a mechanical cleaning and chemical **antisepsis** (inhibiting the growth of causative microorganisms).

Chemical antisepsis is accomplished with an antimicrobial soap. Applying the proper technique and using **antimicrobial** (microorganism growth inhibitor)

PROCEDURE

6-1 Handwashing

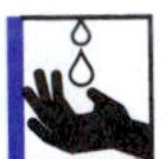
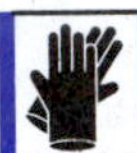
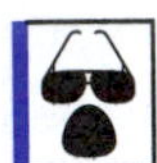

The procedure is performed by all clinical dental team members.

EQUIPMENT AND SUPPLIES

- Liquid antimicrobial handwashing agent
- Soft, sterile brush or sponge (optional)
- Sink with hot and cold running water
- Paper towels

PROCEDURE STEPS

At the beginning of each day (two consecutive thirty-second handwashes)

1. Remove jewelry (rings and watch).
2. Adjust water flow and wet hands thoroughly.
3. Apply antimicrobial handwashing agents with warm water; bring to a lather.
4. Scrub hands together or with a sterile brush or sponge, making sure to get between each finger, the surface of the palms and wrists, and under the finger nails.
5. Rinse and repeat Steps 3 and 4.
6. Final rinse with cool water for ten seconds to close the pores.
7. Dry with paper towels, the hands first and then the wrist area.
8. Use paper towels to turn off the hand-controlled faucets.

Routine Handwashing: Thirty-second handwash before and after patients, donning gloves, and taking breaks. Routine handwashing must be completed at the end of each day and any other time the hands become contaminated.

1. Complete the handwashing steps for the beginning of each day, except Step 5.

handwashing products add additional protection to ensure that microorganisms are reduced each time the hands are washed.

At the beginning of each day, every member of the dental team should complete two consecutive thirty-second handwashes. It is important to use plenty of antimicrobial soap and water while rubbing all areas of the hands. Getting between the fingers, rubbing each finger and thumb, and cleaning beneath the fingernails is essential. A final rinse with cool water is necessary to close the pores in the skin. Dry the hands completely with paper towels, and use the paper towels to turn off the hand-controlled sink faucets and wipe the area clean.

A minimal thirty-second handwashing should be completed before and after patient care, donning and removing gloves, breaks, ending each day, and at any other time the hands become contaminated.

Personal Protective Equipment (PPE)

The dental assistant has constant exposure to saliva and blood during intraoral/invasive dental procedures. Even with the maintenance of good health and immunizations, it is essential for dental team members to ensure better protection against pathogenic microorganisms with constant use of personal protective equipment (PPE). The employer must provide this equipment according to OSHA regulations. Barriers are used to prevent potential pathogens, encountered during patient care, from contacting dental personnel. Barriers such as protective eyewear, face masks, disposable gloves, and appropriate uniforms should be used routinely to minimize exposure.

Protective Eyewear. It is essential that dental team members wear protective eyewear during dental treatment. The splatter of blood and saliva can transfer infectious diseases, such as hepatitis and herpes simplex viruses, to the mucous membranes of the eye. Aerosol droplets that contain pathogenic microorganisms can cause an eye infection known as pink eye (conjunctivitis). Also, during some dental procedures, particles of gold, amalgam, and tooth fragments can be embedded in the eye, causing damage. Dental offices provide protective eyewear for patients to wear during dental treatment. These glasses, like the ones worn by the dental personnel, can be disposable or sterilized after use.

Protective eyewear should provide front, top, and side protection; several choices are available. Dental team members who wear corrective lenses may choose to wear goggles that fit over their glasses or side shields that fit on their own eyewear. Others wear glasses designed for dental personnel that incorporate top and side shields. In addition, a face shield can be worn that covers the entire face. A mask must be worn with a face shield.

Eyewear is also utilized to protect the eyes from high intensity lights used for curing dental materials. These glasses or shields are usually colored orange for protection.

Gloves. Gloves are used as a barrier to microorganisms. Any time a dental team member anticipates contact with saliva or blood, gloves should be worn. This includes saliva- or blood-contaminated surfaces, instruments, or mucous membranes. Numerous gloves are on the market that meet FDA regulations. The FDA regulates the gloves specific for the healthcare industry. Five primary types of gloves are used in the dental office (FDA regulated*):

1. Latex gloves (nonsterile and sterile)*
2. Vinyl gloves (nonsterile and sterile)*
3. Overgloves (nonsterile)
4. Utility gloves (nonsterile)
5. Polynitrile, nitrile (autoclavable)

Both the **latex** and **vinyl gloves** are ambidextrous, used interchangeably for the right or left hand. They are supplied in a variety of sizes to provide the proper fit for most individuals. Many individuals feel that latex gloves provide a better fit. Latex-sensitive individuals use vinyl gloves as an alternative to latex. The vinyl gloves, however, are more rigid, therefore tearing more easily and lacking tactile sensitivity. Gloves (latex and vinyl) can be ordered with powder on the inside to aid in donning (placing the gloves on). Both types of gloves are supplied as nonsterile, referred to as examination gloves, and sterile, referred to as sterile surgical gloves. Most procedures in the dental office require only the use of the nonsterile gloves. They provide the minimal barrier protection needed for the dental personnel. Sterile surgical gloves are only used in specific surgical procedures requiring a sterile environment, such as oral, periodontal, and implant surgery.

Both latex and vinyl gloves need to be changed with each new patient. If, during the procedure, they become torn or punctured, they should be removed, the hands washed, and the gloves replaced with new gloves to complete the procedure. *Gloves should never be washed and reused.*

Harmful Reactions to Latex Gloves and Other Latex Products

Symptoms	Condition
Hands become dry, red, itchy, and sometimes cracked	Irritant contact dermatitis
Redness, initial itching, and vesicles appear in areas of contact within twenty-four to forty-eight hours, followed by dry skin with fissures and sores	Type IV hypersensitivity (delayed hypersensitivity)
Runny nose, sneezing, itchy eyes, scratchy throat, asthma, and, in rare cases, anaphylaxis	Type I hypersensitivity (immediate-type hypersensitivity)

Overgloves, also known as food handlers' gloves, are worn over the latex or vinyl gloves during a procedure to prevent cross-contamination if the dental assistant has to reach inside a drawer, write on a chart, or touch an area that is not contaminated. Overgloves are big, loose gloves that do not have the tactile touch that the latex and vinyl gloves have; however they quickly fit over the gloves to obtain something in a sterile area. They are not to be used as examination gloves. Overgloves can be placed on rapidly to accomplish the secondary task needed, such as opening a container. They must be discarded after each use.

Utility gloves are thicker gloves used during disinfection and cleanup procedures. An assistant carries the tray to the sterilization area, removes the latex or vinyl gloves, washes his or her hands, and dons the utility gloves to complete the cleanup. The utility gloves can be washed and reused. If they do become cracked or punctured, they should be discarded and new gloves used.

Masks. Masks are worn at any time the possibility for splatter or aerosol of saliva or blood can occur. The dental assistant must wear a mask to protect the mucous membranes of the nose and the mouth. The aerosol mist that remains suspended in the air may come from the use of the dental handpiece, the ultrasonic scaler, or the air-water syringe. At times, due to the use of the air-water syringe, splatter occurs where a concentrated amount of saliva or blood projects from the oral cavity to the dental health worker. Proper placement of the high volume evacuator and the air-water syringe aids in the reduction of splatter; however, it can still occur. Wearing a mask, covering the nose and mouth, protects dental personnel in such cases.

Utilization of the dental mask also protects the patient and the dental assistant from the transmission of communicable diseases.

Masks During Dental Treatment

- Use a new mask for each patient.
- Replace the mask if it becomes moist or wet.
- Never let the mask dangle around the neck or from the ear; remove and discard after use.

The mask should be placed along with the eyewear, prior to washing hands and donning gloves (Figure 6–1). It is important that the mask be placed properly so it fits snugly against the face and stays in place during the procedure. The face mask has an outside and an inside (next to the face); place it according to the manufacturer's directions. Often, a color is on the outside surface for quick identification. Masks are also available in a variety of designs for a positive practice image.

The mask is secured with elastic that goes around the head or over the ears, or with ties that are fastened behind the head. Some masks can be pinched above the nose to fit better and not allow the breath to fog the

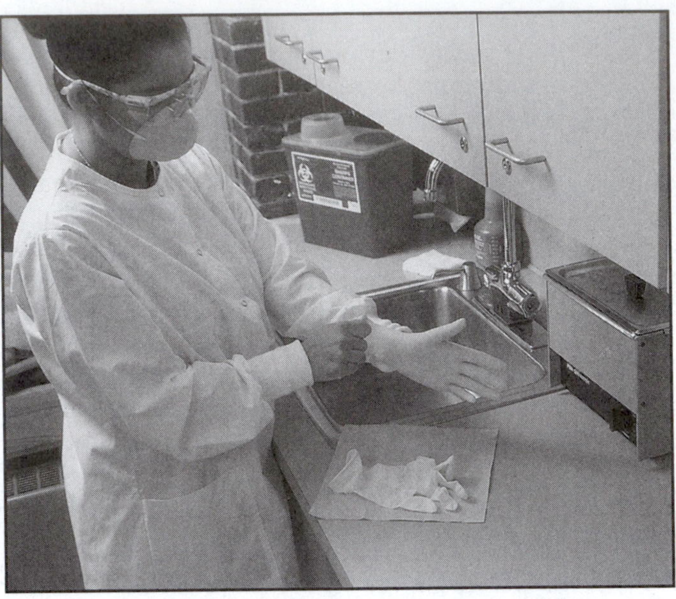

FIGURE 6–1 Dental assistant putting on PPE prior to performing dental procedures.

protective eyewear. Masks should be removed after the procedure by grasping the ties or attachments. Never reuse a mask; replace after every patient or during the procedure if the mask becomes moist. Never slip the mask down on the neck area or let it dangle from the ear after treatment is over. Remove the mask and dispose of it.

Protective Clothing. Special protective clothing worn only in the dental office is regulated by OSHA. Protective clothing includes uniforms, laboratory coats, gowns, and clinic jackets. The dentist must provide protective clothing that is worn and laundered in the office or by a commercial laundering service. One uniform for each staff member each day is appropriate. Dental personnel enter the office and change into uniforms or other PPE overgarments. The employer is required to clean, launder, and dispose of PPE at no cost to the employee. The uniforms or other PPE overgarments, such as laboratory coats, should be removed if the dental assistant is going out to lunch or going into the staff lounge for lunch.

Long isolation gowns are worn by the dental team members who fall in Category 1 or 2. Gowns and uniforms cover the arms and fit closely around the neck and the wrists and provide the greatest protection if impermeable to fluids. During the time the gloves are on, the gloves fit over the cuffs of the uniform.

Protective clothing should be changed daily or immediately if splattered with body fluids. Special attention to the design of the protective clothing should be taken. Buttons, zippers, and ornamental design should be kept to a minimum, because they can harbor pathogens. Disposable outer gowns are an option for dental personnel.

Protective Clothing Worn in the Dental Office

- Worn only in the dental offices (not in staff lounges or lunch rooms)
- Must close tightly at neck and around cuff area
- Must be knee length when sitting
- Must be removed at the end of the day, prior to going home
- Must be laundered in the office or sent to a laundry service

Barriers

Barriers are used in all aspects of the dental office, where possible. In the operatory, the patient dental chair, the light (handles and operating switch), the handpieces, air-water syringe, high volume evacuator, saliva ejector, tubing, writing utensils, and surfaces are covered with barriers (Figure 6–2). Any area that can be covered where contamination is possible during dental treatment should be covered. Barriers have been made specifically for areas that have been hard to disinfect or sterilize in the past, such as tubing and hoses for the handpieces. The patient should wear protective eyewear and a napkin or bib for protection from splatter and debris.

Disinfection

Areas that do not lend themselves to the use of barriers must be disinfected if they cannot be sterilized. Some dental offices use barriers and also **disinfect.** When all surfaces are disinfected and/or protected by a barrier, the requirement of asepsis is met.

Cleaning the Area

All areas where dental procedures are performed must be cleaned prior to disinfection and sterilization. **Cleaning** is the physical removal of organic matter, such as blood, tissue, and debris. The process of cleaning decreases the number of microorganisms in the area and removes substances that may hinder the processes of disinfection and sterilization.

If something is **sanitized,** the process is much like cleaning. Sanitization means the area has been decontaminated, but it does not mean that all microorganisms in the area have been destroyed.

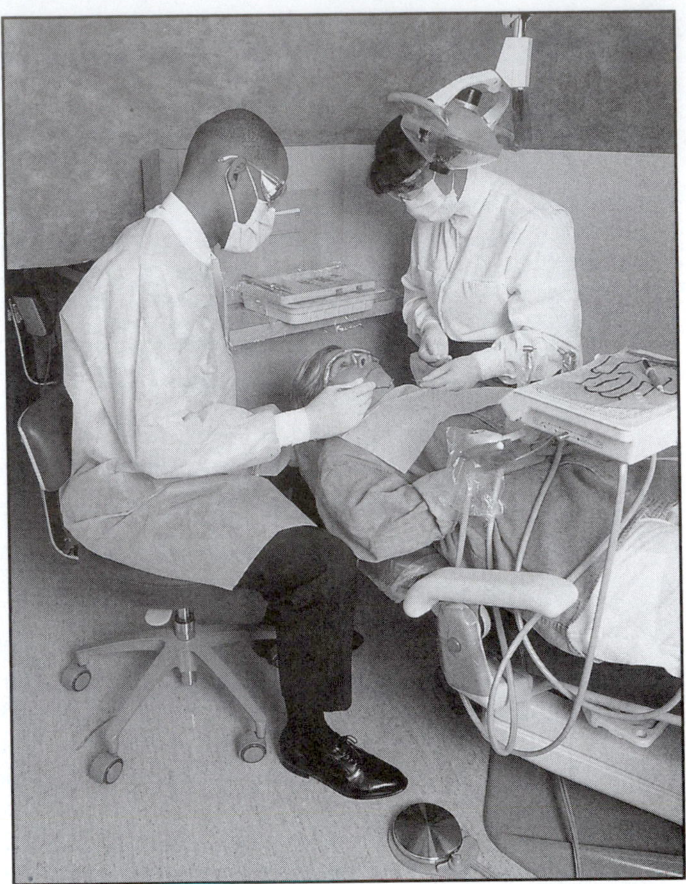

FIGURE 6-2 Barriers in place in a dental treatment room. Doctor, patient, and assistant with PPE.

Environmental Protection Agency Approval

The **Environmental Protection Agency** (EPA) approves disinfection and sterilization solutions only after the products have undergone careful testing. Disinfecting and sterilization solutions must have EPA approval on their labels. Each product registered with the EPA must have a determination as to whether a solution sterilizes or disinfects and what types of microorganisms it will destroy. **Sterilization** means that all forms of microorganisms are destroyed; disinfection occurs when *some* microorganisms are destroyed. The contact time needed for each product is also described on the label. Some products disinfect after ten minutes but need to have ten hours of submersion to sterilize. The disinfection levels according to the EPA are rated as *high, intermediate,* and *low.*

- **High-level disinfection** is a tuberculocidal that kills most but not all bacterial spores. If it is extremely strong and can kill all the bacterial spores, it is noted as a sporicidal on the label.

- **Intermediate-level disinfection** is a tuberculocidal that usually does not kill bacterial spores.
- **Low-level disinfection** kills some viruses and fungi and most of the bacteria microorganisms. It does not kill tuberculosis or bacterial spores.

Products for disinfection and sterilization for the dental office have advantages and disadvantages for use with specific materials. Staining and corrosiveness to instruments and equipment, along with the toxicity of the material, should be considered when selecting solutions.

Chemical Disinfectants

A universally accepted technique for cleaning and disinfecting surfaces is the **spray-wipe-spray-wipe technique.** First, the surface is sprayed then wiped to eliminate debris to accomplish initial surface cleaning. The second spray, which must be a surface disinfectant, is left on the item and/or surfaces for the specific time indicated by the manufacturer (normally ten minutes) and wiped or left to dry (Table 6–1).

Ultrasonic Cleaning

If the dental assistant is not able to recycle the instruments immediately after the procedure, the instruments should be submerged in a holding bath (precleaning), a solution that loosens hardened debris from the instruments prior to cleaning and sterilizing. It also prevents contamination from airborne bacteria and begins the process of disinfection. The instruments remain in the holding bath until the dental assistant is ready to proceed with processing.

After the dental assistant has removed the treatment tray from the operatory and disinfected the area and/or placed the instruments in a holding bath, he or she returns to the sterilizing area to process the instruments. The utility gloves remain on during this procedure as the dental assistant takes the instruments from the tray or holding bath and places them in an ultrasonic cleaner. Metal or plastic containers sometimes are used to hold instruments as they pass from the tray to the different solutions for processing and then on to storage. The use of the utility gloves, along with the containers and ultrasonic cleaning instead of hand cleaning significantly reduces the high risk to the dental assistant. When ultrasonic cleaning is complete, the instruments are rinsed thoroughly and dried. All instruments, both loose and remaining in containers, are rinsed and dried prior to sterilization. They may be placed in an alcohol bath to aid the drying process. It does not matter which method is used to prepare the instruments for sterilization. What is important is that all the debris, blood, saliva, and tissue are removed from the instruments to ensure that the sterilization can be completed on all surfaces. The ultrasonic cleaner should be drained each night, rinsed out with water, and refilled with fresh ultrasonic solution each morning. It should be emptied and refilled any time the ultrasonic cleaning solution becomes exhausted, which varies depending on individual offices.

TABLE 6–1 DISINFECTANT COMPARISON

Disinfectant	Level	Advantages	Disadvantages	Time Required for Effectiveness
Chlorine dioxide	high	Rapid disinfection	Corrosive to metals Requires ventilation Irritating to eyes and skin	5–10 minutes
Glutaraldehyde	high	Used to disinfect some impressions Instrument can be submerged Many have a twenty-eight-day useful life	Some are corrosive to metal Requires ventilation Irritating to eyes and skin	10–90 minutes
Iodophors	intermediate	Used as holding solution for impressions	May discolor white or pastel vinyls Surface disinfectant or holding solution Irritating to eyes and skin	10 minutes on surface
Sodium hypochlorite	intermediate	Rapid disinfection	Corrosive to metals Irritating to skin and eyes Diluted solution unstable, must be mixed daily	5–10 minutes
Phenolics	intermediate	Available as sprays or liquids	Skin and mucous membrane irritation Cannot be used on plastics	10 minutes
Alcohol	cleaner only	NA	NA	NA

Packaging and Loading Instruments into the Sterilizer

Most sterilizers achieve effective sterilization when instruments are loaded loosely into the chamber. The problem, however, occurs after the sterilization cycle is completed and the instruments are removed into an unsterile environment, where they soon become recontaminated. Therefore, it is desirable to wrap instruments in cassettes, pouches, bags, or sealed packs (by procedure) prior to placing them into the sterilizer. This helps ensure sterility following completion of the cycle, during storage, and until opened in the presence of the patient at the time of the appointment.

Before inserting the instrument pack into the sterilizer, the dental assistant must take care to properly label the instrument pack for ready identification afterward. Labeling is written in pencil so when moisture occurs (in steam and chemical sterilizers) the information remains readable. Preprinted indicator tape is designed for instrument setups in the sterilizer bag. Preprinted labels are also available describing the procedure for which instruments are to be used, for example, "perio," "exam," "cementation," "amalgam," and "composite."

Many dental practices use cassette **instrument sterilizing systems** (Figure 6–3), in which the instruments are contained through ultrasonic cleaning, rinsing, and drying; then the cassette is wrapped in penetrable paper or

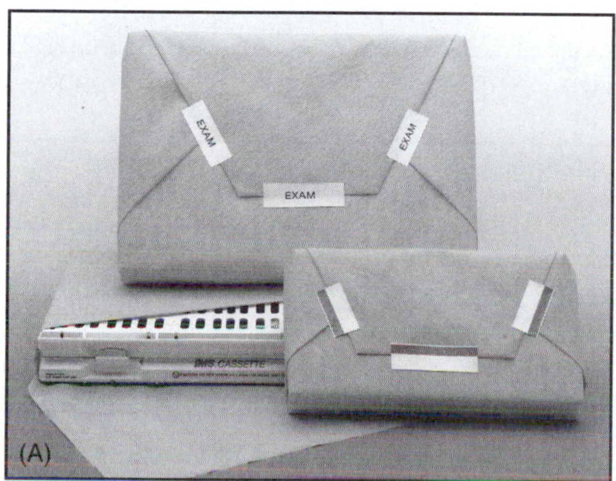

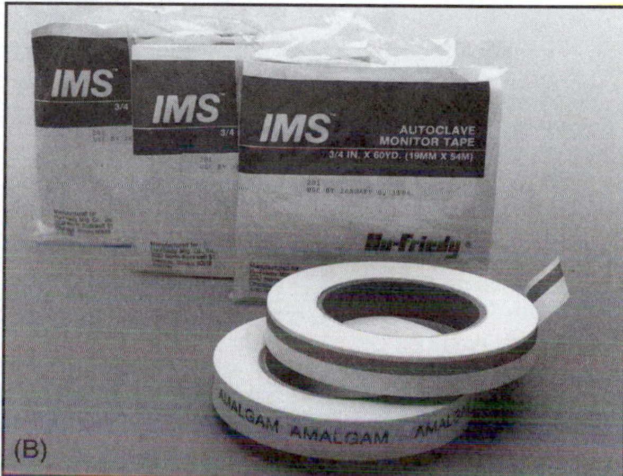

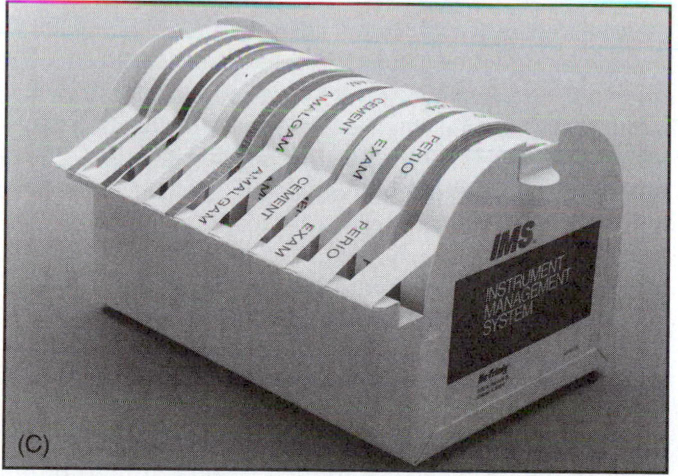

FIGURE 6–3 Cassette instrument sterilizing system. (A) Cassettes wrapped for sterilization. (B) Autoclave monitor tape. (C) Instrument Management System tape. *(Courtesy of Hu-Friedy Mfg. Co., Inc.)*

TABLE 6–2 METHODS OF STERILIZATION

Sterilization	Temperature/Time	Ability to Monitor	Special Considerations
Liquid chemical sterilization	Room temperature/ 6–10 hours	Difficult	Proper ventilation required Does not remain sterile after process
Ethylene oxide sterilization	Heated unit 120°F/ 2–3 hours Room temperature 12 hours	Difficult	Proper ventilation Additional 24 hours to dissipate gas after sterilization
Glass bead sterilizer	450°F/20–30 seconds	Not available	Limited size and use Special beads or salt required
Dry heat sterilization	340°F/1 hour	Easily monitored	Limited rust or corrosion of equipment
Chemical vapor sterilization	270°F/20 minutes	Easily monitored	Proper ventilation Special solution required
Steam under pressure sterilization	250°F/5 minutes wrapped	Easily monitored	Requires distilled water
Steam (flash) autoclave sterilization	270°F/3 minutes unwrapped	Easily monitored	Requires distilled water

biofilm/paper pouches, sealed, labeled, and sterilized. Sealed cassettes, which do not require wrapping, are color-coded for instant procedure recognition.

The dental assistant must ensure that sterilization bags or pouches are not overfilled, because this hampers proper sterilization. The dental assistant must also be sure to avoid overpacking the sterilizer chamber as too many instrument packs may impair sterilization by not allowing the steam or chemical vapor to circulate properly.

The routine use of **sterilization indicators** helps to ensure that all batches of instruments are properly sterilized.

STERILIZATION

All forms of microorganisms are destroyed during the process of sterilization. The dental assistant is most often the staff member who is responsible for ensuring that all items used during invasive oral procedures are sterilized. Any instruments or devices that touch the skin or oral mucosa, or are involved in

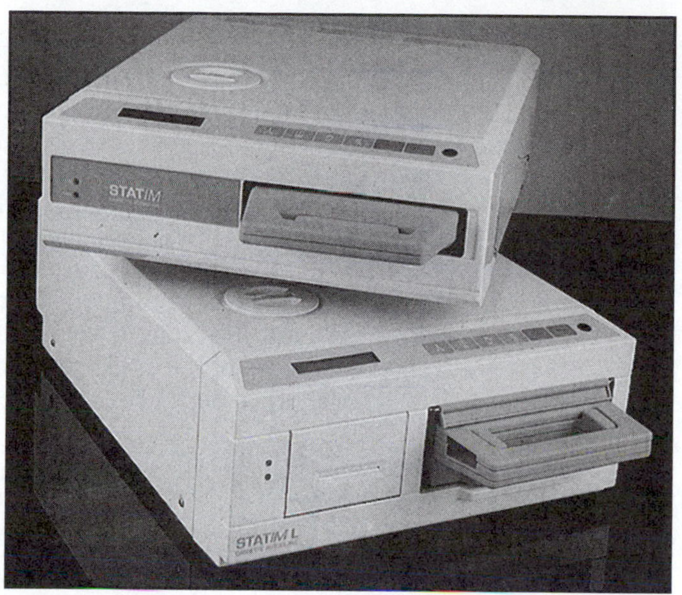

FIGURE 6–4 Steam (flash) sterilizer—Statim. (*Supplied by Sci-Can, Inc., Pittsburgh, PA 15222*)

invasive dental procedures, must be sterilized. Several suitable methods of sterilization are available for use in the dental office (Table 6–2).

Steam Autoclave (Flash) Sterilization. Most dental offices have a steam autoclave sterilizer (Figure 6–4). These units use steam under pressure to quickly sterilize items. The effectiveness of this unit can be monitored, and it is very reliable. Items must be wrapped, bagged, or placed in pouches and sealed to remain sterile after removing them from the sterilizer. The unit takes fifteen minutes at 250°F (121°C) at fifteen pounds of steam pressure at sea level. Careful packing of the unit so that the steam can penetrate all areas is essential. The steam pressure, along with the temperature, allows for rapid sterilization to occur. When unwrapped at 270°F (132°C) at fifteen pounds of steam pressure, sterilization for immediate use can be achieved in three minutes.

The high temperature, along with the steam, may cause plastics to melt, corrosion and rust to occur, and instruments to dull after repeated use. Most dental offices sterilize their dental handpieces exclusively in the steam sterilizer. The handpieces should be properly lubricated and wrapped prior to sterilization. Improper care of the dental handpiece diminishes its life span. Because dental equipment is expensive, a rapid sterilization turnaround time is beneficial so that multiple handpieces need not be purchased. Many steam sterilization units require distilled water to be used in the machine. The dental assistant should always read the manufacturer's directions before using any sterilization equipment.

Instrument Storage

The best way to store instruments is in the packages in which they were sterilized. This limits the amount of package handling after sterilization. If packages become torn, wet, or contaminated, they must be reprocessed. It is also important that "clean" and "dirty" areas in the sterilization room be identified. To avoid contamination, nothing from the dirty side should be placed on the clean side. This aids in the process of maintaining the integrity of the sterilization.

Sterile packs should be stored in an area that has protection from recontamination, is dry, and is away from heat. Most instruments used in dentistry have a quick turnaround time due to the expense and limited quantity of the instruments. The shelf life of the packages is indefinite as long as the packaging material remains intact and uncontaminated.

Sterilization Monitoring

Heat sterilizers are very reliable. It is important, however, that the sterilization process be monitored continually due to many factors that can diminish effectiveness. For example, the dental assistant could wrap instruments improperly, overload the unit, improperly set the time and temperature, or the sterilizer could malfunction.

Ongoing monitoring of the sterilization process is important to ensure proper technique and operation. Documentation reflecting the date monitoring was concluded and the outcome must be completed. Records for each sterilizer should be maintained. Several types of monitors available for use include: biological monitors, process indicators, and dosage indicators.

Clinical Asepsis Protocol

Routine steps should be followed in all treatment areas to maintain absolute clinical asepsis (Procedures 6–2 and 6–3). Shortcuts should never be an option for asepsis in dentistry. The dental assistant must ensure that infectious diseases are not spread from patient to patient, healthcare worker to patient, patient to healthcare worker, or healthcare worker to family (Procedures 6–4 and 6–5).

PROCEDURE

6-2 Preparing the Dental Treatment Room

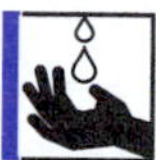 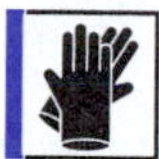 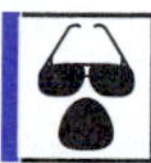

The procedure is performed by the dental assistant prior to seating the dental patient in the treatment room. By following a routine procedure that meets the regulations and the protocol set forth by the dentist and the regulatory agencies discussed earlier in the chapter, the dental assistant prepares the operatory and equipment.

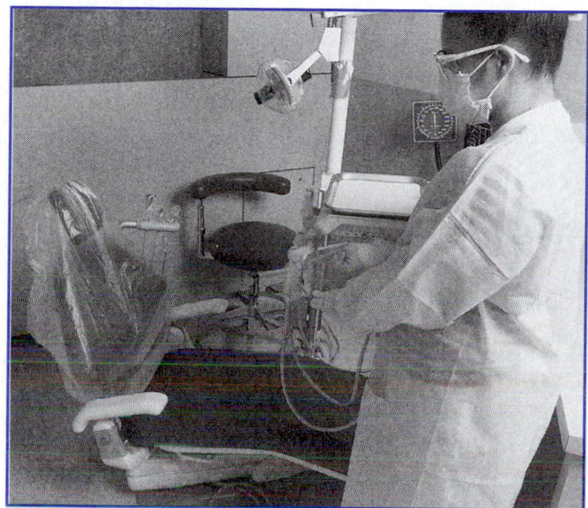

FIGURE 6–4 Dental assistant placing barriers.

EQUIPMENT AND SUPPLIES

- Patient's medical and dental history (including dental radiographs)
- Barriers for dental chair, hoses, counter, light switches, and controls
- PPE for dental assistant and dentist (protective eyewear, mask, gloves, and overgloves)
- Patient napkin, napkin chain, and protective eyewear
- Sterile procedure tray

PROCEDURE STEPS *(Follow aseptic procedures)*

1. Wash hands.
2. Review the patient's medical and dental history, place the radiographs on the viewbox, and identify the procedure to be completed at this visit. Patient's medical and dental history can be placed in a plastic envelope barrier or under a surface barrier.
3. Place new barriers on all potential possible surfaces that can be contaminated (for example, dental chair, hoses, counter, light switches and controls) (Figure 6–5).
4. Bring the instrument tray with packaged sterile instruments into the operatory with patient's napkin and protective eyewear.
5. Don PPE (protective eyewear, mask, gloves, and overgloves).

PROCEDURE

6-3 Completion of Dental Treatment

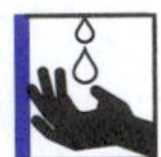 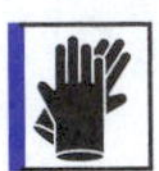 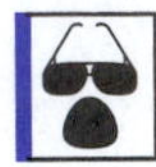

The procedure is performed by the dental assistant at the completion of the dental treatment. By following a routine procedure that meets the regulations and the protocol set forth by the dentist and the regulatory agencies discussed earlier in the chapter, the dental assistant completes the procedure and dismisses the patient.

EQUIPMENT AND SUPPLIES

- Patient's medical and dental history (including dental radiographs)
- Barriers for dental chair, hoses, counter, light switches, and controls
- Dental handpiece
- Air-water syringe tip (disposable)
- Patient napkin
- Contaminated instruments on tray, including HVE tip

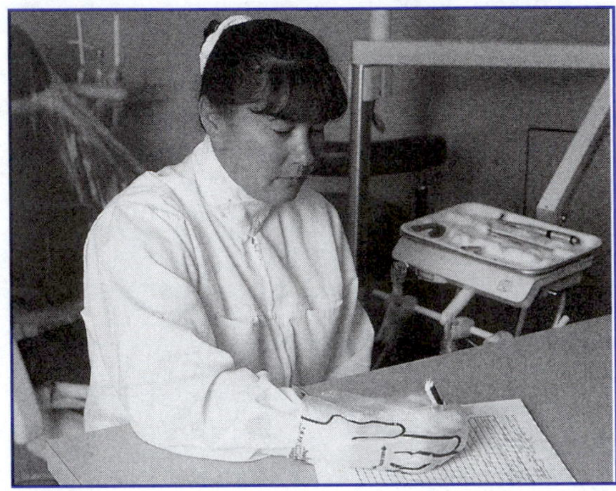

FIGURE 6–6 Wearing overgloves while writing on a patient's chart.

PROCEDURE STEPS *(Follow aseptic procedures)*

1. Remove the handpieces, HVE tip, and air-water syringe tip and place on the treatment tray.
2. Put on overgloves to document information on the chart or on the computer and assemble radiographs and chart, preventing cross-contamination (Figure 6–6).
3. Remove patient napkin and place over the treatment tray prior to dismissing patient.
4. With glove in place, complete Steps 5 through 11.
5. Place the handpiece, HVE, and air-water syringe back on the unit and run for twenty to thirty seconds to clean the lines and flush the system. Remove handpiece and air-water syringe and place back on the treatment tray.
6. Discard sharps into puncture-resistant sharps disposal container if sharps disposal containers are kept in the dental treatment room. Sharps should be discarded in the treatment room to prevent any possible mishaps or in the sterilization area.
7. Remove the chair cover from the patient dental chair, inverting it so any splatter or debris remains on the inside of the bag.
8. Remove all contaminated barriers and place them in the inverted bag. All disposables can be placed in the bag as well.
9. Carry the treatment tray with all items from the treatment area to the sterilizing area. Nothing that is to be sterilized is to be left in the operatory at this time.
10. Remove treatment gloves and place them in the inverted bag. Dispose of the bag.
11. Wash hands.

PROCEDURE

6-4 Final Treatment Room Cleaning and Disinfecting

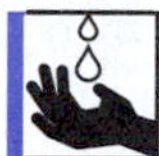
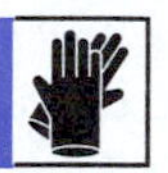
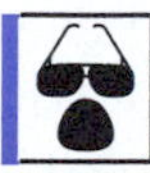

The procedure is performed by the dental assistant after the treatment has been completed and the patient has been dismissed. By following a routine procedure that meets the regulations and the protocol set forth by the dentist and the regulatory agencies discussed earlier in the chapter, the dental assistant completes the procedure.

Use a small utility carry tote to hold and transport items such as disinfecting solutions, HVE solution, 4 × 4 gauze, towels, and disinfectant.

EQUIPMENT AND SUPPLIES

- Utility gloves
- Necessary disinfecting solutions (intermediate level)
- Wiping cloths
- 4 × 4 gauze

PROCEDURE STEPS *(Follow aseptic procedures)*

1. Wash hands, put on utility gloves.
2. Bring the necessary solutions and wiping cloths, including 4 × 4 gauzes, to the operatory.
3. Have a routine procedure established for disinfection to ensure that nothing is missed. All surfaces need to be sprayed and cleaned first, then wiped to remove debris (Figures 6–7A and B). The surfaces are then sprayed a second time and the solution is left on for a designated time according to the manufacturer's directions (normally this time is about ten minutes) and left to dry.

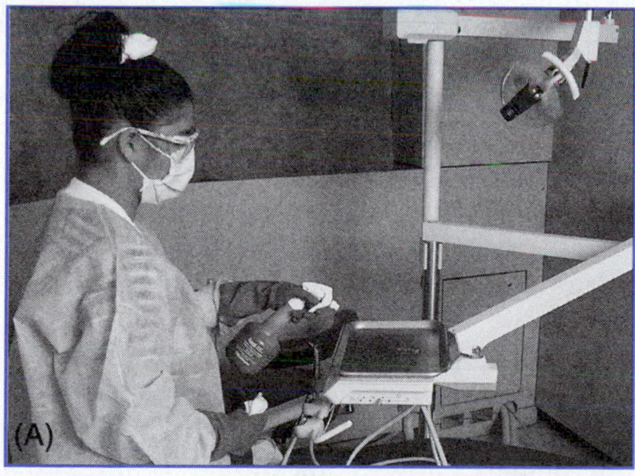
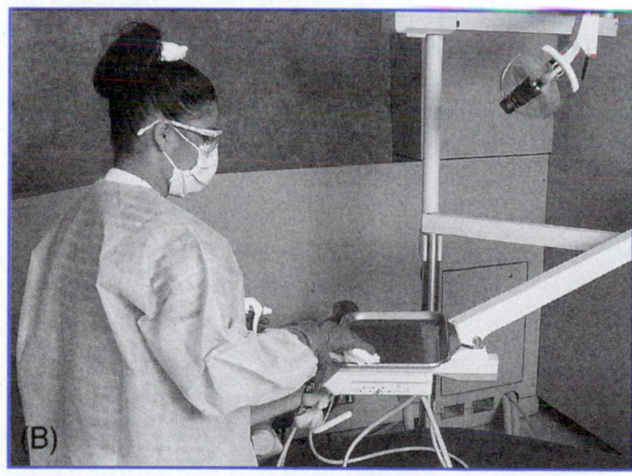

FIGURE 6–7 (A) Spraying the area. (B) Wiping and spraying the area with disinfectant again.

(continued)

PROCEDURE 6-4 *continued*

4. Another method to accomplish the initial spray wipe is to use saturated "wiping devices." Lay out several pieces of 4 × 4 gauze on the counter, spray them with disinfectant, and wipe each surface carefully.
5. Spray on the disinfectant and leave for the correct time to accomplish disinfection (normally ten minutes).
6. Rewipe all surfaces.
7. It is critical that all surfaces that could have been contaminated are disinfected. Areas that are sometimes missed include the amalgam cradle (holding device for amalgam capsule in the triturator), the chair adjustments, the curing light, and the radiographic viewbox switch.

Disinfecting Procedure

- Spray.
- Wipe. (The "Spray and Wipe" technique also can be accomplished by wiping with a disinfectant-saturated "wiping device.")
- Spray and leave (normally ten minutes).
- Rewipe or allow disinfectant to air dry.

Dental Laboratory

The dental laboratory should be disinfected in the same manner as other rooms. Use the spray-wipe-spray technique on all the surfaces. If the dental assistant is polishing with pumice on the rag wheel, PPE should be worn. Extra care should be used when wearing gloves while using the rotary equipment for polishing, because gloves easily can become caught in wheels or motors.

After polishing, discard the pumice and disinfect the pan. (Many dental offices mix the pumice with disinfectant.) Rinse off the rag wheel and cycle it through the autoclave. Many disposable buffing wheels are available as an alternative and can be discarded after one use.

Thoroughly disinfect any contaminated dental laboratory cases before being handled in the office or sent to an outside laboratory. An effective method is to place all acrylic appliances in a diluted sodium hypochlorite disinfection solution. Cases with any metal parts must be placed in another solution, such as glutaraldehyde. Check the manufacturer's directions to identify solutions that meet the criteria for this process.

Dental impressions also must be disinfected prior to sending them out. Check the manufacturer's directions regarding the correct procedure to perform this task. Alginate impressions cannot be immersed in any solution, because this can cause distortion. Alginate impressions should be sprayed and then placed in a sealed plastic bag.

Final impression materials such as polysulfide and silicone can be immersed in most disinfecting solutions according to the manufacturer's

PROCEDURE

6-5 Treatment of Contaminated Tray in the Sterilization Center

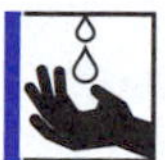 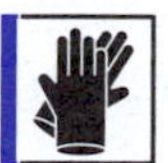 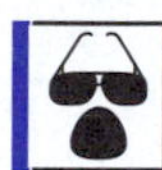

The procedure is performed by the dental assistant in the sterilization center. By following a routine procedure that meets the regulations and the protocol set forth by the dentist and OSHA regulatory agencies discussed earlier in the chapter, the dental assistant completes the procedure.

EQUIPMENT AND SUPPLIES

- Utility gloves
- Disinfecting solutions
- Wiping cloths
- 4 × 4 gauze
- Contaminated procedure tray

PROCEDURE STEPS *(Follow aseptic procedures)*

1. Place the treatment tray in the contaminated area of the sterilization center immediately following dental treatment. Sterilization can be taken care of immediately or after the operatory is disinfected and prepared for another patient.
2. If there will be a long time before the tray is taken care of, immerse the instruments in a disinfecting holding solution. This prevents debris from drying, begins the process of killing the microorganisms, and prevents any airborne microorganisms from being transmitted.
3. Wear utility gloves during the entire procedure.
4. Dispose of sharps in a sharps container if not already done while in the dental operatory.
5. Discard all disposable items. If they are biohazard waste, they must be placed in an appropriately labeled waste container.
6. Place the instruments in the ultrasonic cleaner, either open method or in a cassette. A small strainer is used for items that may become lost. Burs, dental dam clamps, and other such items are placed in this small container. After the timed cleaning is completed in the ultrasonic unit (three to ten minutes), rinse the items off thoroughly.
7. After the instruments are rinsed, towel dry, bag, and place in the appropriate sterilizer (Figure 6–8). If they are in a cassette, they can be dipped in an alcohol bath and left to air dry before being placed in a sealed bag and in the sterilizer.
8. Rinse off or wipe off the dental high-speed handpiece with isopropyl alcohol. Then, lubricate, bag in an instrument pouch with indicator tape, and place in the sterilizer (follow manufacturer's directions). The sterilizer used is normally the steam under pressure sterilizer due to the quick turnaround time.
9. The tray and other items on the tray must be spray wiped, sprayed again, left for ten minutes or a time designated by the manufacturer of the disinfectant, and rewiped or allowed to air dry before assembling them for another tray setup.
10. Clean the area, wash and dry the utility gloves, remove them, and wash and dry hands.
11. After the sterilizer indicates that the time has lapsed and that the instruments are sterile, remove the instruments from the sterilizer using forceps.

(continued)

PROCEDURE 6-5 *continued*

PPE for a Contaminated Tray

- Utility gloves are required when handling contaminated trays.
- Protective eyewear is required when handling contaminated trays.
- Masks are only required if cleaning causes splash, aerosols, and/or splatter to occur.

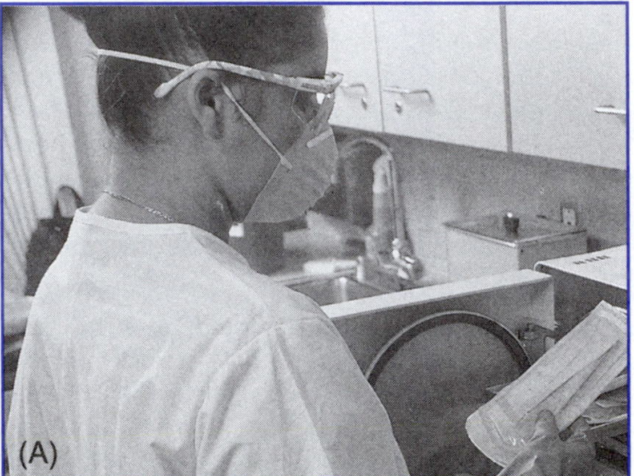

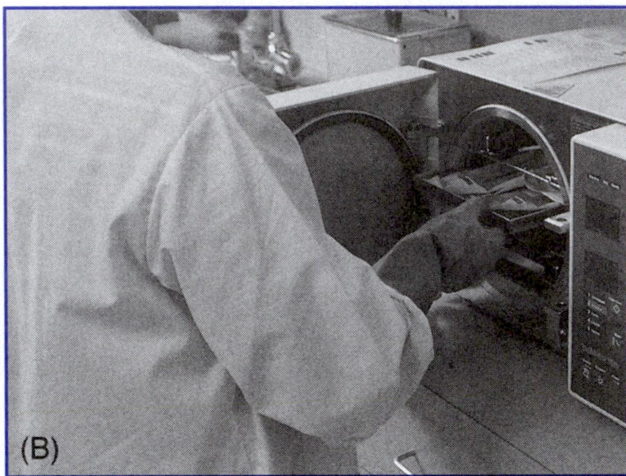

FIGURE 6–8 (A) Dental assistant placing the bagged instruments in the sterilizer. (B) Sliding tray with bagged instruments into sterilizer.

directions without distortion. Procedures for disinfecting polyether and polysiloxane impression materials vary. Some polyether impressions cannot go through the disinfecting procedure until a final set time of thirty minutes has elapsed. If the impression has not been disinfected prior to sending it to the dental laboratory, place it in a leak-proof bag to transport and identify that it has not been disinfected by a biohazard label on the bag.

CHAPTER 7

Management of Hazardous Materials

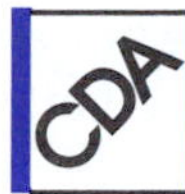

OBJECTIVES

The student should strive to meet the following objectives and demonstrate an understanding of the facts and principles presented in this chapter:

1. Identify the scope of the OSHA Bloodborne/Hazardous Materials Standard.
2. Identify physical equipment and mechanical devices provided to safeguard employees.
3. Demonstrate safe disposal of sharps.
4. Describe the importance and content of MSDS manuals.
5. Describe employee training required to meet the OSHA standard for hazardous chemicals.

KEY TERMS

material safety data sheets (MSDS) (p. 94)
National Fire Protection Association's color and number method (p. 104)
Occupational Safety and Health Administration (OSHA) (p. 94)
other potentially infectious materials (OPIM) (p. 100)
parenteral (p. 100)
pericardial (p. 101)
peritoneal (p. 101)
pleural (p. 101)
synovial (p. 101)

INTRODUCTION

This chapter discusses the requirements of the **Occupational Safety and Health Administration (OSHA)** Bloodborne/Hazardous Materials Standard, such as engineering controls labeling, **material safety data sheets (MSDS)**, housekeeping, laundry, and the disposal of hazardous materials. Dental assistants must understand the complete standard and how compliance is accomplished (Figure 7–1). Dental assisting students do not fall under OSHA guidelines because they are not employees; however, following the same safety standards that are practiced in the workplace is preparation for employment. The scope of the standard covers:

- Employee training, safety, and documentation requirements
- Exposure determination
- Infection control, universal precautions, and standard measures used to control possible exposures
- Post-exposure follow-up
- Labeling/material safety data sheets (MSDS)
- Housekeeping/laundry
- Disposal of biohazardous waste

Scope and Application

- The Standard applies to all occupational exposure to blood and other potentially infectious materials (OPIM) and includes part-time employees, designated first aiders, and mental health workers, as well as exposed medical personnel.
- OPIM includes saliva in dental procedures, cerebrospinal fluid, unfixed tissue, semen, vaginal secretions, and body fluids visibly contaminated with blood.

Methods of Compliance

- General—Standard precautions.
- Engineering and work practice controls.
- Personal protective equipment.
- Housekeeping.

Standard Precautions

- *All* human blood and OPIM are considered infectious.
- The *same* precautions must be taken with all blood and OPIM.

FIGURE 7–1 Understanding OSHA's Bloodborne/Hazardous Materials Standard. *(continued)*

Engineering Controls

- Whenever feasible, engineering controls must be the primary method used to control exposure.
- Examples include needleless IVs, self-sheathing needles, sharps disposal containers, covered centrifuge buckets, aerosol-free tubes, and leak-proof containers.
- Engineering controls must be evaluated and documented on a regular basis.

Sharps Containers

- Readily accessible and as close as practical to work area.
- Puncture resistant.
- Labeled or color coded.
- Leak proof.
- Closeable.
- *Routinely replaced* to prevent overflow.

Work Practice Controls

- Handwashing following glove removal.
- No recapping, breaking, or bending of needles.
- No eating, drinking, smoking, and so on in work area.
- No storage of food or drink where blood or OPIM are stored.
- Minimize splashing, splattering of blood, and OPIM.
- No mouth pipetting.
- Specimens must be transported in leak-proof, labeled containers. They must be placed in a secondary container if outside contamination of primary container occurs.
- Equipment must be decontaminated prior to servicing or shipping. Areas that cannot be decontaminated must be labeled.

Personal Protective Equipment (PPE)

- Includes eye protection, gloves, protective clothing, and resuscitation equipment.
- Must be readily accessible and employers must require their use.
- Must be stored at work site.

Eye Protection

- Is required whenever there is potential for splashing, spraying, or splattering to the eyes or mucous membranes.
- If necessary, use eye protection in conjunction with a mask or use a chin-length face shield.
- Prescription glasses may be fitted with solid side shields.
- Decontamination procedures must be developed.

FIGURE 7–1 *(continued)*

Gloves

- Must be worn whenever hand contact with blood, OPIM, mucous membranes, nonintact skin, or contaminated surfaces/items may occur or when performing vascular access procedures (phlebotomy).
- Type required—Vinyl or latex for general use.
  —Alternatives must be available if employee has allergic reactions.
  —Utility gloves for surface disinfection.
  —Puncture resistant when handling sharps.

Protective Clothing

- Must be worn whenever splashing or splattering to skin or clothing may occur.
- Type required depends on exposure. Prevention of contamination of skin and clothes is the key.
- Examples—Low-level-exposure lab coats.
  —Moderate-level-exposure, fluid-resistant gown.
  —High-level-exposure, fluid-proof apron, head and foot covering.
- *Note:* If PPE is considered protective clothing, the *employer must* launder it.

Housekeeping

- There must be a written schedule for cleaning and disinfection.
- Contaminated equipment and surfaces must be cleaned as soon as feasible for obvious contamination or at end of work shift if no contamination has occurred.
- Protective coverings may be used over equipment.

Regulated Waste Containers (Non-Sharp)

- Closeable.
- Leak proof.
- Labeled or color coded.
- Placed in secondary container if outside of container is contaminated.

Laundry

- Handled as little as possible.
- Bagged at location of use.
- Labeled or color coded.
- Transported in bags that prevent soak-through or leakage.

FIGURE 7–1 *(continued)*

Laundry Facility

- Two options:
  1. Standard precautions for all laundry (alternative color coding allowed if recognized).
  2. Precautions only for contaminated laundry (must be red bags or biohazard labels).
- Laundry personnel must use PPE and have a sharps container accessible.

Hepatitis B Vaccination

- Made available within ten days of employment to all employees with occupational exposure.
- At no cost to employees.
- May be required for student to be admitted to college health program.
- Administered in accordance with United States Public Health Service guidelines.
- Employee must first be evaluated by healthcare professional.
- Healthcare professional gives a written opinion.
- If the vaccine is refused, the employee signs a declination form.
- Vaccine must be available at a future date if initially refused.

Post-Exposure Follow-Up

- Document exposure incident.
- Identify source individual (if possible).
- Attempt to test source if consent obtained.
- Provide results to exposed employee.

Labels

- Biohazard symbol and word *Biohazard* must be visible.
- Fluorescent orange/orange-red with contrasting letters must be used.
- Red bags/containers may be substituted for labels.
- Labels required on—Regulated waste.
  —Refrigerators/freezers with blood of OPIM.
  —Transport/storage containers.
  —Contaminated equipment.

Information and Training

- Required for all employees with occupational exposure.
- Training required initially, annually, and if there are new procedures.
- Training material must be appropriate for literacy and education level of employee.
- Training must be interactive and allow for questions and answers.

FIGURE 7–1 *(continued)*

Training Components

- Explanation of bloodborne pathogens standard.
- Epidemiology and symptoms of bloodborne disease.
- Modes of HIV/HBV transmission.
- Explanation of exposure control plan.
- Explanation of engineering, work practice controls.
- How to select the proper PPE.
- How to decontaminate equipment, surfaces, etc.
- Information about hepatitis B vaccine.
- Post-exposure follow-up procedures.
- Label/color code system.

Medical Records

Records must be kept for each employee with occupational exposure and include:

- A copy of employee's vaccination status and date.
- A copy of post-exposure follow-up evaluation procedures.
- Healthcare professional's written opinions.
- Confidentiality must be maintained.
- Records must be maintained for thirty years plus the duration of employment.

Training Records

Records are kept for three years from date of training and include:

- Date of training.
- Summary of contents of training program.
- Name and qualifications of trainer.
- Names and job titles of all persons attending.

Exposure Control Plan Components

- A written plan for each workplace with occupational exposure.
- Written policies/procedures for complying with the standard.
- A cohesive document or a guiding document referencing existing policies/procedures.

FIGURE 7–1 *(continued)*

Exposure Control Plan

- A list of job classifications where occupational exposure control occurs (e.g., dental assistant, dental hygienist).
- A list of tasks where exposure occurs (e.g., dental assistant who performs sharps disposal).
- Methods/policies/procedures for compliance.
- Procedures for sharps disposal.
- Disinfection policies/procedures.
- Procedures for selection of PPE.
- Regulated waste disposal procedures.
- Laundry procedures.
- Hepatitis B vaccination procedures.
- Post-exposure follow-up procedures.
- Training procedures.
- Plan must be accessible to employees and be updated annually.

Employee Responsibilities

- Complete required training.
- Obey policies.
- Use universal precautions.
- Use PPE.
- Use safe work practices.
- Use engineering controls.
- Report unsafe work conditions to employer.
- Maintain clean work areas.

Cooperation between employer and employees regarding *The Bloodborne Pathogen Standard* facilitates understanding of the law, thereby benefiting all persons who are exposed to HIV, HBV, and OPIM by minimizing the risk of exposure to the pathogens.

Complying with the OSHA standard is not optional, and failure to comply can result in fines.

FIGURE 7–1

Engineering/Work Practice Controls

The physical equipment and mechanical devices that employers provide to safeguard and protect the employees at work are known as engineering and work practice controls. Examples of these are the splash guards on model trimmers, puncture-resistant sharps containers, and ventilation hoods for hazardous fumes. The employer must provide this equipment to meet OSHA standards and provide a safe environment for employees. The employer must ensure that employees wash their hands immediately after gloves are removed and flush their eyes with water at an eye-wash station if contact with microorganisms or hazardous materials is suspected (Figure 7–2). The employer must ensure that employees flush any mucous membranes immediately if there has been possible contact with blood or **other potentially infectious materials (OPIM)** in the office.

The employer sets up work practice controls to diminish harmful occupational exposure. OSHA defines occupational exposure as reasonably anticipated eye, skin, mucous membrane, or parenteral contact with blood or other OPIM that may result from the performance of an employee's duties. It further defines **parenteral** as piercing mucous membranes or the skin barrier through such events as needlesticks, cuts, and abrasions.

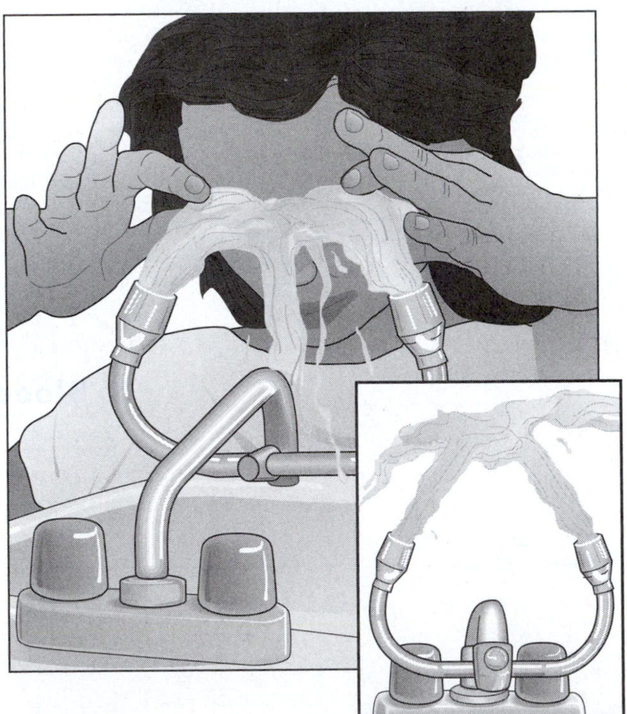

FIGURE 7–2 Flushing eyes at an eye-wash station.

OSHA and the Centers for Disease Control and Prevention define the following human fluids as blood and OPIM according to the standard:

- Blood and anything that is visually contaminated with blood
- Saliva in dental oral procedures
- Cerebrospinal fluid (brain and spinal fluid)
- Amniotic fluid (fluid around the fetus)
- **Synovial** fluid (joint and tendon fluid)
- **Pleural** (lung fluid)/**peritoneal** fluid (abdominal fluid)/**pericardial** fluid (heart fluid)
- Semen and vaginal secretions
- Unfixed tissue or organ (other than intact skin) from a human (living or dead)
- HIV-containing cell or tissue cultures, organ cultures, and HIV- or HBV-containing culture medium or other solutions
- Blood, organs, or other tissues from experimental animals infected with HIV or HBV

SHARPS

Upon completion of a procedure, contaminated sharps and needles must be discarded immediately in a labeled, leak-proof, puncture-resistant container. Other sharps that are placed routinely in the sharps disposal container are blades from knives used in surgery, broken glass, anesthetic capsules, and orthodontic wires. When the sharps disposal containers are full, they are sealed, sterilized using an autoclave if possible, and sent to an outside biohazard agency for safe disposal.

Occupational Exposure to Bloodborne Pathogens

Any employee who sustains an occupational exposure incident must report it immediately. The employer must make available immediately to the exposed employee a confidential medical evaluation and follow-up. The medical evaluation and follow-up is made available to the employee at no cost. The dentist refers the exposed employee to a licensed healthcare professional to have the most current medical evaluation and procedures performed that are in accordance with the United States Public Health Service. OSHA standards do not dictate the procedures to be performed but allow for the most current recommendations to be applied. Reporting the incident immediately allows the dentist to carefully evaluate the circumstances surrounding the incident and to find ways to prevent the situation and exposure incident from happening again.

Documentation of the Exposure Incident. The dentist documents the information of the exposure incident on a report. This report includes the route(s) of exposure, the circumstances that surrounded the exposure incident, and (if known) the identity of the source patient. The exposure incident report is placed in the employee's confidential medical record and a copy of this report is provided to the healthcare professional providing the evaluation.

The employer is required to provide the licensed healthcare professional with a description of the employee's job duties and his or her relation to the incident; information about the route of the exposure; the circumstances surrounding the incident; relevant employee medical records, including vaccination status; a copy of the bloodborne pathogen standard; and the results of the source patient's blood testing (if available).

If the employer has eleven or more employees, the employer may be required to complete the OSHA forms 200 (Log and Summary of Occupational Injuries and Illnesses) and 101 (Supplemental Record of Occupational Injuries and Illnesses) to meet the "recordable occupation injury" requirement.

In a bloodborne pathogens exposure, the dentist must identify and document in writing the source patient, if known. Further, the dentist must contact the source patient and request his or her consent to be tested for HBV and HIV and then further to disclose the results of these tests to the exposed employee. If the source patient does not give consent for the testing, the dentist must document this on the report of the exposure incident. If the source patient agrees to be tested, the tests should be completed as soon as feasible. When the results are disclosed to the exposed employee, information regarding the source patient's rights to disclosure must be discussed.

Exposed Employee Blood (Collection and Testing). The employee has the right to decline testing after an exposure incident or to delay the testing for up to ninety days. The employee may consent to have a baseline blood test to determine the HBV and HIV serological status. The employee may choose to be tested only for HBV and not give consent for HIV testing at that time. The employee's blood sample must be saved for ninety days in case the employee elects to consent to the HIV testing. All tests must be performed by an accredited laboratory at no cost to the employee. The healthcare professional will notify the employee directly of all test results.

Post-Exposure Follow-Up Procedures. The employer must provide to the exposed employee counseling, prophylaxis to prevent sexual transmission of any possible infection, and evaluation of reported illnesses. The counseling provided aids the employee in interpretation of all tests and discussions about the potential risk of infection and the need for further post-exposure prophylaxis. The employee should also be counseled on the necessary use of protection during sexual contact.

Treatment may include, but is not limited to, HBV vaccine if the employee has not had it or chemoprophylaxis for high risk cases of HIV transmission.

The healthcare professional also evaluates any reported illnesses that the exposed employee develops. The healthcare professional can evaluate the

> The post-exposure prophylaxis is provided according to the current recommendations of the United States Public Health Service. OSHA did not define this procedure in the bloodborne standard due to the ongoing changes that have developed in this area.

symptoms in relation to the HBV and HIV infection. This allows the exposed employee to have immediate medical evaluation and referral for medical treatment to take place so treatment can be started as soon as possible. This does not mean that the employer is responsible for any costs associated with the treatment of the disease.

The healthcare professional sends the dental employer a written opinion about the evaluation and notification that the employee was informed of the test results of the evaluation and of the further follow-up. The dentist, however, may not receive the results of the testing. The dentist provides the employee with a copy of this written opinion and evaluation of the exposed employee within fifteen days of the completion of the evaluation. The original document is placed in the employee's confidential record. The employer must maintain employee records in a confidential manner for the duration of employment plus thirty years in accordance with OSHA's standard on Access to Employee Exposure and Medical Records, 29 CFR 1910.20.

Employee Work Site

The employer must provide a work site that is clean and sanitary. Each office must have a written schedule for infection control and decontaminating procedures for each area. Wastepaper baskets, floors, and all other surfaces that may have been contaminated with blood or OPIM must be included. The assistant must wear utility gloves while cleaning contaminated surfaces. All disposable items that are contaminated, including gloves, must be discarded in a biohazard container.

Hazardous Chemicals

The OSHA hazard communication standard requires that employees receive training about the risks of using hazardous chemicals and the safety precautions required when handling them. Employees must be trained in identification of hazardous chemicals and personal protective equipment to be utilized for each chemical. This training must occur within ten days of employment or prior to the employee using any chemicals, and annually thereafter.

Employees must have a certificate available or in their personnel files that shows they have had the proper training. The certificate must identify that the employer has trained the employee in the proper handling of hazardous substances in the dental office.

As with the bloodborne pathogen standard, a written plan identifying employee training and detailing specific control measures used in the workplace must be compiled for hazardous chemicals. If the office is not in compliance, penalties may be imposed on the employer.

All hazardous chemicals must be identified on a written form, such as a chemical inventory form. Other information required about the chemicals includes the quantity stored (each month or year), the physical state of the substance (liquid, solid, or gas), the hazardous class (health problem, fire hazard, reactive), what PPE is required, and the manufacturer's name, address, and phone number.

Material Safety Data Sheets

Each office must have a material safety data sheet manual that is alphabetized, indexed, and available to all employees. These manuals may be in hard copy or on a computer. The manual contains the MSDS. These sheets come from the manufacturer. If the MSDS is unavailable, the employer or a designated employee (the safety assistant) must request it from the manufacturer. The **National Fire Protection Association's color and number method** is used to easily identify information about various hazardous ingredients on the MSDS and product labels.

Chemical Warning Label Determination. The National Fire Protection Association's color and number method is used to signify a warning to employees using the chemicals. Four colors are used:

- Blue identifies the health hazard.
- Red identifies the fire hazard.
- Yellow identifies the reactivity or how stable the chemical is.
- White indicates the PPE needed when using this chemical.

The level of risk for each category is indicated by the use of numbers 0–4. The higher the number, the greater the danger. Letters are used to identify the PPE needed.

A chemical warning label, a diamond-shaped symbol, displays the four colors with a place for the numbers to be written on each. The employee quickly can identify the hazard category, the risk for each, and the PPE equipment required. All hazardous chemicals must be labeled unless they are poured into separate containers for *immediate use.*

CHAPTER 8

Preparation for Patient Care

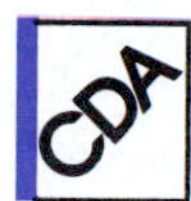

OBJECTIVES

The student should strive to meet the following objectives and demonstrate an understanding of the facts and principles presented in this chapter:

1. Review a medical and dental history.
2. Perform vital signs on the patient, including temperature, pulse, respiration, and blood pressure.

KEY TERMS

asymmetric (p. 107)
baseline vital signs (p. 107)
brachial artery (p. 111)
exhalation (p. 109)
inhalation (p. 109)
sphygmomanometer (p. 111)
stethoscope (p. 111)
symmetric (p. 107)
vital signs (p. 107)

Introduction

Preparation for patient care is an important part of providing quality dental service to each patient. The dental assistant can begin the process of patient preparation by obtaining personal, medical, and dental history from each patient. After history forms are completed, the dental assistant reviews the information and alerts the dentist to any areas of concern.

Once the patient is seated in the treatment room, the dental assistant performs or assists the dentist in an evaluation of the patient. This clinical evaluation includes obtaining vital signs and performing both an internal and an external evaluation of the oral cavity.

Patient History

The dental team members must thoroughly review a patient's medical history to treat the patient effectively. The information must be reviewed and updated at each visit. Most dental offices have a broad questionnaire for patients to complete. The information is confidential and should be as thorough as possible so that the best possible care is rendered. Sensitive topics such as medications being taken, medical treatment, and other factors contributing to the patient's health should be discussed in private.

Personal Information

One of the first steps in caring for patients is to have them complete a patient history. The patient is requested to fill out a personal history that includes the following: full name, address, phone number, Social Security number, insurance, emergency contacts, and physician's name and his or her phone number.

Medical Information

The patient also is requested to fill out a medical history. The medical history contains questions about past surgeries, systemic diseases, injuries, and/or allergies. It is critical for the dental team to know about any allergies that may affect treatment. Allergies of concern are related to anesthetics, latex, and/or antibiotics. The patient also should disclose any medical conditions such as epilepsy, diabetes, or a heart condition. Allergies and medical alerts are to be noted on the chart and highlighted to bring them to the attention of dental team members. Any drugs the patient has taken recently or is currently taking, including over-the-counter medications and food supplements, should be recorded on the medical history. Often, a variety of questions are asked to gain the information needed. The assistant should tactfully question any abnormalities. Usually, any "yes" answers on a questionnaire require further inquiry.

Dental Information

Questions regarding the patient's dental history are included in the patient's history. This information alerts the dental assistant to any concerns the patient has regarding his or her current dental health. It also provides insight into any concerns the patient may have had regarding previous dental care. The last dental examination is noted, as well as the patient's last dental appointment and how often the patient seeks dental treatment. Some questions are asked regarding the patient's attitude toward dentistry and how he or she maintains his or her own personal oral health.

Upon completion of the patient history, the patient signs and dates the form. This record provides the dentist and staff with useful information so that they may provide better care for the patient. The dentist and/or dental assistant reviews the answers prior to initiation of treatment. The personal and medical history should be reviewed prior to each treatment series. It is the dentist's ethical and legal responsibility to obtain information about the patient's medical history prior to dental treatment. The highest degree of confidentiality must be maintained by the dental team regarding the patient's history.

Clinical Observation

The dental assistant observes patients as they are escorted into the treatment room. If the patient displays any deviation from the normal, such as walking with an abnormal gait, further probing into the health history may be required. The assistant may notice speech or behavior problems that should be brought to the dentist's attention. Looking at the patient's face for symmetry is the first step in the oral inspection. Although most individuals do not have faces that are **symmetric** (meaning that if the face was divided in half, the other half would be a mirror image), each side of the face should look fairly similar. If one eyelid droops, for example, or if the face is **asymmetric**, this should be noted on the patient's chart. The dental assistant also evaluates the patient's eyes and facial skin for any scars or abnormalities in color or texture.

VITAL SIGNS

The measuring and recording of vital signs is an important part of the health evaluation, and it should be done with every patient before starting any dental treatment. After the patient's history is completed and the patient is seated, the dental assistant can obtain vital signs. Vital signs give the dental operator specific information about the physical and emotional condition of the patient. They may point out previously undetected abnormalities. Vital signs aid in the planning of the patient's dental treatment and are essential during emergency treatment.

Vital signs are the basic signs of life. They include body temperature, pulse, blood pressure, and respiration rate. **Baseline vital signs** are the initial measurements of vital signs. Baseline vital signs help the dentist compare subsequent measurements with the initial measurements.

PROCEDURE

8-1 Taking an Oral Temperature Using a Digital Thermometer

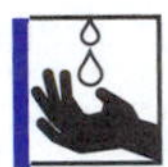

This procedure is performed by the dental assistant to obtain the patient's body temperature.

EQUIPMENT AND SUPPLIES

- Digital thermometer
- Probe covers
- Biohazard waste container

PROCEDURE STEPS *(Follow standard precautions)*

1. Wash hands.
2. Assemble the thermometer and probe cover.
3. Seat patient in the dental treatment room and position him or her comfortably in an upright position.
4. Verify that the patient has not had a hot or cold drink or smoked within the last half hour. (This may give a false temperature reading.)
5. Explain the procedure to the patient.
6. Position the new probe cover on the digital thermometer.
7. Insert the probe under the tongue to either side of the patient's mouth.
8. Instruct the patient to carefully close his or her lips around the probe without biting down on it.
9. Leave the probe in position until the digital thermometer beeps.
10. Remove the probe from the patient's mouth.
11. Read the results from the digital thermometer display window.
12. Dispose of the probe cover in a hazardous waste container.
13. Wash hands.
14. Document the procedure and record the results on the patient's chart.

Body Temperature

Measurement of body temperature (Procedure 8–1) is an essential component of every patient's health evaluation. Body temperature is compared to the normal body temperature range and, if higher or lower, it should be further investigated. A range is used when identifying the normal body temperature, because temperature varies from person to person and at different times of the day. It is well known that after exercise, emotional excitement, and eating, the temperature increases. A person's face may turn red and blush due to excitement, increasing the body temperature. Temperature in young children and young infants will vary more than in adults. Normal temperature ranges are as follows:

◗ Normal range in Fahrenheit	99.5° 98.6° (Average) 96.0°
◗ Normal range in Celsius	37.5° 37.0° (Average) 35.5°

Pulse

The pulse is the intermittent beating sensation felt when the fingers are pressed against an artery. A pulse rate is determined by **palpation** (feeling with the fingers or hand). Do not use the thumb to palpate, because it has a pulse of its own and could distort the readings. Pulse may be palpated on one of several arteries: radial, carotid, or temporal. The dental assistant most commonly uses the radial artery.

Radial Pulse Site. The radial pulse site is located on the radial artery on the thumb side of the wrist (Procedure 8–2). It can be found approximately one inch above the base of the thumb. This is the most common site used for obtaining pulses in the dental office.

◗ Normal pulse rate for adults	Sixty to ninety beats per minute
◗ Normal pulse rate for children	Ninety to one hundred and twenty beats per minute

Respiration

Respiration is one breath taken in (**inhalation**) and one breath let out (**exhalation**). To ensure an accurate reading—where the patient is unaware that the respiration is being measured—take it after obtaining the pulse rate. Leave the fingers over the pulse site and count the breaths in and out for one minute. The patient will assume that the pulse is still being taken.

Normal respiration rates are as follows:

◗ Normal respiration rate in adults	Twelve to eighteen respirations per minute
◗ Normal respiration rate in children	Twenty to forty respirations per minute

PROCEDURE

8-2 Taking a Radial Pulse and Measuring the Respiration Rate

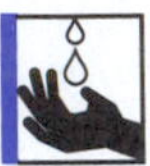

This procedure is performed by the dental assistant to obtain the patient's pulse and respiration rate.

EQUIPMENT AND SUPPLIES

- Watch with a second hand

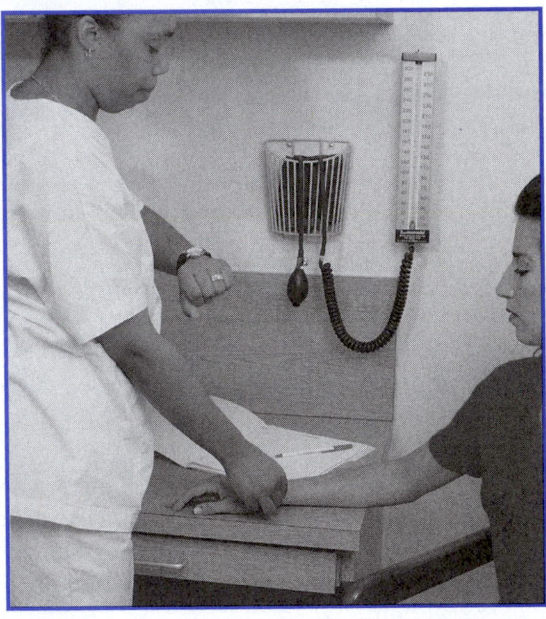

FIGURE 8–1 Taking patient's radial pulse and respiration.

PROCEDURE STEPS *(Follow standard precautions)*

1. Wash hands.
2. Position the patient in a comfortable position, upright in the dental chair (same position used for taking the temperature).
3. Explain the procedure.
4. Have the patient position the wrist resting on the arm of the dental chair or counter.
5. Locate the radial pulse by placing the pads of the first three fingers over the patient's wrist.
6. Gently compress the radial artery to feel the pulse.
7. Using the watch with the second hand, count the number of pulsations for one full minute (Figure 8–1).
8. Record the number of pulsations.
9. Note any irregular rhythm patterns.
10. While still keeping the finger pads placed on the radial pulse, count the rise and fall of the chest wall for one minute. This allows the patient to breath normally due to the fact that he or she believes the pulse is still being recorded.
11. Record the number of respirations. Note any irregularities in the breathing.
12. Wash hands.
13. Document the procedure and the pulse and respiration rates on the patient's chart.

Blood Pressure

Blood pressure is an important indicator of the health of a patient's cardiovascular system. A patient may have heart disease and still feel well and look outwardly healthy; however, the fear of dental treatment may be sufficiently stressful to induce a heart attack. Therefore, taking and recording a patient's blood pressure is very important.

Blood pressure is measured by placing a **sphygmomanometer**, the blood pressure apparatus, around the **brachial artery**. This apparatus is a cloth-covered inflatable rubber bladder used to control the flow of blood in the artery. A rubber hand bulb and pressure control valve are attached to one tube; a pressure gauge is attached to the other tube. The dental assistant uses the **stethoscope**, an instrument used to hear and amplify the sounds produced by the heart. The stethoscope has two earpieces that must be placed in the ears in a forward position. At the end piece of the stethoscope is a diaphragm, which amplifies and sends the sounds up the tubing to the ears.

Two measurements, the first (systolic) and the last (diastolic) sounds heard, are always recorded when taking blood pressure (Procedure 8–3). They are recorded as a fraction: The systolic pressure is the upper figure and the diastolic pressure is the lower figure. They are always recorded in even numbers (the gauge has indications for even numbers only). A measurement of 120 over 80 is average for an adult.

◗ Normal systolic pressure	100 to 140 mm Hg
◗ Normal diastolic pressure	60 to 90 mm Hg

PROCEDURE

8-3 Measuring Blood Pressure

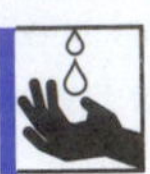

This procedure is performed by the dental assistant to obtain the patient's blood pressure.

EQUIPMENT AND SUPPLIES

- Stethoscope
- Sphygmomanometer
- Disinfectant and gauze

PROCEDURE STEPS *(Follow standard precautions)*

1. Wash hands.
2. Assemble the stethoscope and sphygmomanometer and disinfect the earpieces of the stethoscope.
3. Position the patient in a comfortable position, upright in the dental chair (same position used for taking the temperature), for a minimum of five minutes.
4. Explain the procedure.
5. Have the patient position the arm resting at heart level on the counter or the arm of the dental chair.
6. Have the patient remove any outer clothing that is restrictive to the upper arm. Bare the upper arm and palpate the brachial artery.
7. Center the bladder of the cuff securely, about two inches above the bend of the elbow.
8. Position the earpieces of the stethoscope in a forward manner, into the ears.
9. Place the diaphragm of the stethoscope over the brachial artery and hold it in place with a thumb. Place other fingers under the elbow to hyperextend the artery. (By extending the elbow, the artery can be accessed more easily and enable better reading of the blood pressure.)
10. Inflate the cuff using the bulb and the control valve on the sphygmomanometer. If the cuff is not inflating, recheck the control valve on the sphygmomanometer to ensure that it is closed. Air should not be escaping. The inflation should be to a level of 160 for a normal adult.
11. Deflate the cuff at a rate of two to four millimeters of mercury per second by rotating the control valve just slightly (Figure 8–2).
12. Listen for the first sound and note its measurement on the scale. This sound is the systolic blood pressure.
13. Continue to deflate the cuff and listen to the pulsing sounds. Note when all sounds disappear, this sound is the diastolic blood pressure. Continue deflating for another ten millimeters to ensure that the last sound has been heard.
14. Deflate the cuff rapidly and remove it from the patient's arm.
15. Disinfect the earpieces of the stethoscope.
16. Wash hands and record the procedure and the measurement on the patient's chart. (Blood pressure is recorded in even numbers in a fraction format with the systolic measurement on top.)

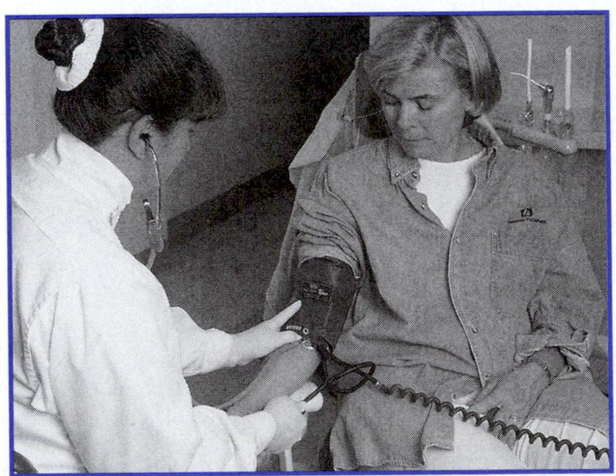

FIGURE 8–2 Taking patient's blood pressure.

SECTION 

Clinical Dental Procedures

CHAPTER 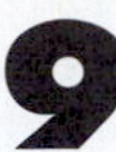

Chairside Assisting Skills

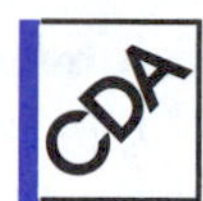

OBJECTIVES

The student should strive to meet the following objectives and demonstrate an understanding of the facts and principles presented in this chapter:

1. Explain the basic concepts of chairside assisting.
2. Describe the steps necessary to prepare a patient for treatment.
3. Explain the steps necessary to seat the patient for treatment.
4. Describe the position of the assistant at chairside.
5. Describe the necessary steps to dismiss the patient after treatment is completed.
6. Describe the grasps, positions, and transfer of dental hand instruments.
7. Define and demonstrate how to maintain the oral cavity and the equipment utilized in treatment of the oral cavity.

KEY TERMS

activity zones (p. 124)
air compressor (p. 122)
air-water syringe (p. 118)
amalgamator (p. 121)
central vacuum system (p. 122)
curing light (p. 121)
dental unit (p. 117)
four-handed dentistry (p. 124)
fulcrum (p. 129)
handpieces (p. 119)
high volume evacuation (HVE) (p. 119)
intraoral camera (p. 121)
mobile carts (p. 118)
modified pen grasp (p. 129)
operating light (p. 120)
palm grasp (p. 130)
palm-thumb grasp (p. 130)
pen grasp (p. 129)
reverse palm-thumb grasp (p. 130)
rheostat (p. 119)
saliva ejector (p. 119)
six-handed dentistry (p. 124)
subsupine position (p. 117)
supine position (p. 117)
triturates (p. 121)
ultrasonic scaler (p. 119)

Dental Office Design

The dental office is composed of several basic components designed to meet the individual dentist's preferences and needs. The office may be small with two or three treatment rooms or may be a clinic setting with any number of treatment rooms. Most offices are designed with a reception area, a business area, treatment rooms, a sterilizing area, a laboratory, an x-ray processing room, a restroom, and the dentist's private office. The size and number of these rooms varies. Dental offices may also include the following: consultation rooms/areas, staff lounge, prevention and/or patient education area, storage area, office for the office manager, space for panoramic radiograph machine, shower/change room, and laundry room.

Treatment Rooms

Dental treatment rooms are also called **operatories** (Figure 9–1). Most dentists have a minimum of three treatment rooms. The type and size of practice also dictate the number of operatories. The treatment rooms in a general practice are usually designated for either operative dentistry or dental hygiene and are equipped accordingly.

A dental treatment room contains a dental chair, dental unit, operating stools, cabinets, sinks, x-ray machine, x-ray viewbox, and mobile carts.

The Dental Chair

The dental chair is the center of all clinical activity. The chair is designed for the operator and the assistant to treat the patient in a comfortable and efficient

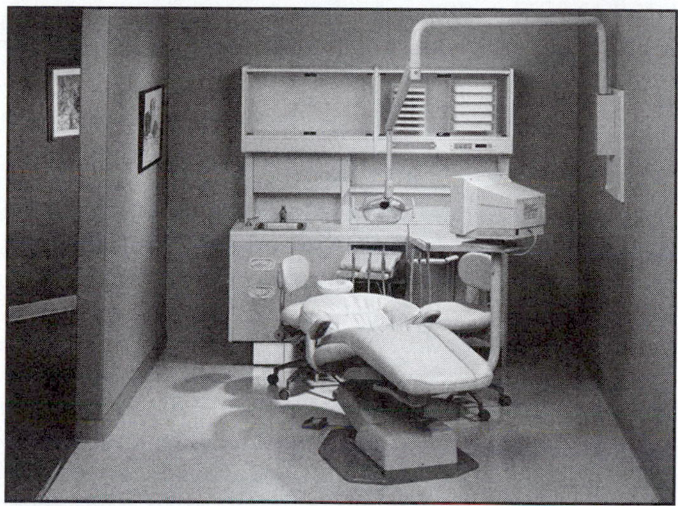

FIGURE 9–1 Treatment room. *(Courtesy of A-dec, Inc., Newberg, OR)*

manner. The dental chair supports the patient's entire body, in either an upright, **supine position** (reclined position with the nose and knees on the same plane) or a **subsupine position** (reclined position with the head lower than the feet). The head rest is narrow to allow the dentist and the assistant to be positioned close to the patient's head: It is adjustable to provide support. The dental chair has arm rests designed to lift or move out of the way when the patient is being seated or dismissed.

It has controls to move the chair up and down, recline the back rest, and raise the seat and a combination button that automatically reclines or raises the patient. The controls are either on the sides of the chair back or on the floor (the floor controls are becoming more popular because they eliminate the need for barriers). The chair also has a control on the floor that allows it to be rotated left and right. To prevent cross-contamination, the head rest and controls located on the chair are covered with barriers.

The dental chair is covered in a material that is comfortable, easy to clean, and coordinates with the office color theme. The base of the chair is secured to the floor. The chair base must be cleaned and disinfected routinely.

The Dental Unit

The **dental unit** consists of handpieces, an air-water syringe, a saliva ejector, an oral evacuator (HVE), an ultrasonic scaling unit, and numerous other options. The dental unit may be fixed to the wall, the cabinets, or on mobile carts. The unit is positioned according to the preference of the dentist, whether the dentist is left- or right-handed, if he or she routinely works with an assistant, and according to the design of the treatment room. The dental unit is available in three basic modes of delivery:

1. The **rear delivery system** is designed with the equipment located behind the patient's head.
2. The **side delivery system** is designed with the equipment located on the dentist's side. The unit is mounted to a moveable arm or a mobile cart.
3. The **front delivery system** is designed so that it can be pulled over the patient's chest and is located between the dentist and the assistant.

Mobile Carts. Sometimes **mobile carts** are used to hold delivery systems, including the air-water syringe, oral evacuator (HVE), handpieces, and saliva ejector. One cart may be used by both the operator and the dental assistant with the instrumentation on the appropriate side. Two carts, one on each side of the dental chair, may be equipped and used. The **operator's cart** is usually set up for two or three dental handpieces plus an air-water syringe. The **assistant's cart** is usually set up with the air-water syringe, saliva ejector, and HVE.

Air-Water Syringe. The **air-water syringe** provides air, water, or a combination spray of air and water (Figure 9–2). The tip of the syringe is removable and made of either disposable plastic or autoclavable metal. New barriers are placed on the syringe handle and the tubing for each patient. The controls for the syringe are on the handle and should be easy to operate using the thumb of one hand. Air, water, and the combination spray help keep the oral cavity clean and dry and protect the tooth from the heat produced by the handpieces.

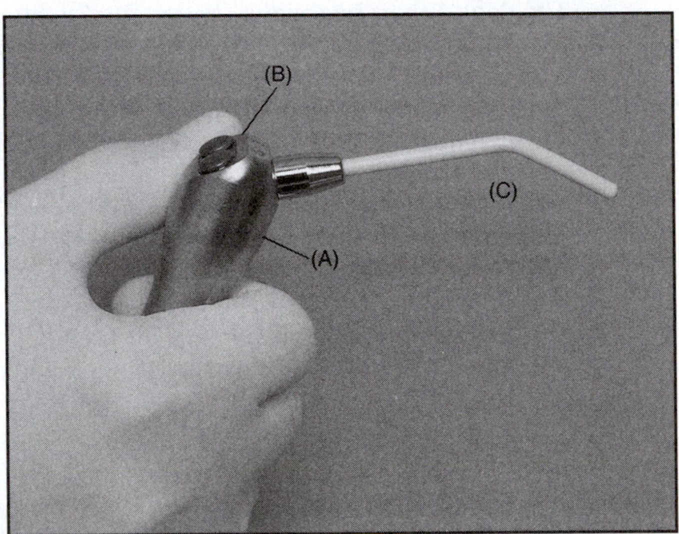

FIGURE 9–2 Air-water syringe. (A) Handle. (B) Air-water controls. (C) Removable and disposable tips.

For easier use, the syringe tips are supplied in several lengths and are slightly angled. To reduce the risk of retaining oral fluids, the dental assistant flushes the air-water syringe with water between patients and at the beginning and end of the day.

Dental Handpieces. There are usually two dental **handpieces** on the dentist's unit: low and high speed. The handpieces are attached to hoses that are part of the dental unit. It is important that these hoses are not bent or tangled. Each handpiece has two controls. The hose attachment has an on/off switch to prevent more than one handpiece from running at once. The speed of the handpiece is controlled by a foot pedal called a **rheostat** (**REE**-oh-stat). The dental handpieces are removed after each patient's treatment and are sterilized. (Prior to removal from the unit, like the air-water syringe, caution should be taken to flush oral fluids from the handpieces.) At the beginning and end of the day, the handpiece should be run for several minutes. Between patients, the dental assistant runs the handpieces for at least one minute to flush the system. Some dental manufacturers provide a water reservoir for the handpieces and air-water syringe on the unit.

Ultrasonic Scaler. The **ultrasonic scaler** is attached to the dental unit. The scaler is used during prophylaxis and periodontal procedures. Small tips attach to the ultrasonic scaler. The scaler has a vibrating action that removes hard deposits, such as calculus, and other debris from the teeth.

Saliva Ejector. The **saliva ejector** is used to remove saliva and fluids from the patient's mouth slowly. It has a low volume suction that is used during certain procedures, such as fluoride treatments and under dental dams. The saliva ejector tip is a thin, flexible, plastic tube that is disposed of after each patient's treatment. This plastic tip slides into the opening of the saliva ejector hose that is part of the dental unit. There is a small trap located in the saliva ejector that must be cleaned routinely by the dental assistant.

High Volume Evacuation (HVE). **High volume evacuation (HVE)** is also called the oral evacuator. It is used by the assistant to remove fluids from the patient's mouth. Evacuation tips are wider tubes that are often beveled at both ends. Some of the tips are metal and can be sterilized; however, most offices use plastic tips that can be sterilized or disposed of. The evacuation tips fit into the handle of the hose, which is covered with a protective barrier during procedures. The on/off control for the HVE is on the handle. Each unit has a trap that collects debris from the evacuator. This trap must be changed or cleaned weekly or as needed. Cleaning systems are available to flush the HVE at the end of the day and week.

Dental Stools

Dental stools are required by the operator and the assistant during most four-handed dental procedures. Ergonomic studies have resulted in the improved design of dental stools to provide comfort and prevent fatigue during dental procedures.

Dental Assistant's Stool. The dental assistant's stool features the following characteristics:

- **Adjustable height**—The stool should adjust to a variety of different levels to accommodate the height of the assistant. The assistant is positioned four to eight inches higher than the operator, with feet resting on the foot ring and thighs parallel to the floor.
- **Adjustable back rest**—The stool back rest should provide support for the lumbar region and be easily adjustable. Some stools have an extended arm for support of the abdomen or side areas. The arm moves easily into place and locks to stabilize the assistant when leaning or reaching.
- **Comfortable seat**—The seat of the stool has a broad, flat surface with no seams or hard edges.
- **Mobility**—The assistant's stool should be designed to move freely. Five casters are recommended to provide stability.
- **Broad base**—The base of the stool should be broad and well balanced. It should be heavy and stable to prevent tipping.
- **Foot rest**—The foot rest gives the assistant support so that good circulation is maintained.
- **Easy to adjust**—All parts of the assistant's stool should be easy to adjust.

Operating Light

The **operating light** is attached to the dental chair or mounted to the ceiling. Both the operator and the assistant should be able to adjust the position of the light. Operating lights have improved in many ways: They are easier to move, more flexible, and direct less heat on the patient. The light has a control switch for high and low intensities, an on/off switch, and handles on both sides. The light is attached to extension arms for positioning over the patient's face to view either the maxillary or mandibular arch.

The handles and on/off switch are covered with barriers during procedures. The barriers are changed between each patient. Maintenance includes changing the lightbulb occasionally and keeping the heat shield clean.

Small Equipment in the Treatment Room

There may be a variety of equipment in the treatment room depending on the primary use of the room. Most rooms have an x-ray viewbox, curing light, amalgamator, communication system, computerized intraoral dental camera, and a computer.

X-ray Viewbox. The x-ray viewbox is used to read and diagnose radiographs. The viewbox may sit on a counter or be installed in a wall or cabinet.

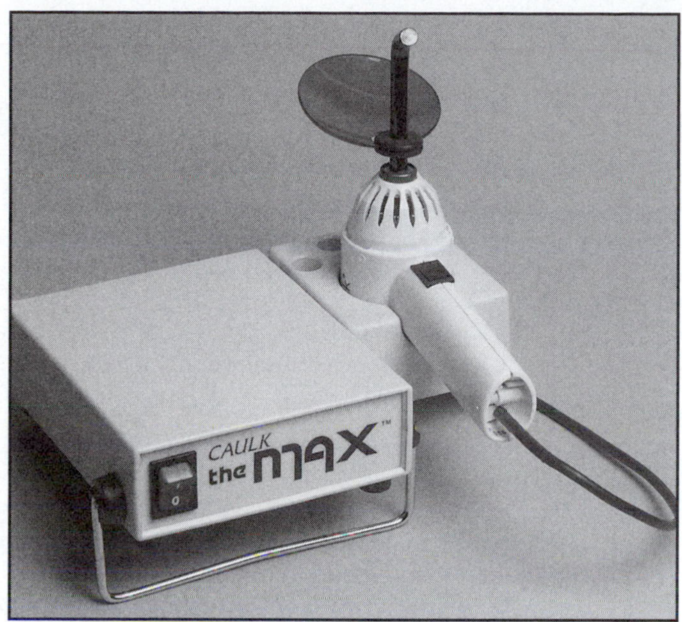

FIGURE 9–3 Dental curing light. *(Courtesy of Lasermed, Inc., Salt Lake City, UT)*

It consists of a bright light source covered with a frosted surface. X-rays are placed on the frosted surface for clear viewing.

Dental Curing Light. A dental **curing light** is used to "cure" or "set" light-cured materials (Figure 9–3). Many dental restorative products are light cured. The curing light has a small motor that produces the high intensity light, a wand, a protective shield, a handle, and a trigger to turn the light on and off. To determine if the light is working at full capacity, the curing light should be tested periodically. A small, handheld instrument tests the light and gives a reading to determine the strength of the light. The curing light uses halogen bulbs. Follow the manufacturer's instructions when changing the bulb.

Amalgamator. The **amalgamator** is a machine that mixes (**triturates**) dental amalgam and some dental cements. It is placed near the assistant, either on the counter or in a drawer.

Computerized Equipment. Computerized equipment includes a computer terminal and **intraoral camera**. The intraoral wand contains a small camera that transmits to the television monitor. The wand is placed in the patient's mouth, and the image is displayed on the monitor. The computer freezes a picture on the screen or prints it out. The intraoral computer allows patients to see areas and conditions in their mouths while the dentist explains them.

Dental Air Compressor and Central Vacuum System

The **air compressor** provides compressed air for the handpieces and air for the air-water syringes. The size of the air compressor depends on the number of dental units utilized by the office. The compressor is stored away from the main office because of its size and noise level.

The **central vacuum system** provides suction for saliva ejectors and oral evacuators at each dental unit. The filters or traps must be cleaned regularly to keep the system working to capacity. This system is also stored away from the main office.

Dental office staff and dental service companies must follow the manufacturer's instructions for maintenance and repairs on the air compressor and the vacuum system.

Routine Office Care

The dental assistant is often responsible for providing routine office care. This includes opening the dental office, preparing for the day's schedule, and closing the office to prepare for the next day (Procedures 9–1 and 9–2).

PROCEDURE

9-1 Daily Routine to Open the Office

These tasks are done by the assistant each morning. The assistant arrives to the office early to open the office and prepare for the day's schedule.

PROCEDURE STEPS

1. Turn on master switches to lights, each dental unit, vacuum system, and air compressor.
2. Check the reception room, turn on lights, straighten the magazines and the children's area, and unlock the patients' door to the office.
3. Turn on the communication system, check the answering machine or the answering system, start the computers, unlock the files, and organize the business area.
4. Post copies of patient schedules in designated areas throughout the office.
5. Turn on all equipment in the x-ray processing area. Change the water in the processing tanks and replenish solutions, if necessary.
6. Change into appropriate clinical clothing, following OSHA guidelines.
7. Review the daily patient schedule.
8. Prepare the treatment rooms for the first patients. Check supplies, place barriers, and review patient records. Then, prepare the appropriate trays and lab work for the first patients.
9. Turn on any sterilizing equipment and check solutions levels. Prepare new ultrasonic and disinfecting solutions. Complete overnight sterilization procedures.
10. Replenish supplies needed for the day.

PROCEDURE

9-2 Daily Routine to Close the Office

These tasks are done by the assistant at the end of the day. The office evening routine includes closing the office down for the evening and preparing for the next day. Each office has specific details; the following are general tasks.

PROCEDURE STEPS

1. Clean the treatment rooms. This may include an in-depth cleaning of the dental chair and dental unit. Flush the handpieces and air-water syringes, run solutions through the evacuation hoses, and clean traps/filters.
2. Position the dental chair for evening housekeeping.
3. Turn off all master switches.
4. Process, mount, and file x-rays. Follow manufacturer's instructions to shut down automatic processors. Turn off water supply to manual processing tanks.
5. Wipe counters and turn off the safe light.
6. Sterilize all instruments and set up trays for the next day. Empty ultrasonic solutions and turn off all equipment. Restock supplies.
7. Make sure all laboratory cases have been sent to the lab and early-morning cases have been received from the lab.
8. Confirm and complete appointment schedule for the next day, insurance forms, and daily bookkeeping responsibilities. Pull charts for the next day.
9. Turn off business office equipment and turn on the answering machine or service. Lock patient and business office files.
10. Straighten the reception room. For the security of the office, all doors and windows should be locked.
11. Change from uniform to street clothes, following OSHA guidelines.
12. Turn off machines in the staff lounge and clean tables and counters.

With the amount of equipment being operated in the dental office, a routine schedule needs to be in place to ensure proper maintenance control. Often this responsibility is given to the dental assistants. Usually, the office is cleaned professionally, but the assistant should periodically check the overall appearance of the office.

Weekly or monthly maintenance tasks may include the following: changing x-ray processing solutions, cleaning the inside of the sterilizers, changing ultrasonic solutions, performing monitoring activities to check the effectiveness of the sterilizers, and making miscellaneous repairs. It is necessary to keep replacement parts on hand for equipment that needs routine care.

Concepts of Dental Assisting

Originally, the dentist and the dental assistant worked standing on either side of the dental chair. Although some dentists still may stand occasionally, both the dentist and assistant now sit during procedures the majority of time. Many studies and research in ergonomics found that sit-down dentistry was the best for both the dentist and the assistant, creating less strain and increasing efficiency. When both the dentist and assistant work at the dental chair together, it is called **four-handed dentistry**. The assistant assists the dentist throughout the entire procedure, passing instruments, mixing materials, and observing the patient. Sometimes, an additional assistant is needed to bring items to the treatment room, assist the assistant in mixing materials, or help with a patient. This is called **six-handed dentistry**. Four- and six-handed dentistry have proven to be efficient and effective in providing patients with quality care.

Activity Zones

When the dentist and the assistant are positioned around the patient, it is vital that there is:

- Good visibility of the patient's mouth
- Easy access to all areas of the patient's mouth
- Easy access to dental equipment, instruments, and materials
- Safety and comfort for the patient, the operator, and the assistant

The area around the patient's mouth is divided into four **activity zones: operating zone, assisting zone, static zone,** and **transfer zone.** These activity zones are determined by visualizing the patient's head as the center of a clock (Figure 9–4).

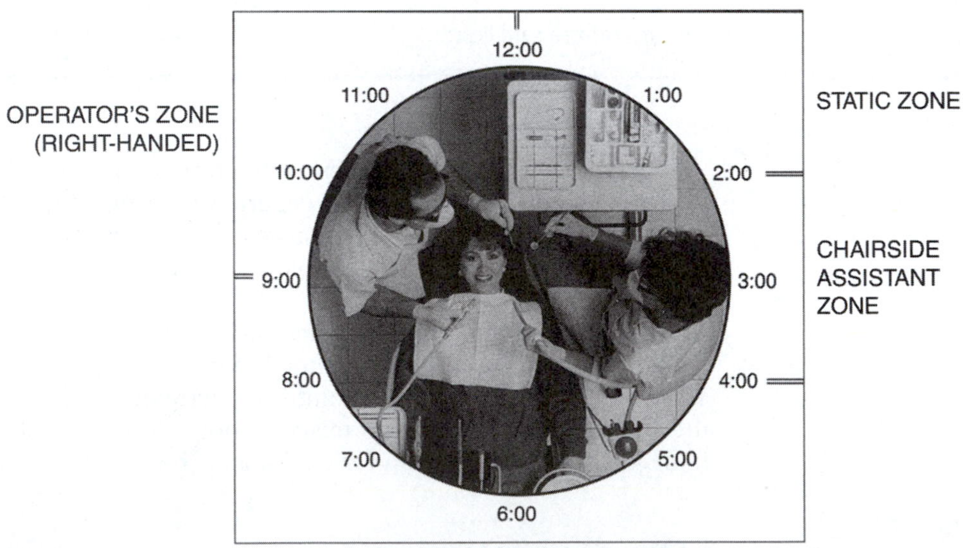

FIGURE 9–4 Working zones. *(Photo courtesy A-dec, Inc., P.O. Box 111, Newberg, OR)*

The operating zone is the area where the operator is positioned to access the oral cavity and have the best visibility.

The assisting zone is the area where the assistant is positioned to easily assist the dentist and have access to instruments, the evacuator, and the dental unit or cart without interference. Dental instruments and equipment used at the chair are located in the static zone.

The transfer zone is the area below the patient's nose where instruments and materials are passed and received. The operator and the assistant transfer instruments between the area that is below the patient's nose and above the upper chest.

Seating the Dental Patient

Greet and Escort the Patient

The dental assistant greets the patient by stepping into the reception area and identifying him or her by name. If you have not met the patient before, introduce yourself and ask the patient to follow you into the treatment room.

Seat and Prepare the Patient

Ask the patient to be seated in the dental chair (Procedure 9–3). The patient's back should be against the back rest and his or her legs completely supported. Once the patient is in the chair, lower the arm of the chair and offer a drink of water, tissue to remove lipstick, or lip lubricant. Place the **napkin** or **bib** on the patient and secure it with the napkin chain (bib clips). Give the patient **safety glasses** for protection during the procedure.

Recline the patient to the **supine position**, with the patient's nose and knees at about the same level. Sometimes the chair height needs to be adjusted so the patient is at the height of the operator's elbow; this is about eight inches above the seat of the operator's chair. Adjust the head rest and ask the patient if he or she is comfortable.

Position the dental light for maximum illumination of the area where the dental procedure is being performed. This is accomplished by bringing the light three to five feet from the patient's mouth and tilting the light downward toward the patient napkin. Then turn the light on. After the light is on, slowly raise it to the arch being treated:

- For the **mandibular teeth,** the light is raised and the beam is directed downward.
- For the **maxillary teeth,** the light is lowered and the beam is directed upward (Figure 9–5).

After the light is adjusted, the assistant turns the light off until the operator is seated. During the procedure, the light may need to be adjusted periodically. The assistant must be observant to keep the field of operation well lit and the light out of the patient's eyes.

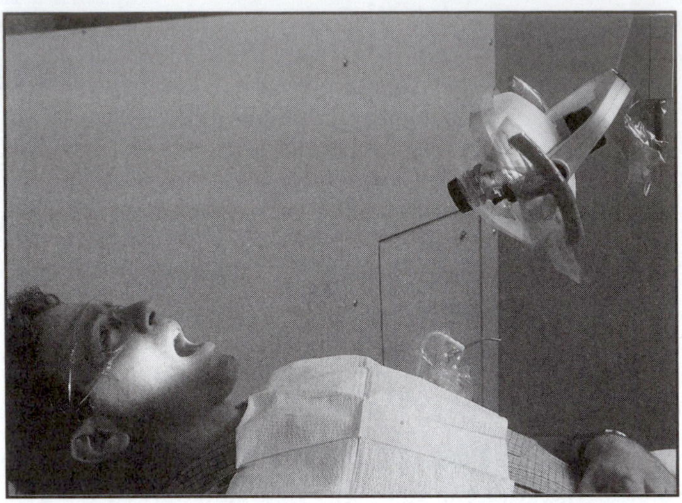

FIGURE 9–5 Patient seated and light adjusted for maxillary arch.

Positioning the Assistant

The assistant is positioned across from the operator on the opposite side of the patient. The assistant must also have good visibility and easy access to the oral cavity. The tray setup and other necessary instruments should be close at hand.

1. The assistant's stool is positioned 4 to 6 inches above the operator's for good visibility.
2. The assistant is positioned on the stool so his or her weight is distributed evenly over the seat.
3. The front edge of the assistant's stool is even with the patient's mouth.
4. The assistant's feet rest on a flat ring around the base of the stool and his or her thighs are parallel to the floor.
5. The assistant is positioned as close as possible to the side of the patient.
6. The assistant's back is straight, with support in the lumbar region; on some assistant's chairs there is an arm support that extends around in front of the assistant. This arm supports the assistant when he or she leans forward slightly or when reaching. The arm is adjusted to fit the assistant at the level of the abdomen.
7. After the assistant is correctly positioned on the chair, the cabinet top or mobile cart is placed over the thighs as close as possible for convenience and efficiency.

PROCEDURE

9-3 Seating the Dental Patient

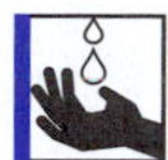 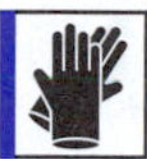 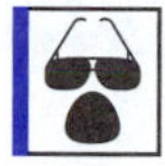 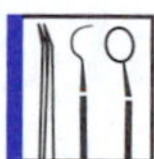

This procedure is performed by the dental assistant to prepare the patient for the dental treatment. The dental assistant has reviewed the patient's medical and dental records, cleaned and prepared the treatment room with appropriate barriers, readied the tray setup, and removed any possible obstacles from the patient's pathway. After being greeted by name in the reception area, the patient is escorted to the treatment room by the dental assistant.

EQUIPMENT AND SUPPLIES

- Patient's medical and dental records
- Basic setup: mouth mirror, explorer, and cotton pliers
- Saliva ejector, evacuator (HVE), and air-water syringe tip
- Cotton rolls, cotton-tip applicator, and gauze sponges
- Lip lubricant
- Patient bib and bib clip
- Tissue
- Safety glasses

PROCEDURE STEPS *(Follow aseptic procedures)*

1. Greet and escort the patient to the treatment room. Show the patient where to place his or her personal items, such as a purse, backpack, or coat. Some offices offer mouth wash to the patient at this time.
2. Seat the patient in the dental chair. Have the patient sit all the way back in the chair. (At this time, the dental assistant may offer the patient a tissue to remove lipstick and ask if he or she would like lubricant for his or her lips.)
3. Place the bib on the patient, and give the patient safety glasses to wear during the procedure.
4. Review the patient's medical history for any changes since his or her last visit. Ask the patient if he or she has any questions, and give a brief explanation or confirmation of the dental treatment to be completed at this appointment. Place x-rays in viewbox.
5. Position the patient for treatment, adjust the head rest, and adjust the dental light for the appropriate arch.
6. Position the operator's stool and the rheostat.
7. Position the assistant's stool. Put on mask and protective eyewear, then wash hands and put on gloves before being seated at chairside.
8. Position the tray setup. Prepare the saliva ejector, evacuator tip, air-water (three-way) syringe tip, and dental handpieces (Figure 9–6).

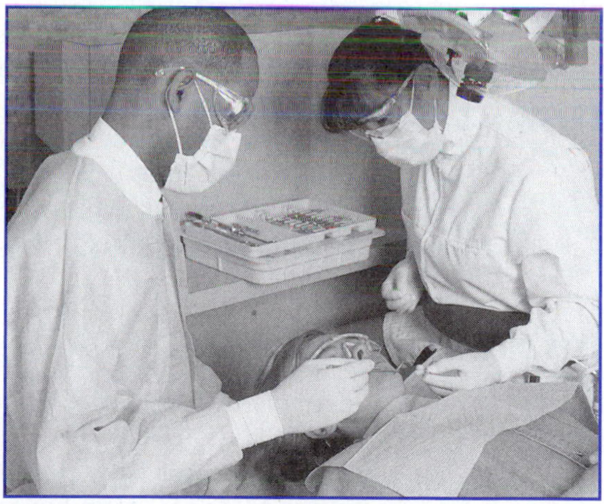

FIGURE 9–6 Operator and assistant positioned correctly with patient reclined and ready for treatment.

PROCEDURE

9-4 Dismissing the Dental Patient

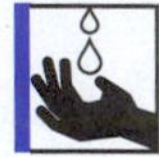
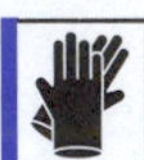
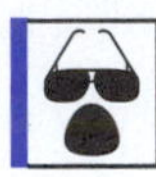
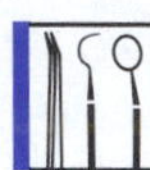

This procedure is performed by the dental assistant after the dental procedure has been completed.

PROCEDURE STEPS *(Follow aseptic procedures)*

1. When the operator has completed the procedure, the dental assistant thoroughly rinses and evacuates the patient's mouth. The dental light is positioned out of the patient's way.
2. Return the patient to an upright position. Remove any debris from the patient's face. (The patient may wish to double-check his or her appearance in a mirror before leaving the treatment room.)
3. Remove the patient's soiled bib and place it face down over the contaminated tray setup.
4. Remove the HVE tip, saliva ejector, and air-water syringe tip.
5. Position the dental light out of the patient's way. Move the operator's stool and the rheostat out of the patient's way.
6. Remove the treatment gloves, wash hands, and don overgloves. Document the procedure on the patient's chart or onto the computer at the terminal. Gather the patient's chart and radiographs.
7. Give postoperative instructions to the patient.
8. Return the patient's personal items and escort the patient to the business office or counter in the reception area.

Dismissing the Patient

After the treatment is completed, the light is turned off and moved out of the way. The dentist leaves the operatory and the assistant begins the process of dismissing the patient (Procedure 9–4).

Instrument Transfer

Instrument transfer or exchange is one of the basic functions in **four-handed, sit-down dentistry.** The assistant must learn to pass and receive instruments to the operator with confidence and skill. Efficient instrument transfer allows the operator to keep his or her eyes focused on the oral cavity and requires little movement of the operator's hand. A smooth transfer of instruments and materials occurs when the assistant is able to anticipate the operator's needs. This takes practice and cooperation between the operator and the assistant. When the transfer skills are accomplished, the operator and assistant work as one.

The transfer of instruments between operator and assistant takes place in the **transfer zone,** the area just below the patient's nose, near the chin. The assistant brings the instrument to the operator so the operator does not have to move his or her hand from the established **fulcrum** to exchange the instrument. The **tactile** sensation allows the operator to know the exchange has taken place without his or her eyes moving from the area. The assistant should pass the instrument with pressure firm enough for the operator to feel the instrument in his or her hand.

Fulcrum

A fulcrum is a point of rest on which the fingers are stabilized. When working on the mandibular first molar, the fingers rest on the occlusal surface of the mandibular bicuspids, providing the fulcrum.

Tactile Sensation

Tactile sensation is the feeling sensed by touch. For example, the pressure of the instrument exchanged during an instrument transfer is tactile sensation.

Transfer Hand

To aid the assistant in the delivery of instruments, the fingers and thumb of the hand are identified as follows: the thumb, the index finger or the first finger, the middle finger or the second finger, the ring finger or the third finger, and the little finger or the fourth finger.

The assistant passes and receives instruments with the **left hand** when working with a right-handed dentist and with the right hand when assisting a left-handed operator. Using one hand for instrument transfer frees the other hand for evacuation and retraction.

Instrument Grasps

The way an instrument is held influences how efficiently the instrument can be used. The way an instrument is grasped also dictates how it is exchanged. There are several instrument grasps that are commonly used in operative dentistry: pen, modified pen, palm, palm-thumb, and reverse palm-thumb.

Pen Grasp. The **pen grasp**, as the name indicates, is when an instrument is grasped in the same manner as a pen or pencil (Figure 9–7). The pen grasp is used to hold instruments that have angled shanks.

Modified Pen Grasp. The **modified pen grasp** is similar to the pen grasp. The instrument is held with the same fingers as the pen grasp, except the pad of the middle finger is placed on the top of the instrument with the index

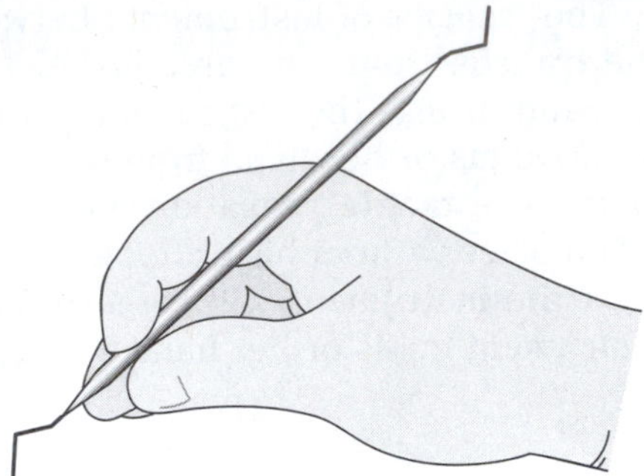

FIGURE 9–7 Pen grasp.

finger. The modified pen grasp is used with the same instruments as the pen grasp—those with angled shanks.

Palm Grasp. With the **palm grasp**, the operator holds the instrument in the palm of the hand and fingers grasp the handle of the instrument. The palm grasp is used with surgical pliers, dental dam forceps, and other forceps.

Palm-Thumb Grasp. Using the **palm-thumb grasp**, the operator grasps the handle of the instrument in the palm of the hand with the four fingers wrapped around the handle while the thumb is extended upward from the palm. The palm-thumb grasp is used with instruments having straight shanks and blades, such as the straight chisel or the Wedelstaedt chisel.

Reverse Palm-Thumb Grasp. The **reverse palm-thumb grasp** is a variation of the palm-thumb grasp that is frequently used to hold the evacuator tip in the patient's mouth. The reverse palm-thumb grasp is sometimes called the **thumb-to-nose grasp.** With this grasp, the evacuator tip is held in the palm of the hand with the thumb directed toward the assistant instead of toward the patient, as with the palm-thumb grasp (Figure 9–8).

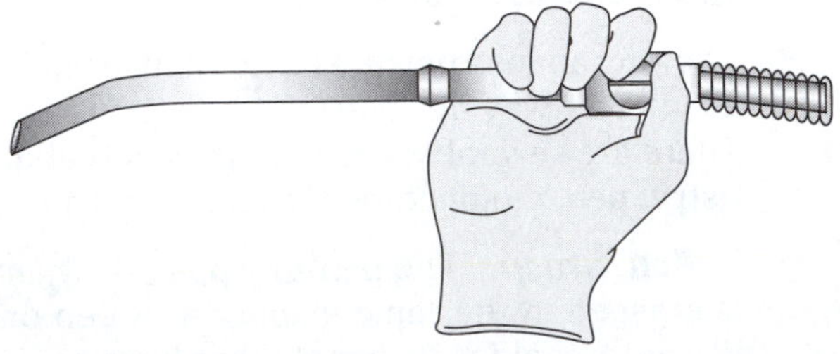

FIGURE 9–8 Reverse palm-thumb grasp.

Instrument Transfer Methods

The assistant selects the next instrument and holds it ready for transfer until the operator signals for the exchange. Usually, this signal occurs when the operator tilts the instrument back away from the patient while still maintaining the fulcrum.

Eight Basic Rules of Instrument Transfer

1. When using angled-shank instruments, the primary working end is placed *away* from the assistant on the tray.
2. When using straight-shank instruments, the primary working end is placed *toward* the assistant on the tray.
3. When using hinged instruments, the beaks are placed toward the assistant, with the beaks up for the maxillary arch and down for the mandibular arch.
4. Hold the instrument between the thumb and the index finger and the middle finger.
5. Pick up the instrument from the tray near the end closest to the assistant. (This is the end opposite from the one that the operator uses.)
6. The assistant's hand is placed on the instrument opposite from the end the operator uses to allow the operator to receive the instrument.
7. Rotate the working end of the instrument until it is directed toward the dental arch being treated, positioned upward for maxillary and downward for mandibular.
8. Hold the instrument to be passed parallel to the instrument held by the operator. Instruments are held as close to one another as possible, without touching during the transfer.

One-Handed Transfer. When using the one-handed transfer, the assistant picks up the next instrument to be transferred with one hand and with the same hand receives the instrument the operator is finished using (Procedure 9–5). Immediately after receiving the used instrument, the dental assistant rotates the new instrument into the operator's hand.

A sequence for instrument transfer includes the following movements: the approach, the retrieval, and the delivery.

Two-Handed Transfer. When using the two-handed transfer, the assistant uses both hands for the transfer. One hand receives the instrument from the operator and the other passes the next instrument. This transfer is used most commonly for surgical forceps or when both hands are free. This transfer is also used for dental handpieces and the air-water syringe.

PROCEDURE

9-5 One-Handed Instrument Transfer

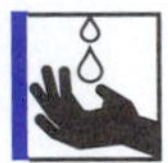 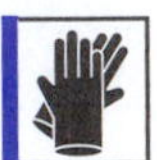 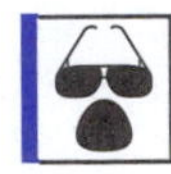 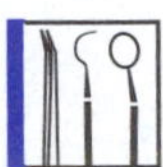

This procedure is performed at the dental unit by the dental assistant and the operator. In this procedure, the dental assistant uses his or her left hand to transfer instruments for a right-handed dentist. This is reversed for a left-handed operator. The dental assistant's free hand may hold the evacuator or retract oral tissues.

EQUIPMENT AND SUPPLIES

- Basic setup: mouth mirror, explorer, and cotton pliers
- Spoon excavator (for pen or modified pen grasp)*
- Straight chisel, forceps, or elevators (for palm grasp)*

**Any instrument combination can be used to provide a variety of instrument grasps and transfers.*

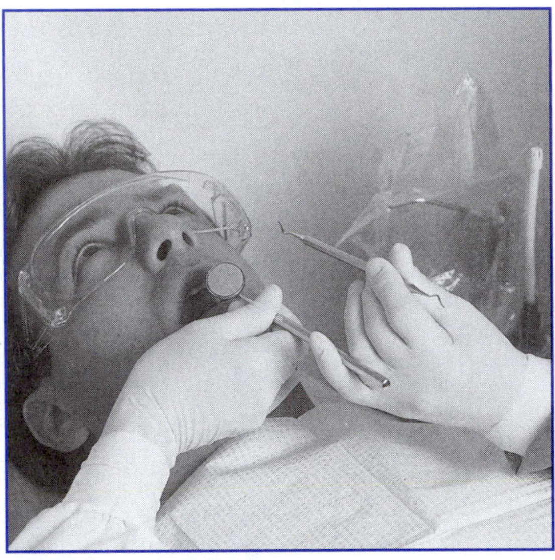

FIGURE 9–9 Operator signals he or she is ready for an exchange. Assistant retrieves the instrument.

PROCEDURE STEPS *(Follow aseptic procedures)*

Approach

1. Lift the instrument from the tray using the thumb, index finger, and second finger, holding it near the non-working end.
2. Turn palm upward into passing position, rotating the nib toward the correct arch.
3. Move toward the operator's hand.

Retrieval

4. Extend the little finger and close around the handle of the instrument the operator is holding (Figure 9–9).
5. Lift the instrument out of the operator's hand and pull this instrument toward the assistant's palm and wrist.

Delivery

6. Rotate the hand toward the operator and place the instrument in the operator's fingers.
7. Once the operator has the new instrument, rotate it to the delivery position for use again or return it to the tray.

Maintaining the Operating Field

Maintaining the operating field is the process of keeping the area directly involved in the treatment clean, visible, as accessible as possible, and comfortable for the patient. A well-maintained field is essential for the procedure to be performed safely.

The dental assistant is responsible to ensure that:

- The operator's vision and access are not obscured by the oral tissues, moisture, or debris
- Fluids do not interfere with the application of dental materials
- There are no fluids or materials for the patient to swallow or aspirate
- There is no interference with the manipulation of the handpiece and the instruments being used by the operator

Maintaining the operating field is accomplished by a combination of the following techniques:

- Use of the dental dam or cotton rolls to isolate the field
- Use of high volume evacuation and the air-water syringe to rinse and clean the oral cavity
- Retraction of oral tissues for clear vision

The following items are used by the dental team for maintaining the operating field:

- Dental light
- High volume evacuator
- Low volume saliva ejector
- Air-water syringe
- Retractors and mouth props

The Evacuation System

A **high volume evacuator (HVE)** is used to remove the water, saliva, blood, and debris. This evacuation system eliminates the need for the patient to sit up and empty his or her mouth.

In Which Hand Is the Evacuator Positioned?

The evacuator is held in the assistant's right hand when assisting a right-handed operator and in the left hand when assisting a left-handed operator.

Grasps for Oral Evacuation (HVE tip). The grasps most commonly used by the dental assistant to hold the HVE tip are the pen, modified pen grasp, or the reverse palm-thumb.

General Guidelines for Oral Evacuation Tip Placement (Procedure 9–6).

- Gently place the HVE tip in the patient's mouth. Avoid bumping the teeth, lips, or gingiva.
- Place the HVE tip in the mouth, and position it before the operator positions the handpiece or an instrument.
- Place the HVE tip approximately one tooth distal to the tooth being treated.
- Hold the bevel of the HVE tip parallel to the buccal or lingual surface of the teeth.
- The middle of the HVE tip opening should be even with the occlusal surface. Position the tip far enough away from the handpiece so that it does not draw the water coolant away from the bur.
- Hold the HVE tip still while the handpiece or instrument is being used. Any movement may startle the operator or the patient and may cause the handpiece or instrument to be bumped.
- Rest the HVE tip on cotton rolls, not the gingival tissue. Cotton rolls are placed in the vestibular area near the tooth being treated before the evacuator tip is placed.
- Avoid placing the HVE tip on the soft palate, the back of the tongue, or the anterior pillar/tonsilar area. Allowing the tip to contact any of these areas could cause the patient to gag.
- Keep the HVE tip far enough away from the mucosal tissue to prevent it from being sucked into the tip and making a noise. If this does occur, either turn it off or rotate the tip to break the seal.

Saliva Ejector

The saliva ejector is the low volume evacuation system. It is a flexible, plastic tube about one-third the size of the high volume evacuation tube. The saliva ejector is bent and then positioned between the tongue and the mandibular teeth or between the cheek and the mandibular teeth.

The saliva ejector is used during procedures such as fluoride treatments, under the dental dam, or during a coronal polish.

The Air-Water Syringe

The air-water syringe, also referred to as the three-way syringe, emits water, air, or a combination of both in a spray. The patient's mouth is rinsed with the air-water syringe and simultaneously evacuated. The assistant can dry an area or

PROCEDURE

9-6 Specific Tip Placements for Evacuation of the Oral Cavity

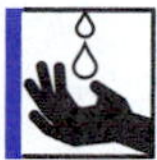
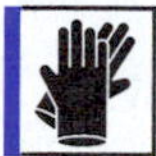
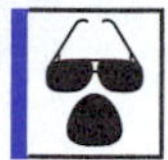
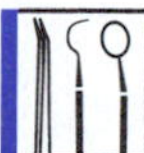

This procedure is performed by the dental assistant during dental treatment. The oral cavity is maintained to keep the area clear for the operator and for the comfort of the patient. Each area of the mouth requires different evacuator tip positioning. The following illustrates how to position the tip for each quadrant when assisting a right-handed operator.

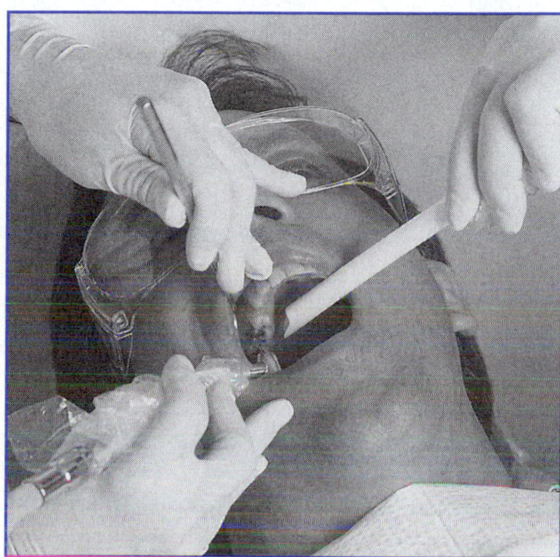

FIGURE 9–10 The tip is placed near the lingual surface just distal to the tooth being worked on. The bevel of the tip is parallel to the lingual surface of the teeth. Notice that the tip is resting on the teeth in the maxillary left quadrant.

EQUIPMENT AND SUPPLIES

- Basic setup: mouth mirror, cotton pliers, and explorer
- HVE tip and air-water syringe tip
- Cotton rolls
- Dental handpiece

PROCEDURE STEPS (*Follow aseptic procedures*)

1. Maxillary right posterior tip placement (Figure 9–10).
2. Maxillary left posterior tip placement. The evacuator tip is positioned on cotton rolls that are placed in the maxillary left vestibule. The handpiece is positioned and mouth mirror is used for indirect vision. The air-water syringe tip is placed near the edge of the mouth mirror to keep the mirror surface clear. The evacuator tip is placed parallel to the buccal surface of the teeth and is resting on the cotton roll.
3. Mandibular right posterior tip placement. The evacuator tip is positioned with the handpiece and mouth mirror in place. The evacuator tip comes across the mandibular left teeth and is positioned between the lingual surface of the teeth and the tongue. The tip is placed parallel to the lingual surface of the teeth. A cotton roll is used for retraction of the tongue.
4. Mandibular left posterior tip placement (Figure 9–11).

(continued)

PROCEDURE 9-6 *continued*

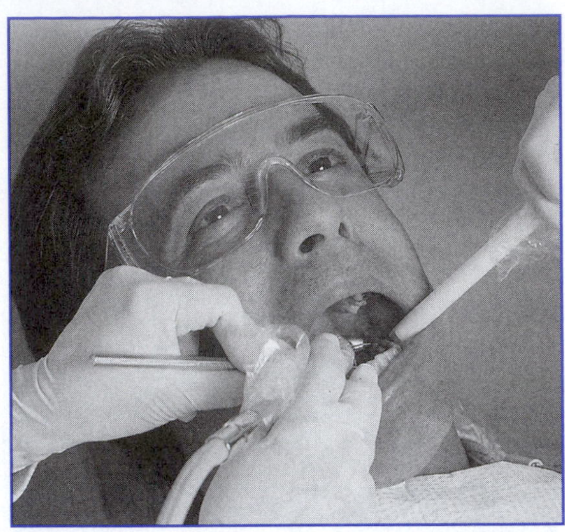

FIGURE 9–11 Evacuator tip placed and handpiece in position. The tip of the bevel of the evacuator tip is positioned parallel to the buccal surface of the teeth.

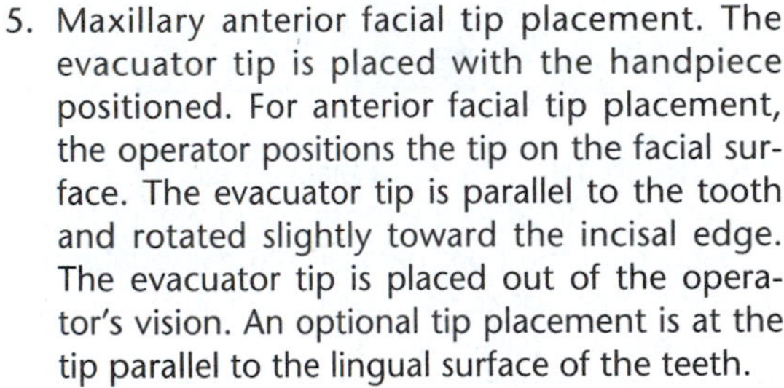

5. Maxillary anterior facial tip placement. The evacuator tip is placed with the handpiece positioned. For anterior facial tip placement, the operator positions the tip on the facial surface. The evacuator tip is parallel to the tooth and rotated slightly toward the incisal edge. The evacuator tip is placed out of the operator's vision. An optional tip placement is at the tip parallel to the lingual surface of the teeth.

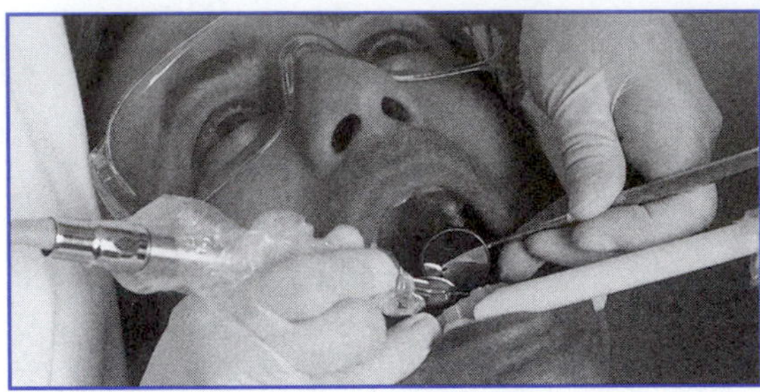

FIGURE 9–12 Tip placed and the handpiece in position. The evacuator tip is positioned on a cotton roll near the facial surface of the teeth. The lip is retracted and the bevel is parallel to the facial surface.

6. Maxillary anterior lingual tip placement. The evacuator tip is placed before the dentist positions the handpiece and mouth mirror. The tip is placed on the lingual surface, out of the dentist's vision, rotated slightly toward the incisal edge. The handpiece and mouth mirror are then readied and the air-water syringe tip is positioned.
7. Mandibular anterior facial tip placement (Figure 9–12).
8. Mandibular anterior lingual tip placement. The evacuator tip is placed and the handpiece and mouth mirror are then positioned. The tip is placed with the bevel parallel to the lingual surface of the teeth.

keep the mirror clean with air for the operator to have clear vision. The air-water syringe is held in the assistant's left hand for a right-handed operator and in the right hand for a left-handed operator.

Guidelines for Use of the Air-Water Syringe.

1. The most effective way to use the air-water syringe is with the air-water spray. A spray is effective and easier to control.

2. When rinsing a patient's mouth, use the evacuator tip to follow the spray. The patient's mouth is rinsed in quadrants, and the evacuator tip and the air-water syringe tip are rotated for correct placement. Rinsing and evacuating the patient's mouth requires practice to achieve efficiency and control.
3. When the operator is using the handpiece and a mirror for indirect vision, water from the handpiece falls onto the mirror and distorts the operator's view. The assistant is expected to keep the mirror surface dry and free from debris. To accomplish this, the assistant places the tip of the air-water syringe tip *close to the edge* of the mouth mirror and directs air across the surface of the mirror without interfering with the operator's view.
4. When the operator stops the handpiece, the assistant completes a quick "rinse and dry" to give the operator a clean, dry mirror for good vision. This is accomplished by first using the spray, followed by the air.

Retraction of Tissues

Retraction of the tongue, cheeks, lips, and tissue is used to increase the field of vision in the oral cavity. Several types of retractors are used, including the mouth mirror, the dental dam, the evacuator tip, cotton rolls, cotton gauze, and specially designed tissue retractors. Retractors are used for better access and lighting and to prevent injury to the tissues.

CHAPTER 10

Dental Instruments and Tray Systems

CDA

OBJECTIVES

The student should strive to meet the following objectives and demonstrate an understanding of the facts and principles presented in this chapter:

1. Identify the parts of an instrument and describe how instruments are used.
2. Identify categories and functions of dental burs.
3. Describe types and functions of abrasives.
4. Explain various dental handpieces and their uses.
5. Describe tray systems.

KEY TERMS

abrasives (p. 151)
air abrasion (p. 154)
bevel (p. 140)
Black's formula (p. 142)
blade (p. 140)
burs (p. 148)
cutting edge (p. 140)
high-speed handpieces (p. 153)
low-speed handpieces (p. 153)
mandrels (p. 152)
manufacturer's number (p. 142)
non-cutting (p. 141)
revolutions per minute (rpm) (p. 153)
rotary instruments (p. 148)
shaft (p. 140)
shank (p. 140)
working end (p. 140)

INTRODUCTION

Most instruments are constructed of stainless steel. However a few are a high-tech plastic/resin or anodized aluminum. Manufacturers of dental instruments provide many designs and sizes and make improvements as new materials become available. The dentist selects the instruments that he or she feels the most confident and comfortable using. Each procedure requires specific instruments to accomplish the task; for example, when examining the pits and grooves of the teeth, the dentist uses an explorer. The ends of all explorers are pointed and sharp but designed with different angles to reach all surfaces of the tooth.

It is the dental assistant's responsibility to keep the instruments sterilized and in working condition. The dental assistant orders new instruments as needed and keeps the instruments in sequence while assisting during the procedure.

Instruments are categorized into hand instruments and rotary instruments. Hand instruments are manually operated and are categorized according to the specific procedure.

INSTRUMENTS FOR BASIC CHAIRSIDE PROCEDURES

Parts of Dental Hand Instruments

The dental instrument is approximately six inches long and is single- or double-ended. The parts of the dental hand instrument include the working end, the shank, and the handle.

The Working End of an Instrument. The **working end** actually performs the specific function of the instrument. The working end may be a point, blade, or nib. A point is sharp and is used to explore, detect, and reflect materials. The **blade** may be flat or curved and have a rounded edge or a cutting edge. The **cutting edge** is formed by a **bevel** (slanted edge or side) on the working end of the instrument. The blade may also be **bi-beveled** (beveled on both sides of the blade). A nib is a blunt end that is either serrated or smooth (Figure 10–1).

The working ends of instruments may also be beaks or rounded ends.

Handle (Shaft). The handle, or **shaft**, of an instrument is where the instrument is held by the operator.

Shank. The **shank** connects the handle to the working end. It narrows or tapers from the handle to the working end. The shank may be angled to reach different areas of the mouth. Instruments used in the posterior areas of the oral cavity have greater angles, while instruments with lesser angles are used in anterior areas.

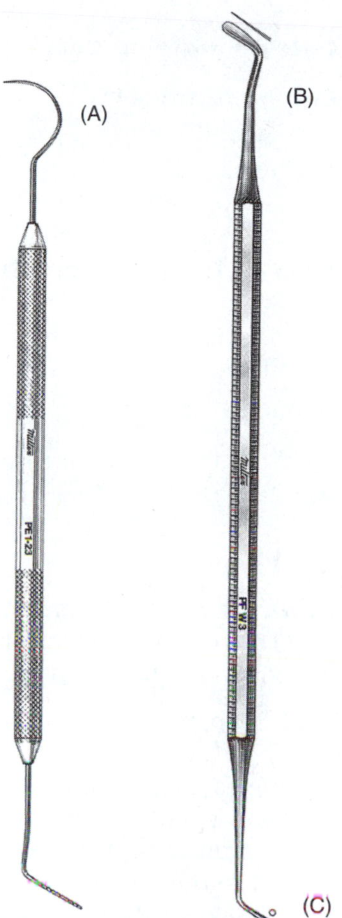

FIGURE 10–1 Various working ends. (A) Point. (B) Blade. (C) Nib. *(Courtesy of Miltex Instrument Co., Inc., Lake Success, NY)*

Classification of Dental Instruments

Dental instruments are classified in many ways, including by number of working ends, function, manufacturer's name and number, and Black's number formula.

Number of Working Ends. The number of working ends an instrument has falls into two categories: single-ended and double-ended instruments.

Instruments Classified by Function. Instruments are classified by function to describe the specific use. Operative hand instruments are divided into cutting and **non-cutting** functional classification. Other instruments are classified according to a specialty, use with a specific material, or a procedure.

Cutting and Non-Cutting Instruments

Cutting Instruments

- Angle formers
- Chisels
- Excavators
- Gingival margin trimmers
- Hatchets
- Hoes

Non-Cutting Instruments

- Basic instruments (mouth mirror, explorer, and cotton pliers)
- Burnishers
- Carriers
- Carvers
- Composite instruments
- Condensers
- Files
- Finishing knives
- Plastic filling instruments

Manufacturer's Number. The **manufacturer's number** is a number engraved on the handle of the instrument. The number is used when ordering the instrument and indicates the instrument's placement in a set of instruments.

Black's Formula. **Black's formula** was developed by G.V. Black to standardize the exact size and angulation of an instrument. This formula minimizes discrepancies in the production of instruments from one manufacturer to another and simplifies the ordering of instruments. Black's formula for hand cutting instruments includes the size of the blade and the angle at which it is positioned to the handle.

Cutting Instruments

Hand cutting instruments are used to assist in the design of the cavity preparation. They refine and define the cavity walls and margins (Figure 10–2).

Chisels. Chisels are used to shape and plane enamel and dentin walls of the cavity preparation.

Hatchets. Hatchets, sometimes called enamel hatchets, are used in a downward motion to refine the cavity walls and to obtain retention in the cavity preparation.

Hoes. A hoe is an instrument used in a pulling motion to smooth and shape the floor of the cavity preparation.

Gingival Margin Trimmers. The gingival margin trimmer (GMT) is similar to the hatchet but has two distinctive differences. First, the blade on the GMT is curved, not as flat as the hatchet. Second, the cutting edge is at an angle, not straight across as is the hatchet. The GMTs are used to bevel the gingival margin wall of the cavity preparation.

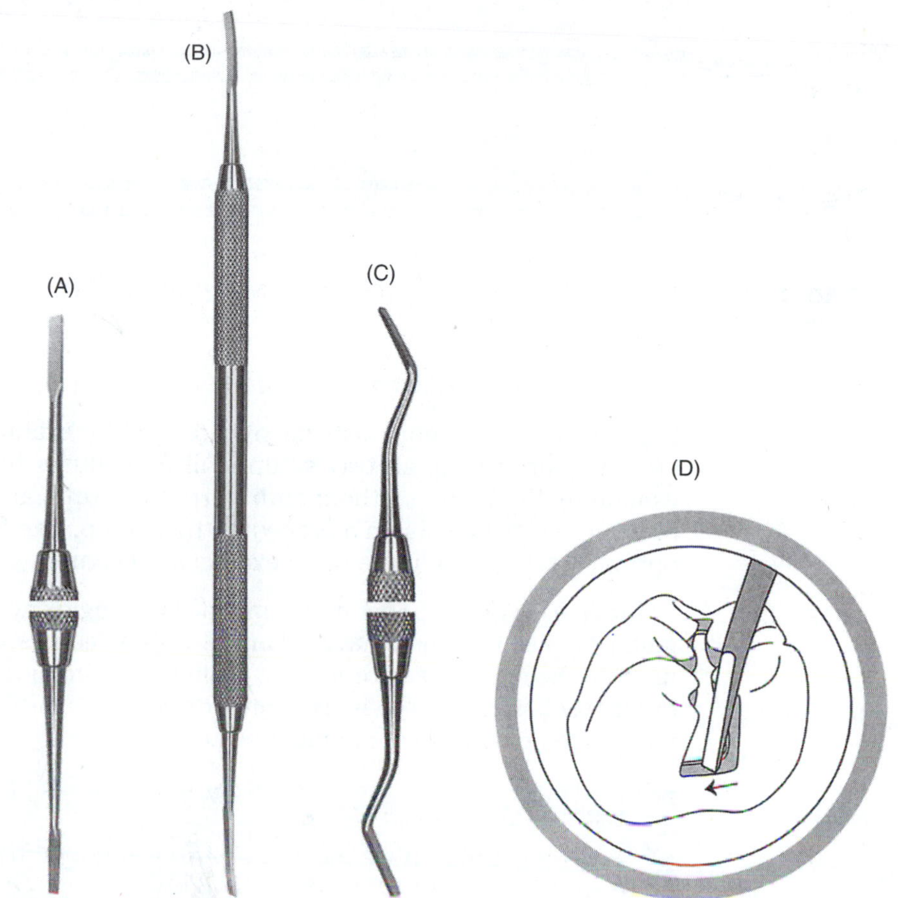

FIGURE 10–2 Chisels. (A) Straight. (B) Wedelstaed. (C) Binangle. (D) Chisel being used to prepare cavity. *(Courtesy of Hu-Friedy Mfg. Co., Inc.)*

Angle Formers. The angle former is used in a downward pushing motion to form and define point angles and to sharpen line angles.

Excavators. Excavators, also known as "spoon excavators," are used to remove carious material and debris from the teeth. They are also used for numerous other tasks, including removing excess dental cement, tucking dental dam material, and packing gingival retraction cord (Figure 10–3).

Non-Cutting Instruments

Non-cutting instruments include the basic examination instruments and instruments used to insert and finish amalgam and composite restorative materials.

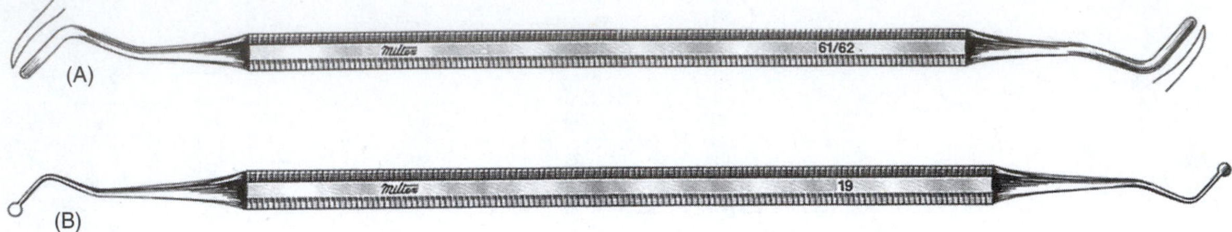

FIGURE 10–3 Excavators. (A) Blade. (B) Spoon. *(Courtesy of Miltex Instrument Co., Inc., Lake Success, NY)*

Basic Examination Instruments

Basic examination setup instruments are used for examination of the teeth and are also common to all tray setups. All procedures begin with the operator examining the teeth, so the mouth mirror, explorer, and cotton pliers are the first three instruments on a procedure tray setup. The periodontal probe is an optional instrument in the basic examination setup.

Mouth Mirrors. The mouth mirror is a single-ended instrument made of metal or plastic. It may have a handle with a "cone socket" for easy replacement of the mirror head or may be available in one piece. Mirrors are available in different sizes and types. The mirror sizes are identified by number, and the most commonly used are numbers 4 and 5.

Uses of the Mouth Mirror

- **Indirect vision**—When the operator uses a mirror to view areas of the oral cavity not seen with direct vision
- **Reflection of light**—Illumination of an area being examined or treated
- **Retraction**—When the cheeks or tongue are retracted for better visibility and to protect tissues
- **Transillumination**—Reflection of light through the tooth surface to detect fractures

Explorers. Explorers are single- or double-ended instruments. The working end is a thin, sharp point of flexible steel. There are a variety of angles of explorers, and often the ends are different to allow the operator access to various areas of the mouth. Several common shapes include the pig tail, the shepherd's hook, the right angle, and the #17.

Uses of Explorers

- **Examination** of the tooth structure for defects or areas of decay
- **Examination** of restorations to check for faulty margins or fractures
- **Removal of excess materials** from around the margins of restorations or from bases and liners in the cavity preparation

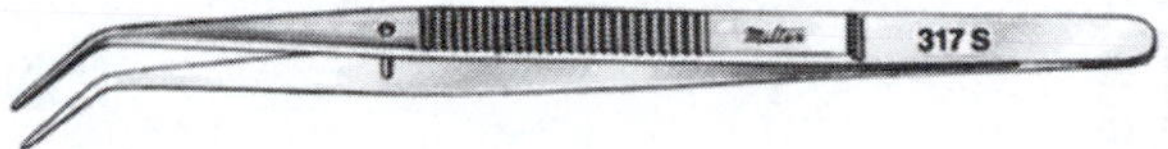

FIGURE 10–4 Cotton pliers. *(Courtesy of Miltex Instrument Co., Inc., Lake Success, NY)*

Cotton Pliers. Cotton pliers are shaped like large tweezers with either smooth surfaces or serrations on the ends of the beaks. They are available in locking or non-locking handles; the tips may be straight or angled (Figure 10–4).

Uses of Cotton Pliers

- **To place** and remove items from the oral cavity, such as cotton rolls, cotton pellets, wedges, and large pieces of debris
- **To grasp** and transfer materials to and from the oral cavity
- **To retrieve** materials from drawers and cupboards to avoid contamination

Periodontal Probes. Periodontal probes are used to measure the depth of the gingival sulcus. They may be single- or double-ended. The working end of the probe is a blade that is rounded or blunted and is marked in millimeters (mm). There are variations in the indication of calibrations, including color coding. A combination instrument that has an explorer tip on one end and a periodontal probe on the other end is known as an **Expro** (Figure 10–5).

Plastic Filling Instruments

Plastic Filling Instruments. Plastic filling instruments are used to place and condense pliable restorative materials and to place cement bases in the cavity preparation.

Amalgam Carriers

The amalgam carrier is designed to carry and dispense amalgam or composite into the cavity preparation. The carriers may be single- or double-ended with small and large ends. Most carriers are made of stainless steel; some have

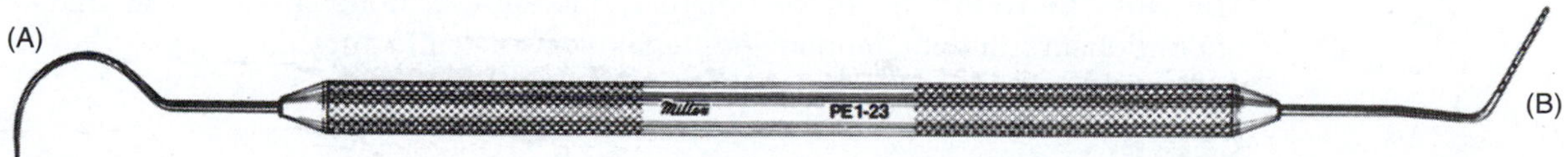

FIGURE 10–5 Expro with (A) explorer and (B) periodontal probe. *(Courtesy of Miltex Instrument Co., Inc., Lake Success, NY)*

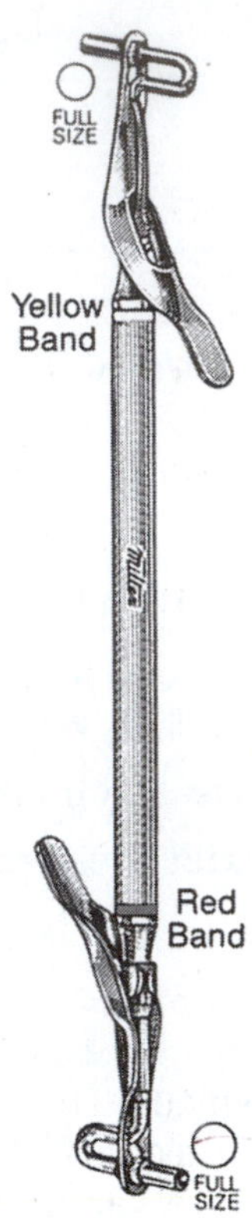

FIGURE 10–6 Double-ended amalgam carrier. *(Courtesy of Miltex Instrument Co., Inc., Lake Success, NY)*

Teflon® or coated barrels to prevent clogging. The dental assistant loads both ends of the carrier with the restorative material and either passes it to the operator or places the material in the cavity preparation and then refills the carrier as needed (Figure 10–6).

Amalgam Condensers (Pluggers)

Amalgam condensers, or pluggers, are used to pack amalgam into the cavity preparation. Hand condensers are usually double ended and have a wide variety of working ends. The working ends may be plain (smooth) or serrated. They may be round, ovoid, rectangular, diamond, or cone shaped. The shanks of condensers may be monangled, binangled, or triple angled.

Carvers

Carvers are used to remove excess restorative material and carve tooth anatomy in the restoration before the material hardens. Carvers are also used to carve wax inlays, onlays, and crowns. There are a wide variety of working ends

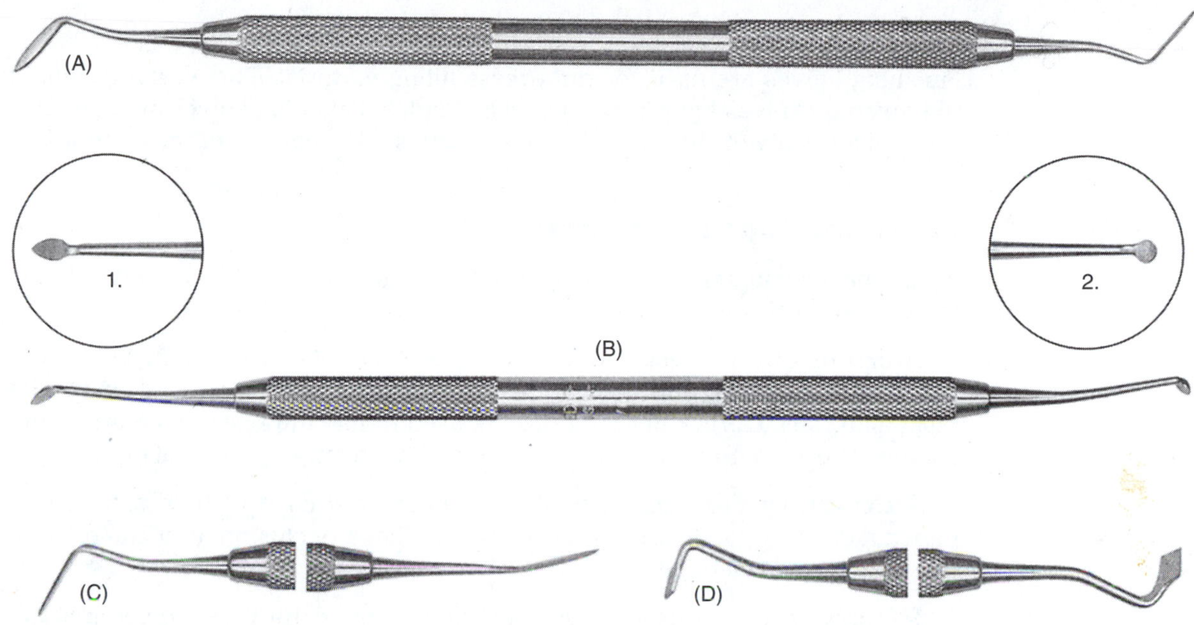

FIGURE 10–7 Carvers. (A) Hollenback. (B) 1. Cleoid/ 2. discoid. (C) Ward's. (D) Frahm. *(Courtesy of Hu-Friedy Mfg. Co., Inc.)*

on carvers, including long-bladed pointed ends and rounded and oval shapes. Usually, carvers are double ended, with some ends having sharp edges and others rounded blades similar to excavators. The operator usually has several favorite carvers; often these include the Hollenback® and the cleoid-discoid. The Hollenback® is a long-bladed carver used to shape the restoration. The cleoid-discoid carver is used to shape amalgam restorations. The cleoid end looks like a claw, and the discoid end is shaped like a round disc (Figure 10–7A through D).

Burnishers

Burnishers are used to smooth rough margins of the restoration and to shape metal matrix bands. Burnishers are blunt, rounded instruments that come in a variety of shapes, including the beavertail, the egg or football shape, the ball shape, and the T-ball. Burnishers may be single- or double-ended instruments.

Files

Files are used to trim excess filling material and to smooth the restoration, especially the margins. They are manufactured in a variety of shapes, with a serrated surface on one side of the blade. The working end is often thin and small enough to reach interproximal spaces. Files are available as either single- or double-ended instruments.

Finishing Knives

Finishing knives are used to trim excess filling material. The working ends of the finishing knives have sharp, knifelike blades. Finishing knives are manufactured in a variety of shapes and angles to access the margins of the restoration.

Miscellaneous Instruments

Additional instruments found on restorative trays include spatulas, articulating forceps, and scissors.

Spatulas. During restorative procedures, **cement spatulas** may be used to mix cements, bases, and liners. **Plastic spatulas** are used to mix composite resin materials. **Laboratory spatulas** are used to mix impression materials and plaster. These spatulas are larger in size and have longer, wider blades.

Articulating Forceps. Articulating forceps are used to hold articulation paper, a colored paper used to check the patient's occlusion after the restorative material has been placed.

Scissors. Scissors used most commonly with restorative procedures are **crown and collar scissors.** These scissors have short blades that may be either straight or curved.

DENTAL ROTARY INSTRUMENTS

Dental **burs** are part of a group of instruments referred to as **rotary instruments**. Rotary instruments include disks and stones and are designed to be used with dental handpieces. They are used in differently speeded handpieces, both at chairside and in the dental laboratory. Burs are used to cut cavity preparations, to finish and polish restorations, for surgical procedures, and for dental appliance adjustments.

Bur groups include cutting burs, diamond burs, surgical burs, laboratory burs, and finishing burs.

Parts of the Bur

All burs have three basic parts: the shank, the neck, and the head (Figure 10–8A).

Shank. The shank of the bur is inserted into the handpiece. To accommodate dental handpieces, there are three styles of bur shanks (Figure 10–8B). The **straight shank** (designated HP when ordering), or long shank, functions with the straight, low-speed handpiece. The **latch-type shank** (designated RA) is shorter than the straight-shanked burs. On the latch-type shank there is a notch that fits into the contra-angle/right-angle handpiece that latches securely in place. The **friction-grip shank** (designated FG) is short, small, and smooth. These burs are used in friction-grip, high-speed handpieces.

Neck. The neck of the bur is the tapered connection of the shank to the head.

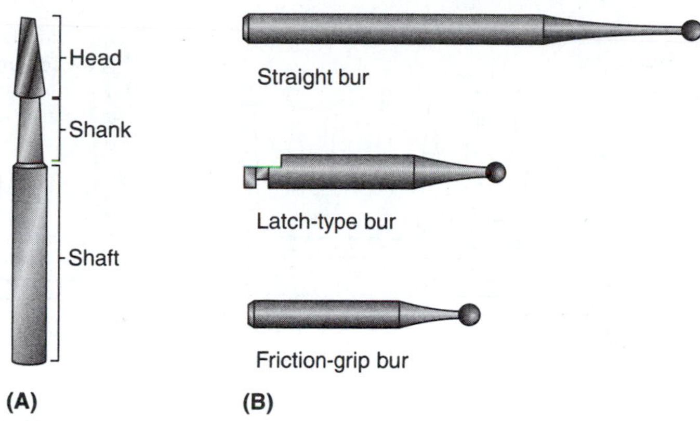

FIGURE 10–8 (A) Parts of a bur. (B) Different shanks: straight, latch type, and friction grip.

Head. The head is the working end of the bur. There are many shapes and sizes of heads on dental burs. A variety of burs are needed to perform the multiple tasks in restoring teeth and specialty procedures.

Cutting Burs

Cutting burs are identified by number ranges. The bur numbers describe the shape, size, and variation of the bur. It is important to know the number ranges, because dentists will ask for a bur by its number (Table 10–1 and Figure 10–9).

TABLE 10–1 BURS, THEIR SPECIFIC FUNCTIONS AND NUMBER RANGES

Name	Function
Round bur	Used first to open the cavity and remove carious tooth structure
Inverted cone bur	Removes caries and makes undercuts in the preparation
Plain fissure straight bur and Plain fissure cross-cut bur	Forms the cavity walls of the preparation
Tapered fissure straight bur and Tapered fissure cross-cut bur	Forms divergent walls of the cavity preparation
End cutting bur	Forms the shoulder for crown preparations
Wheel bur	Forms retention in preparations
Pear bur	Opens and extends the cavity preparation

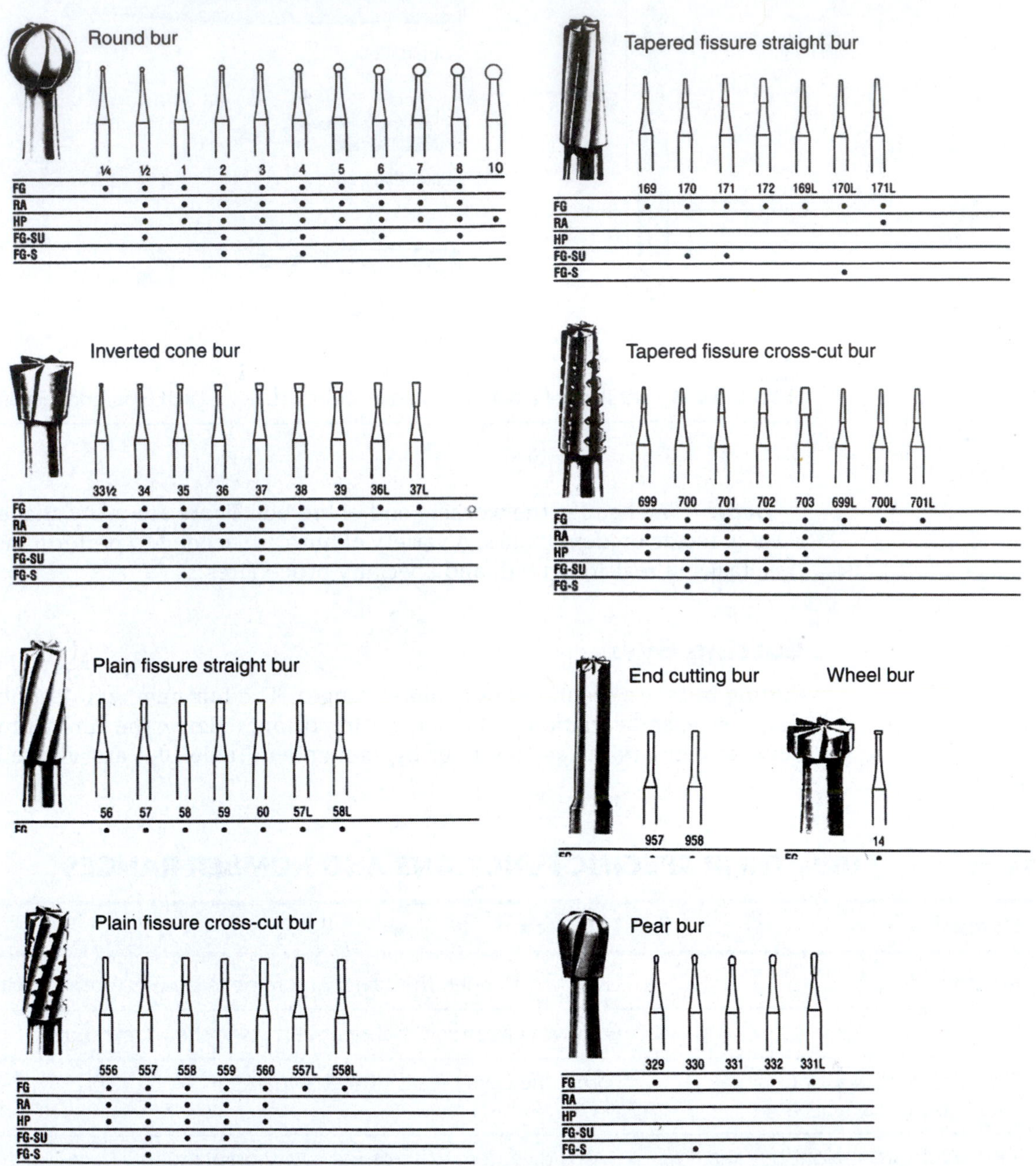

FIGURE 10–9 Bur shapes and number ranges. *(Courtesy of Miltex Instrument Co., Inc., Lake Success, NY)*

Burs have variations in both head and shank design. An example of a change in the head (working end) of the bur is the fissure burs. Fissure burs are flat on the end, however some fissure burs have rounded or dome-shaped working ends. The number range for these burs is different from that for the regular fissure burs.

Diamond Burs

Diamond rotary instruments are categorized as diamond burs or stones. They are used for rapid reduction of tooth structure during cavity and crown preparation, polishing and finishing composite restorations, and occlusal adjustment. Diamond burs are also used for bone and gingival contouring during surgical procedures.

Diamond burs are manufactured in a wide variety of shapes, sizes, and grits.

Finishing Burs

Finishing burs smooth, trim, and finish metal restorations and natural-tooth-colored materials. Finishing burs have thirty or more blades for ultra-fine finishing. These burs are supplied in a variety of shapes and sizes, similar to the cutting burs.

Surgical Burs

Surgical burs are used in a low-speed handpiece to reduce and contour the alveolar bone and tooth structure. The heads of surgical burs are manufactured in various sizes and shapes and have long shanks.

Laboratory Burs

Laboratory burs are used to make adjustments on acrylic materials, such as partials, dentures, and custom trays. They are also used on plaster, stone, and metal materials. Laboratory burs have long shanks and large working ends. These burs are supplied in a variety of sizes and shapes. Sometimes they are referred to as **vulcanite burs.**

ABRASIVES

Abrasives are non-bladed instruments used to finish and polish restorations and appliances. Some abrasives also are used for cutting. Abrasives are supplied in a wide variety and are categorized by their shapes, such as discs, points, and wheels. Abrasives also are categorized by the materials they are made of, such as rubber, stone, and sandpaper (Figure 10–10).

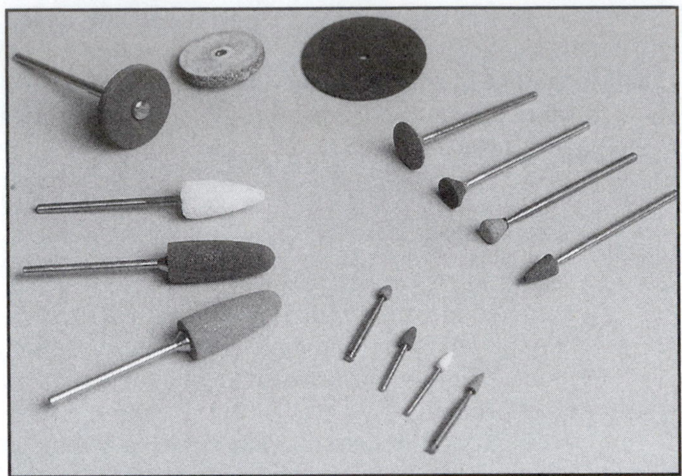

FIGURE 10–10 Various types and grits of stones, wheels, and points.

Mandrels

Mandrels are rods of various lengths that are used in low-speed handpieces. They are used with abrasives. The abrasives are either permanently attached (mounted) to a mandrel or are supplied separately and are placed on a mandrel (unmounted). Mandrels are available in three shanks: latch, friction grip, or straight. The head of the mandrel, where the abrasives attach, is available in snap on, screw on, or pin type.

Discs

Discs are used to polish, smooth, and adjust restorative materials and dental appliances. Discs are circular, abrasive instruments that are usually designed to be mounted to mandrels.

Stones

Stones are available in many sizes, shapes, and grits, similar to discs. They are used for cutting, polishing, and finishing amalgam, gold, composite, and porcelain restorations. Stones are used in the laboratory to adjust and polish appliances and custom trays.

Rubber Points and Wheels

Rubber points and wheels are supplied in a variety of sizes and grits. They are made of rubber material impregnated with abrasive agents. The points and wheels are used for finishing and polishing dental restorative materials.

Sterilization and Storage

Rotary instruments are sterilized or disposed of after each use. Burs that are sterilized are first scrubbed or placed in an ultrasonic unit to remove debris from the blades; if debris remains between the blades, a wire brush is used to remove embedded materials. The burs are then rinsed and sterilized according to manufacturer's instructions.

Bur Blocks. Rotary instruments are stored in a **bur block.** There are many variations and designs, such as round or rectangular shapes. Bur blocks come with covers and may be magnetic. Both friction-grip and latch-type burs can be stored in bur blocks. They are made of metal or plastic.

Some bur blocks can be sterilized with the burs they hold. If the bur blocks cannot be sterilized, the burs are placed in a mesh holder, run through the ultrasonic cleaner, and then placed in the sterilizer.

DENTAL HANDPIECES

Dental handpieces are often divided into two categories: **high-speed handpieces** and **low-speed handpieces**. High-speed handpieces operate at 400,000 **revolutions per minute (rpm)** and higher (Figure 10–11). The low-speed handpieces operate under 30,000 rpm (Figure 10–12).

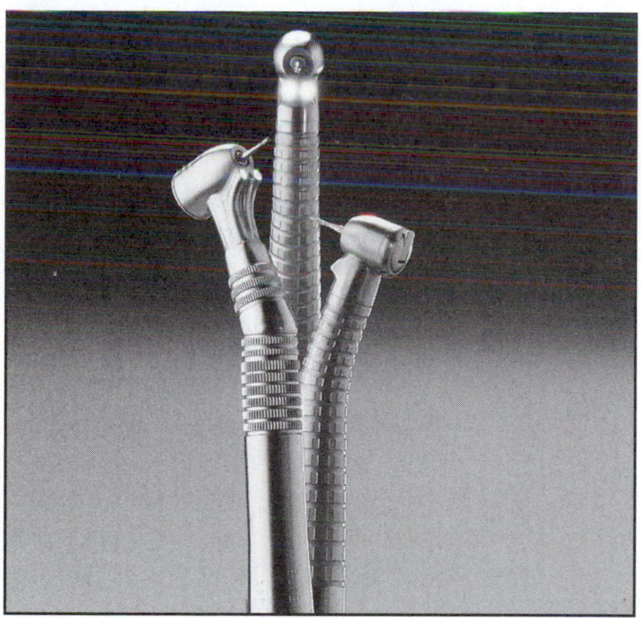

FIGURE 10–11 High-speed handpieces with fiberoptics. *(Courtesy of Midwest Dental Products Corporation, a division of DENTSPLY International)*

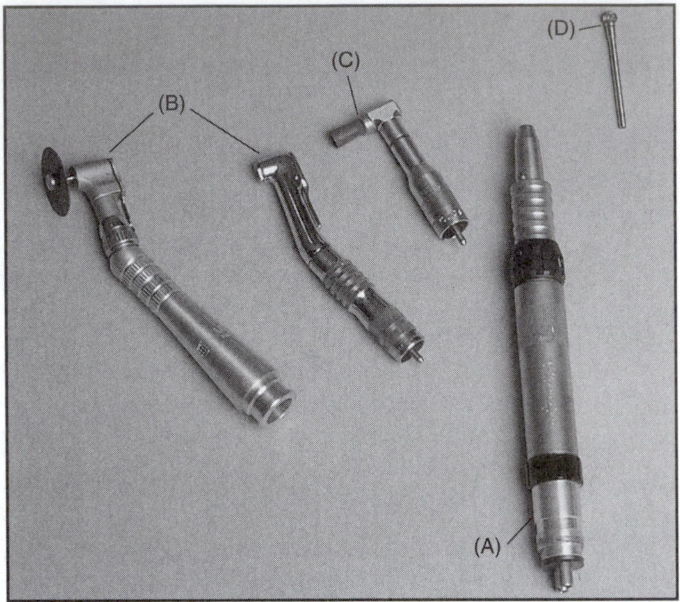

FIGURE 10–12 (A) A low-speed handpiece with attachments. (B) Contra-angle with and without a disk, (C) right-angle with a rubber cup, (D) long shanked bur.

Air abrasion reduces or eliminates the use of anesthetics and dental handpieces. This shortens and/or reduces appointments for the patient. The technology allows various types of cavities to be prepared for restoration, special repairs in restorations, and the inside surfaces of restorations to be roughened before bonding.

High-Speed Handpiece

The high-speed handpiece is used for rapid cutting of tooth structure and finishing of restorations. Because of the high speed of this handpiece, **frictional heat** is produced. Frictional heat can cause pulpal damage to the tooth. To reduce the frictional heat of the handpiece, a coolant such as air, water, or an air-water spray is used.

A **rheostat** (foot control) is used to activate and control the speed of the handpiece.

Low-Speed Handpiece

The low-speed (or slow-speed) handpiece is used both in the dental operatory and the laboratory. At the dental unit, the low-speed handpiece is used to polish teeth and restorations, remove soft carious material, and define cavity margins and walls.

In the dental laboratory, this handpiece is used to adjust, finish, and polish appliances.

Tray Systems

A **preset tray system** is most commonly used in dental offices. It provides an efficient means of transporting instruments to the treatment room, saving time for the dental assistant. Instruments and auxiliary items are placed on a tray in the order of their use during the procedure. The tray is covered and carried to the treatment room when the patient is seated. There are many varieties of systems to choose from, including plastic or metal trays, tubs, or cassettes; trays, tubs, and accessories that are color coded; and systems that can be placed in the ultrasonic and then sterilized in the same cassette or tray.

Positioning on Trays

Every operator has certain preferences of instrumentation for a procedure. However, there are some basic considerations:

- Instruments are placed in order of use, beginning on the left and moving to the right.
- The basic tray setup (mouth mirror, explorer, cotton pliers) is placed first on the left side.
- Instruments should be grouped according to functions; for example, all the carvers are placed together.
- Cotton supplies are usually arranged across the top of the tray.
- Scissors, hemostats, or other hinged instruments are placed on the far right of the tray for easy access.
- Instruments are returned to their original positions after receiving them from the operator. This ensures that an instrument can be found easily if the operator needs to use it again.
- Instruments are kept clean and free of debris before returning them to the tray. Gauze sponges on the tray aid with immediate removal of cement, blood, or debris.

CHAPTER 11

Dental Radiography

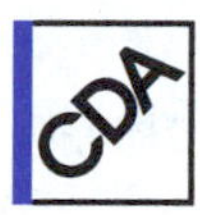

OBJECTIVES

The student should strive to meet the following objectives and demonstrate an understanding of the facts and principles presented in this chapter:

1. Describe safety precautions to be utilized when using radiation.
2. Explain how an x-ray is produced.
3. Describe the composition, sizes, types, and storage of dental x-ray film.
4. Explain intraoral and extraoral x-ray production.
5. Identify means of producing quality radiographs on a variety of patients.
6. Explain the bisecting and paralleling techniques.
7. List common production errors.
8. Describe the processing techniques, the composition of the solutions, and the storage of final radiographs.
9. Explain x-ray mounting procedures.

KEY TERMS

ALARA (p. 159)
automatic processing (p. 185)
blurred images (p. 179)
cone cutting (p. 178)
double exposure (p. 178)
duplication technique (p. 188)
elongation (p. 177)
foreshortening (p. 178)
herringbone pattern (p. 179)
interproximal (p. 165)
kilovoltage (kV) (p. 159)
leakage radiation (p. 158)
milliamperage (mA) (p. 159)
overlapping (p. 178)
primary radiation (p. 158)
radiopaque (p. 179)
reticulation (p. 180)
roentgens (p. 158)
scatter radiation (p. 158)
secondary radiation (p. 158)
short wavelengths (p. 158)
thermionic emission (p. 160)
tube head (p. 160)
x-rays (p. 158)

INTRODUCTION

Wilhelm Conrad Roentgen (ren-ken) discovered **x-rays** in 1895. Roentgen was a professor of physics at the University of Wurzberg in Germany.

The news of the discovery of the x-ray was soon heard around the world. Roentgen was awarded the first Nobel Prize in physics in 1901 for his work. Today, units of x-ray exposure are still expressed in **roentgens** in his honor.

Types of Radiation

The wavelengths desired in dental radiographs are **short wavelengths**, or **hard radiation.** These have high frequency, high energy, and high penetrating power.

There are four types of radiation: primary, secondary, scatter, and leakage (Figure 11–1).

1. **Primary radiation** is the central beam emitted from the x-ray tube head. It consists of high energy, short wavelength x-rays traveling in a straight line. Primary radiation, often called the primary beam, is the useful x-ray that produces the diagnostic image on the x-ray film.
2. **Secondary radiation** is formed when primary x-rays strike the patient or come in contact with matter (any substance). The waves are often transformed into longer wavelengths that lose their energy.
3. **Scatter radiation** is deflected from its path as it strikes matter. Often, secondary and scatter radiation are used interchangeably. This radiation is scattered in all directions and therefore presents the most serious danger to the operator. Due to scatter radiation, the operator must stand at least six feet away from the patient while exposing x-ray film or structural shielding and out of the path of the primary beam.
4. **Leakage radiation** escapes in all directions from the tube or the tube head. The x-ray machine must be checked for leakage and should not be used until the problem is taken care of.

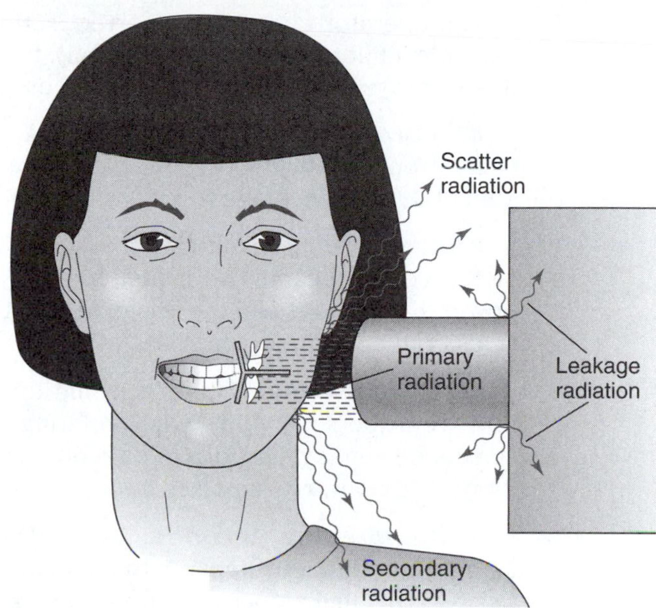

FIGURE 11–1 Primary, secondary, scatter, and leakage radiation identified on an x-ray tube and a patient's face.

Biological Effects of Radiation

X-rays can cause injury to biologic tissues. Some of these injuries heal, but some cause permanent damage.

Low-level radiation normally does not cause damage that cannot be repaired within the cells. Tissues radiosensitive in the dental region are the lens of the eye and the thyroid gland. Because of their location near the oral cavity, the tissues may be exposed to the primary beam (central beam) of the x-ray. Very high radiation dosages (not used in dentistry) have been known to cause cataracts and thyroid carcinoma. It is unlikely that dental x-rays would cause one of these serious effects; however, it is always necessary to utilize the least amount of radiation possible. All dental personnel use the **as low as reasonably achievable** (ALARA) concept for radiation protection. Dental offices use a thyroid shield extension on the lead apron to further protect the patients.

Dental X-Ray Unit/Components

Control Panel

The **control panel** is where the circuit boards and controls are located that allow the operator to adjust the correct setting for each patient. It is where the on/off switch is located, along with the selection for the **milliamperage (mA)** and **kilovoltage (kV)** and the **electronic timer**.

The operator chooses the correct settings according to the individual (for example, children need less radiation), the area of the oral cavity needing diagnostic x-rays, the exposure technique used, and the film speed.

Milliamperage. Milliamperage (mA) determines the amount or quantity of electrons. The higher the milliamperage, the greater the amount of radiation. Milli (1/1,000) amperage is a measurement unit for electrical current.

Kilovoltage. Kilovoltage (kV) determines the quality or penetrating power of the central beam. The higher the kilovoltage, the greater the penetration power of the x-rays and the less exposure time that is required; therefore, there is less radiation to the patient.

Electronic Timer. The electronic timer controls the total time that rays flow from the x-ray tube. It is a rotating dial with which the dental assistant selects how many fractions of a second or impulses are needed to produce the x-ray. It takes thirty impulses to equal one-half of a second.

Milliamperage Seconds. Milliamperage seconds (mAs) determine the amount of radiation exposure the patient is receiving. The dental assistant calculates the milliamperage times the exposure time to determine the milliamperage seconds (mAs).

Arm Assembly and Tube Head

The **arm assembly** is attached firmly to the wall in the x-ray room. The flexible extension of the arm allows the operator to freely position the tube head for the various positions required for dental radiography exposures.

The **tube head** is where x-rays are generated. The tube head is made of a metal casing that is lead lined or lead to limit the amount of radiation leakage.

Safety and Precautions

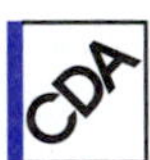

It is the responsibility of the manufacturers and dental team members to follow safety precautions when using radiography equipment. Steps must be used to minimize risk to the patient and all dental personnel.

Radiation Production

X-rays are produced when the operator depresses the exposure switch and starts the process of generating electricity (Figure 11–2). The electricity passes to the control panel by the step-down and step-up transformers, where specified instructions on the quantity and the quality of x-rays have been selected. From the setting of the milliamperage, time, and kilovoltage circuits, the electricity travels to the cathode filament. This current passes through the filament and heats it to an extremely high temperature. This process is called **thermionic emission**. When the filament reaches a certain temperature, electrons are given off. These electrons are negatively charged and therefore attracted to the positively charged anode side of the tube. The electrons travel toward the anode

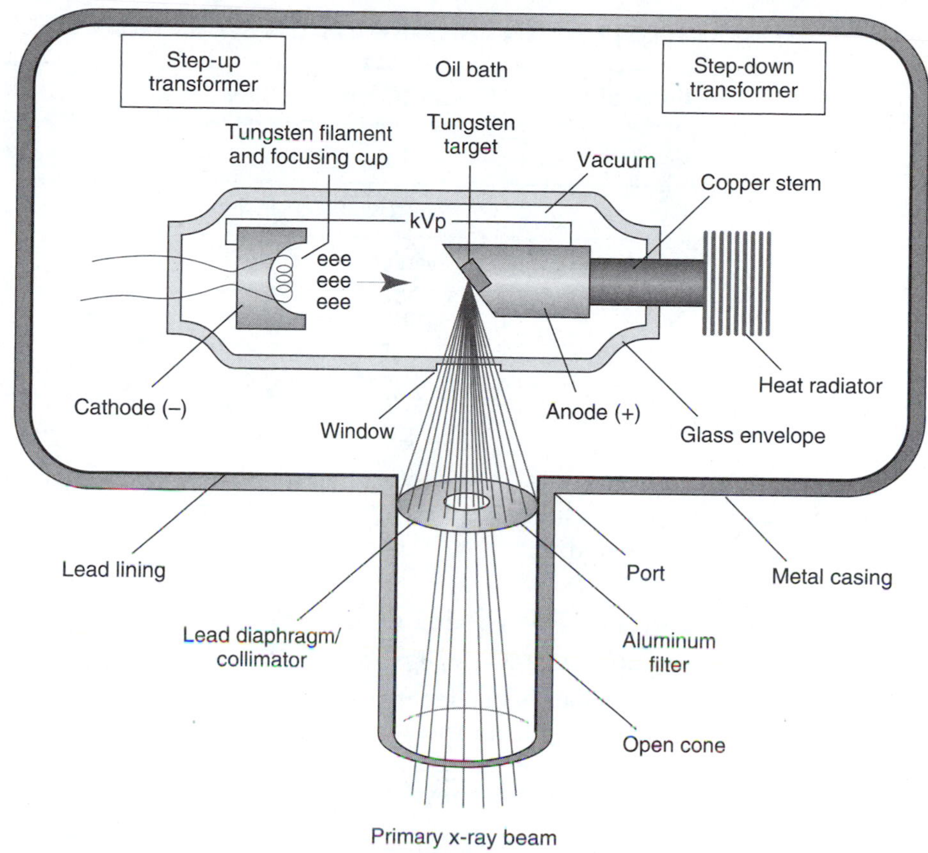

FIGURE 11–2 Production of x-rays within the tube head.

at a rapid speed. The focusing cup on the cathode directs the electrons to a small area (about one square millimeter in size), called the focal spot, on the anode tungsten target. The precise moment of contact is when the x-rays are produced due to the forceful collision of the electrons. At the time of the collision, the x-rays are given off the tungsten target and weaker rays travel in all directions. The useful x-rays travel through the filters and collimator and out the PID (position indicator device) opening.

The excess heat generated by the collision is dissipated by a heavy copper stem that takes it away from the tungsten target and cools it in oil present in the tube head. In addition to the copper stem cooling, a bulb also takes heat into the oil bath chamber of the tube head to increase cooling.

Dental X-Ray Film

Film Sizes

Dental intraoral film packets are supplied in five basic sizes. Each size is used for a specific radiographic exposure, depending on the size of the patient's oral

TABLE 11–1 INTRAORAL FILM SIZES AND USES

Film Size	Description/Uses
No. 0	Child
No. 1	Narrow anterior film
No. 2	Adult
No. 3	Long bite-wing film
No. 4	Occlusal film

cavity and the area to be radiographed (see Table 11–1). The film that produces the best radiographic results with the least radiation exposure for the patient is selected.

Dental Film Packet

The intraoral film packet has a sealed outer plastic wrap (Figure 11–3). Inside the wrapper, a black paper is folded around the film and a lead foil backing is placed away from the x-ray tube. The lead foil absorbs any unused radiation and the scattering of secondary radiation and film fogging. The outer plastic wrap is sealed to prevent moisture from contaminating the film.

PRODUCING QUALITY RADIOGRAPHS

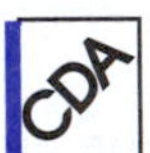

Preparing for X-Ray Exposure

The dental chair should be covered with a plastic bag or at least have a barrier on the head rest and the chair controls. The x-ray units should have barriers covering the dials, the exposure buttons, the cone, the tube head, areas of the extension arm that would be touched, and any other areas that may be contaminated. If there is a door the dental assistant needs to open and close, a barrier should be placed on the door knob. An area for clean and contaminated films should be prepared.

The dental assistant sets up the required materials, for example, components of the sterile Rinn XCP instruments and appropriate x-ray films. The dental assistant should also have a tissue available for the patient and gauze and cotton rolls to facilitate film positioning.

Preparing for Film Exposure

The dental assistant wears gloves, protective eyewear, and a mask during film exposure. After removing each exposed film from the patient's mouth, the dental assistant wipes the saliva from the film and places it in a paper cup or on a

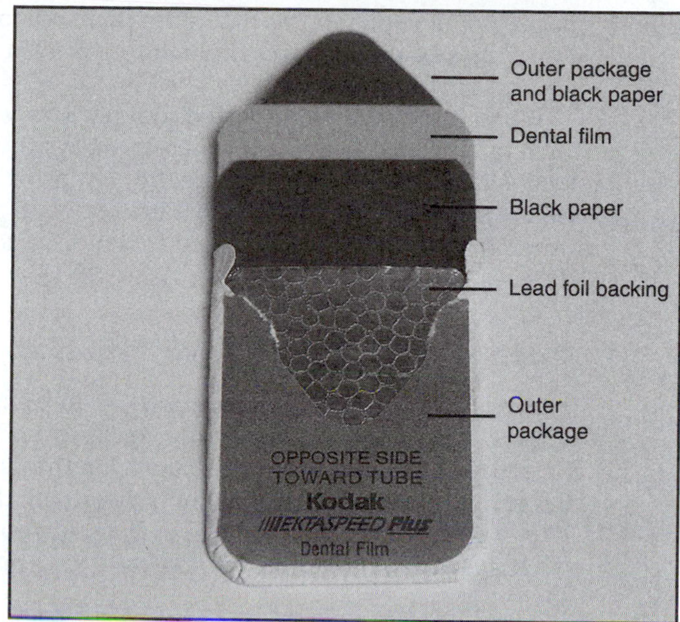

FIGURE 11–3 A film packet.

covered surface out of range of the x-ray beam or scatter radiation (outside the immediate exposure area).

Patient Exposure

The dental assistant reviews the patient's medical history and checks the dental chart to confirm the number and types of x-rays the dentist requires for diagnosis.

The dental assistant escorts the patient into the x-ray room, seats the patient in an upright position, and positions the headrest to secure the patient's head. The assistant asks the patient to remove his or her eyeglasses, full or partial dentures, orthodontic appliances, or any metal objects that may interfere with x-ray image quality.

The dental assistant places a lead apron with a thyroid collar on the patient. The dental assistant explains the procedure to the patient and indicates how the patient can be helpful during the exposure of the x-rays. The dental assistant brings the tube head close to the working area and proceeds with the first film.

Following Film Exposure

After the films are exposed, the dental assistant removes his or her gloves and puts on overgloves. The dental assistant removes the patient's lead apron and makes the necessary chart notations. The dental assistant dismisses the patient. Following appropriate infection control procedures, the dental assistant removes and disposes of the barriers from the dental chair, x-ray unit, and control panel buttons.

When handling contaminated film packets without outer protective barrier jackets, the dental assistant wipes or sprays the packets with disinfectants and leaves them for a full ten minutes to dry, prior to processing. If outer film barriers are used, the dental assistant removes and discards them, along with other contaminated barriers, and transports the films to the processing area or dark room.

Intraoral Techniques for Film Exposures

There are two basic techniques used for film exposures in dentistry: the **bisecting technique** and the **paralleling technique**. The bisecting technique is used for more specific or unique radiographs rather than the routine. The paralleling technique is widely accepted because the detail of the image is more accurate. The American Association of Dental Schools and the American Academy of Oral and Maxillofacial Radiology recommend the paralleling technique.

Paralleling Technique

The paralleling technique is most commonly used in exposing periapical and bite-wing radiographs. It is accurate and produces excellent diagnostic-quality radiographs.

The paralleling technique requires the film packet and the long axis of the teeth to be parallel. The x-ray beam is directed perpendicular to this parallel line formed by the teeth and the film packet.

Holders Used for the Paralleling Technique. There are a variety of film holders available for use with the paralleling technique. The function of the holder is to secure the film away from the lingual surfaces of the teeth and parallel to the long axis of the teeth. Some holders have supports to prevent the film from bending. One example is the Rinn XCP. Some holders have positioning rings that assist the operator in correct cone placement and allow the patient to be in a variety of positions for x-ray exposure.

Film Positioning. When using the paralleling technique, the film should be placed in the patient's mouth with care to keep the patient relaxed and cooperative during film and holder placement. The dental assistant places the film in the film holder evenly and allows no more than one-eighth inch to extend beyond the edge of the occlusal plane once the film/film holder is placed in the patient's mouth. The film packet/film holder should be placed parallel to the long axis of the teeth, encompassing all teeth to be exposed. The film packet should be kept flat and away from the lingual surface of the teeth. Vertical and horizontal angulation is obtained by keeping the cone end even with the positioning ring or following the guide of the handle with the other film holders. The positioning ring guides the cone for correct placement to ensure that the film is exposed.

Types of Film Exposures

Three types of film exposures/radiographs are used most commonly in the dental office: periapical, bite-wing, and occlusal. The type of film used and the number of x-rays taken are determined by the dentist.

Periapical Radiographs. The **periapical radiograph** pictures the entire tooth and surrounding area. Periapical radiographs are used to assess the health of the teeth, bone, and surrounding tissues. Tooth development and eruption stages also appear on periapical radiographs. Abnormalities and pathological conditions are diagnosed by the dentist using these radiographs. The size of the patient's mouth usually determines the size of the x-ray film used and the number of exposures necessary.

Bite-wing Radiographs. The **bite-wing radiograph** depicts the crowns, the interproximal spaces, and the crest area of the alveolar bone of both the maxillary and the mandibular teeth. Bite-wing radiographs usually are taken only on the posterior teeth and are used to detect caries, faulty restorations, and calculus and to examine the crestal area of the alveolar bone. The size of the patient's mouth determines the size of the film used for the bite-wing x-ray.

Occlusal Radiograph. The **occlusal radiograph** depicts large areas of the mandible or maxilla. These radiographs can be used alone or to supplement periapical or bite-wing films. A size 4 film is used on adults; a size 2 film may be used for children.

Full-Mouth Radiographic Survey

A full-mouth radiographic survey (FMX) is composed of periapical and bite-wing radiographs. This survey includes a number of radiographs that collectively display all the teeth and surrounding structures. A full-mouth survey for an adult routinely includes fourteen periapical and four bite-wing films. This number may vary depending on the factors listed and the dentist's directions (Procedure 11–1).

Bite-Wing Series

Bite-wing radiographs are a routine part of the dental exam. They are taken as part of the full-mouth series and also at 6-month or 12-month intervals. These radiographs are used specifically for caries detection but also assist in the evaluation of restorations, calculus detection, assessment of the alveolar crestal bone, tooth eruption, occlusal relationships, and some pulpal pathology. Bite-wing radiographs, also known as **interproximal** radiographs, are taken of the premolar area and the molar area. The film is placed most often in a horizontal position, but in cases where the dentist wants to see more of the tooth root and alveolar bone, the film is placed vertically.

PROCEDURE

11-1 Full-Mouth X-Ray Exposure Using the Paralleling Technique

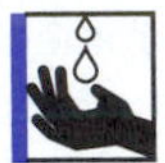 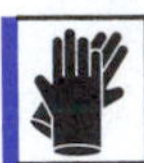 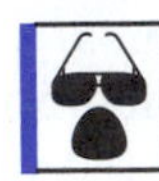 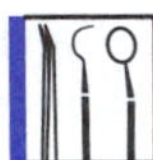

This procedure is performed by the dental assistant when the dentist requests a full-mouth set of radiographs. The dental assistant prepares the equipment (Rinn XCP instruments), the area, and the patient; exposes the radiographs; and processes and mounts the films for viewing according to infection control protocol.

This procedure explains film placement and exposure for the central incisors in each arch and one-half of the maxillary arch and one-half of the mandibular arch. The same technique is used to expose the opposite arches.

EQUIPMENT AND SUPPLIES

- Barriers for the x-ray room and equipment
- X-ray film (appropriate size and number of films)
- X-ray film barriers (optional)
- Cotton rolls (optional)
- Rinn XCP materials (assembled for use) or other paralleling technique aids
- Lead apron with thyroid collar
- Container for exposed film
- Paper towel or tissue

PROCEDURE STEPS *(Follow aseptic procedures)*

1. Review the patient's chart.
2. Wash and dry hands.
3. Place appropriate barriers on dental chair, film, and x-ray equipment.
4. Prepare equipment and supplies needed for the procedure, including the sterile Rinn XCP instruments, tissue or paper towel, and cup or container with patient's name on it.
5. Turn the x-ray machine on and check the mA, kV, and exposure time.
6. Seat and position the patient in an upright position.
7. Have the patient remove any removable appliances, earrings, or eyeglasses that may interfere with the exposing process.
8. Place the lead apron with the thyroid collar on the patient.
9. After the patient is prepared, wash and dry the hands and don treatment gloves.

Positioning for Maxillary Arch

◗ **Maxillary Incisors** (Figure 11–4)

1. To prepare the maxillary incisors for exposure, tilt the back of the film holder slightly and insert the film vertically into the slot on the bite-block. Adjust the ring on the metal rod to cover the film. Pull positioning ring back on the metal rod, away from bite-block.
2. Bring the tube head near the area of exposure.

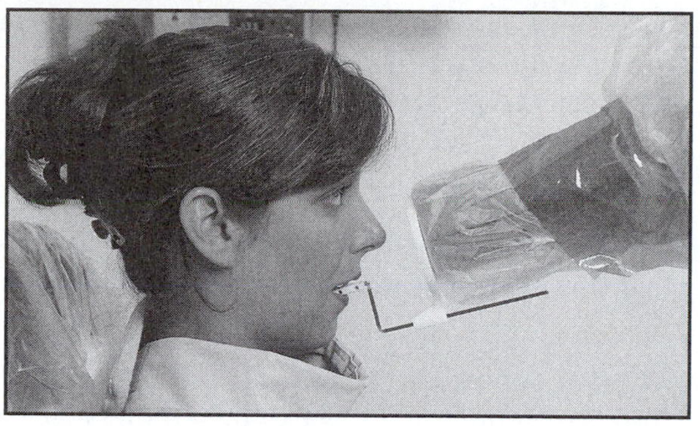

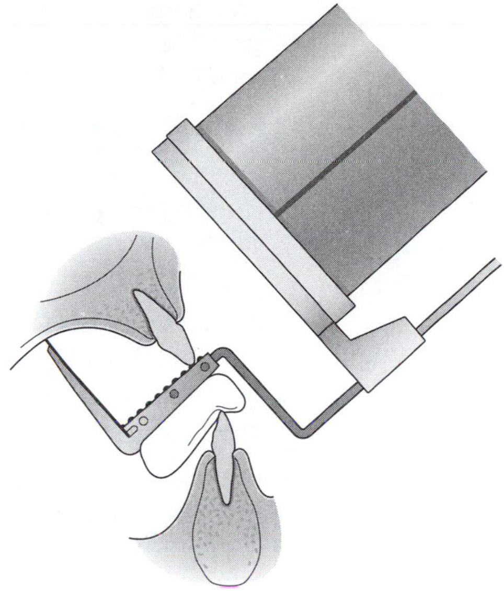

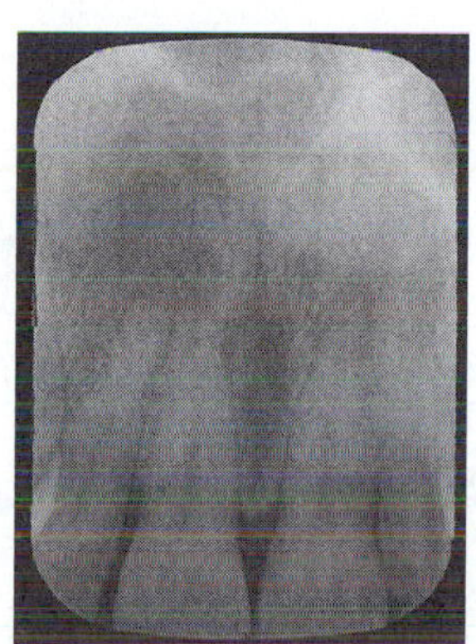

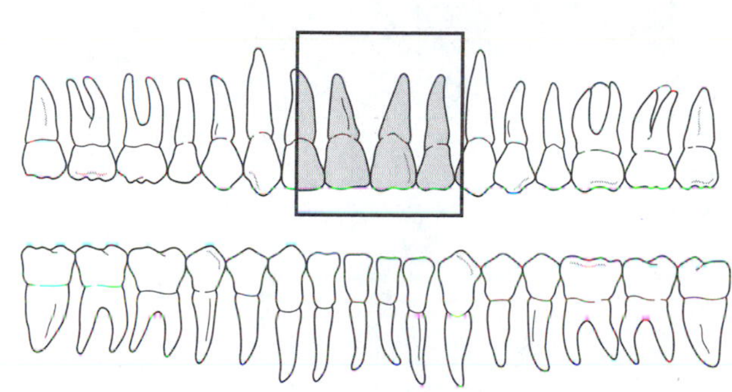

FIGURE 11–4 Maxillary incisors.

3. Tilt the film/film holder downward to place in the patient's mouth. Position in the mouth away from the lingual surfaces and centered behind the incisors. Have the patient close slowly and evenly on the bite-block.
4. Holding on to the metal rod, slide the positioning ring close to the patient's face. Position the cone parallel to the metal indicating rod and place to within one-half inch of the positioning ring. The cone end should be at an equal distance from the positioning ring. This directs the central ray perpendicular to the film. The patient may help hold the metal rod to secure the film holder in position.
5. The incisal edges rest on the flat portion of the bite-block.
6. The diagram shows the film, tooth, positioning ring, and open end of the cone parallel to each other. The central ray is perpendicular to the film.

(No. 2 size film will show all four incisors. Teeth are centered on the radiograph, showing the apices, roots, and crowns. The bite-block may be seen as a radiopaque area near the incisal edge of the film.)

Maxillary Cuspids (Figure 11–5)

1. For the maxillary cuspids, tilt the film/film holder, place it in the patient's mouth, and position it away from the lingual surfaces. The film is placed in the mouth, directly behind the center of the cuspid and positioned toward the midline.
2. Have the patient close slowly and center the cuspid on the bite-block. Holding the metal rod, slide the positioning ring toward the patient's face.
3. Bring the tube head toward the ring, placing the cone end evenly around the positioning ring.
4. All planes are parallel so that the central ray is directed perpendicular to the film plane. Because of the curvature of the maxillary arch, the distal

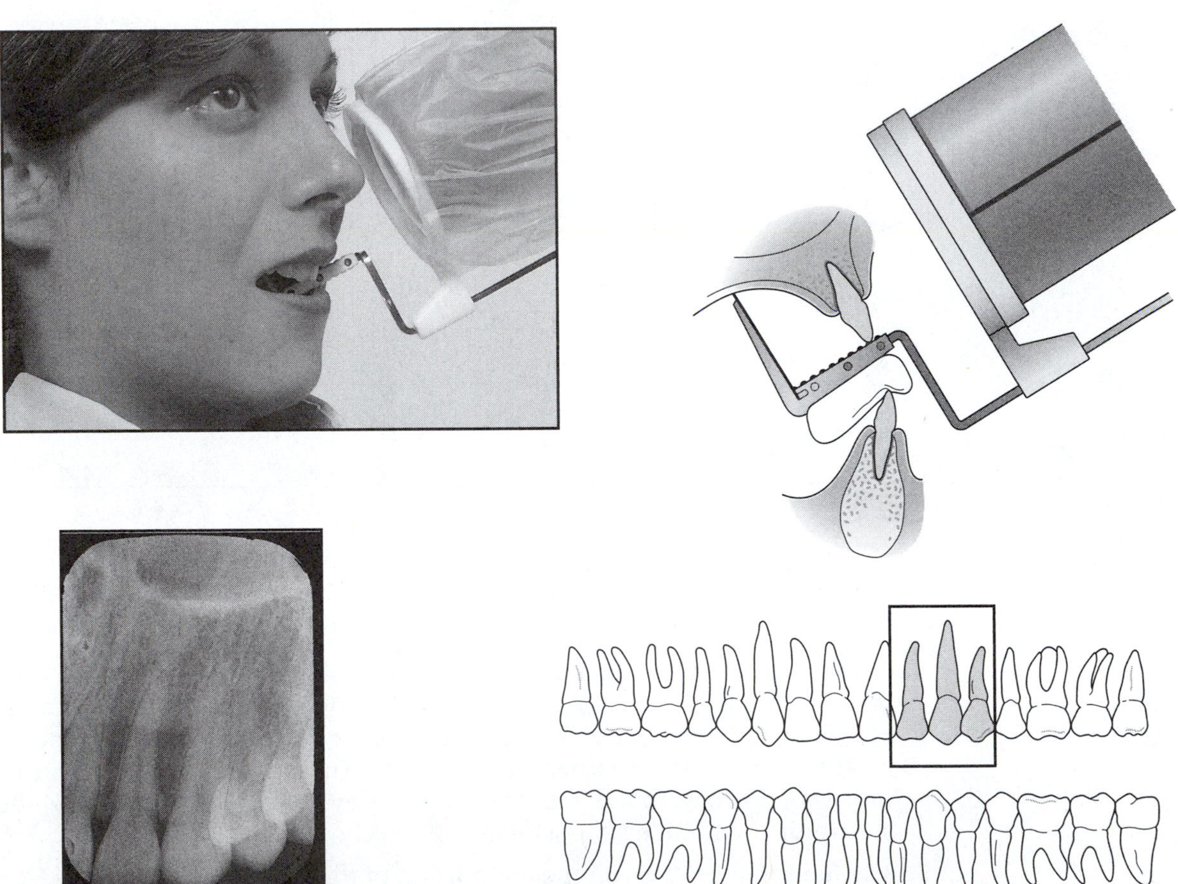

FIGURE 11–5 Maxillary cuspids.

of the cuspid is overlapping the first bicuspid on many cuspid radiographs. Note that the central ray is directed at the center of the cuspid.

Maxillary Premolars (Figure 11–6)

1. For the maxillary premolars, tilt the film/film holder, place it in the patient's mouth, and position it away from the lingual surfaces, toward the middle of the palate.
2. Place the anterior edge of the film behind the middle of the cuspid to ensure that the film will cover the area of the two premolars.
3. While holding the film in place, have the patient close slowly on the bite-block. Hold the metal rod and slide the positioning ring toward the patient's face.
4. Bring the tube head toward the ring, placing the open cone evenly around the ring. Note the angle of the film and the film holder, positioned so that the central ray will pass through the contact point of the first and second premolars.

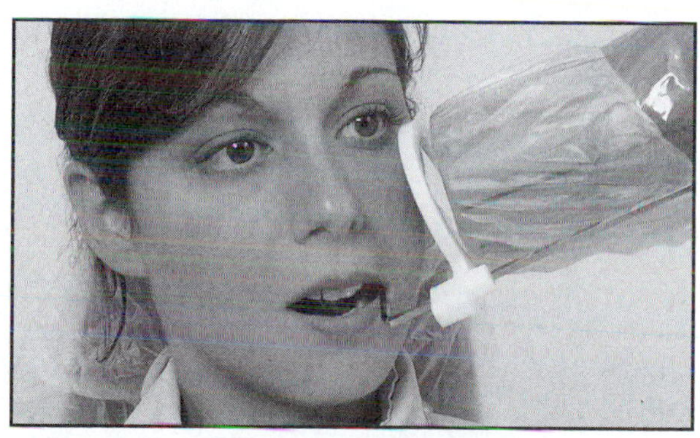

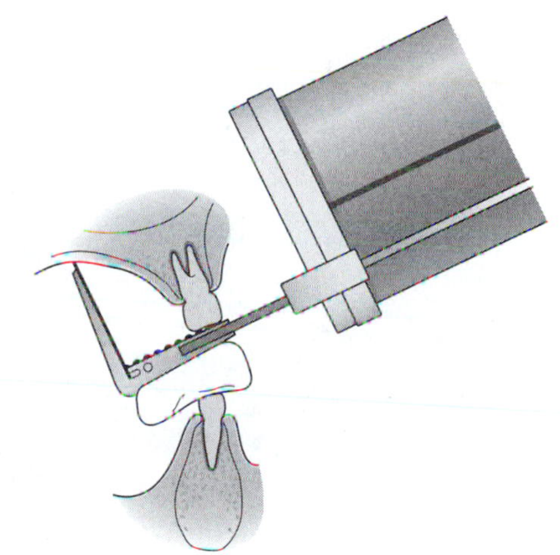

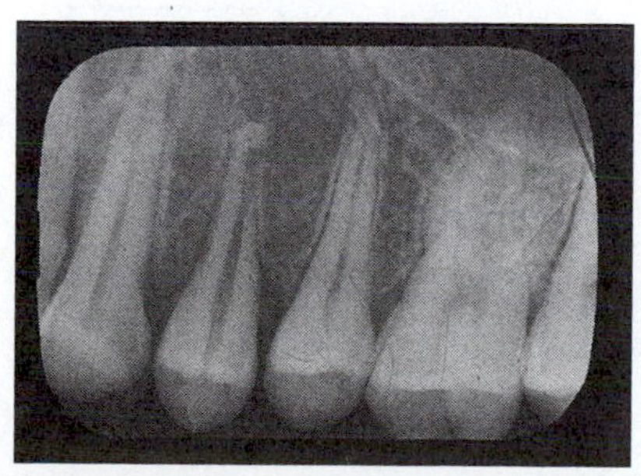

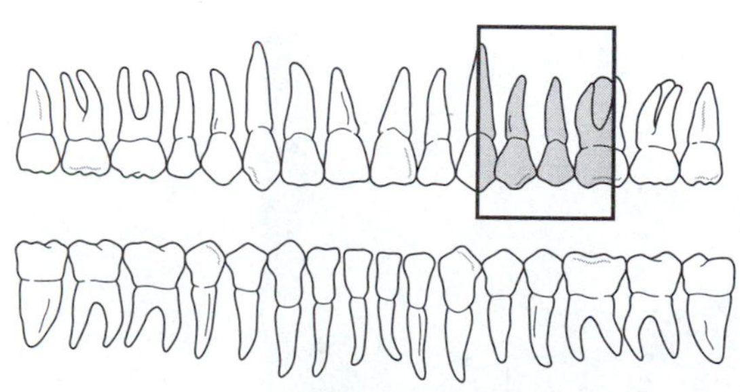

FIGURE 11–6 Maxillary bicuspids (premolars).

5. The bite-block is centered on the premolars. On this radiograph, the distal of the cuspid is seen and the first and second bicuspids show that the contact between them is open.

Maxillary Molars (Figure 11–7)

1. For the maxillary molars, tilt the film/film holder so that it is less vertical when entering the patient's mouth. Place the film in the patient's mouth and position it away from the lingual surfaces of the molars.
2. Center the bite-block on the second molar. Have the patient close slowly on the bite-block.
3. Bring the tube head toward the ring, placing the open end of the cone evenly around the positioning ring.
4. The diagram shows the film, tooth, and cone lined up for correct direction of the central ray. This radiograph shows the open contact between the first and second molars. The distal of the second premolar is seen. Note that the film angles are parallel to the lingual surface of the molars and placed near the middle of the palate.

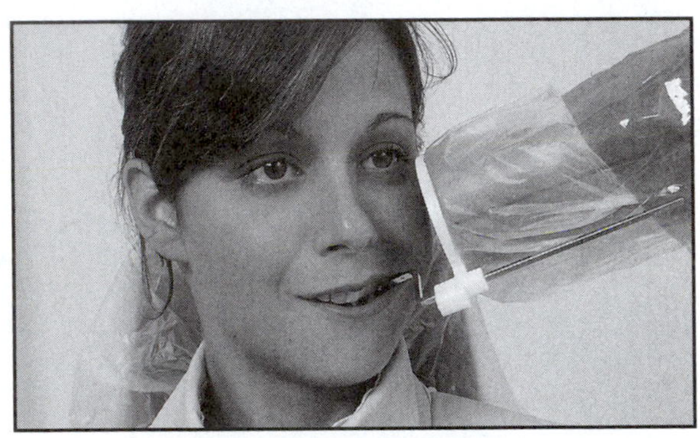

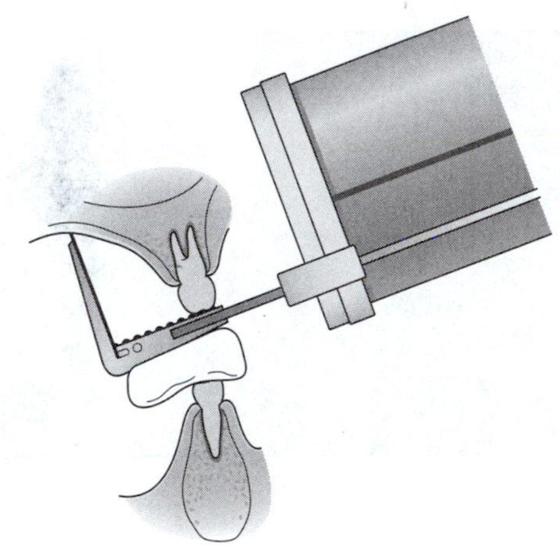

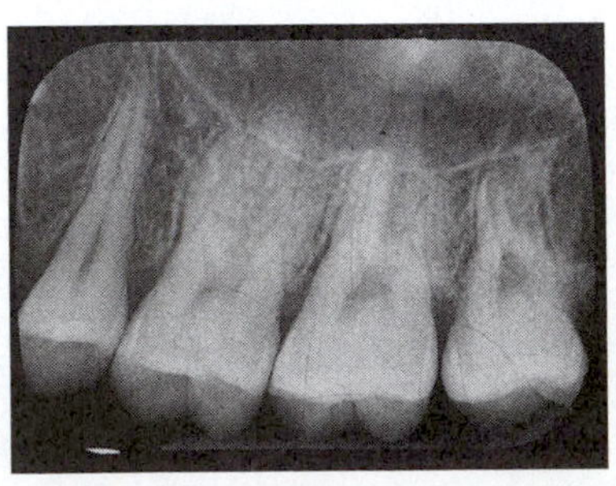

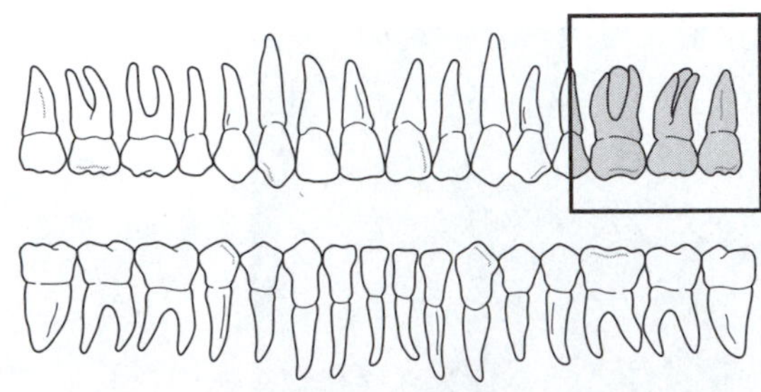

FIGURE 11–7 Maxillary molars.

Positioning for the Mandibular Arch

◗ **Mandibular Incisors** (Figure 11–8)

1. The film holder is assembled in the same way for mandibular and maxillary positions. For the mandibular incisors, tilt the film/film holder and place it in the patient's mouth, gently pressing the film on the floor of the mouth behind the incisors and away from the lingual surface.
2. Have the patient close slowly on the bite-block. Holding the metal rod, slide the positioning ring close to the patient's face.
3. Bring the tube head close and place the cone parallel to the metal rod. The open end of the cone should be even with the ring.
4. The diagram shows how far the film needs to be placed in the mouth to see the entire length of the tooth. Sometimes the tongue is moved when the film is being placed. Being gentle with the placement encourages patient cooperation.

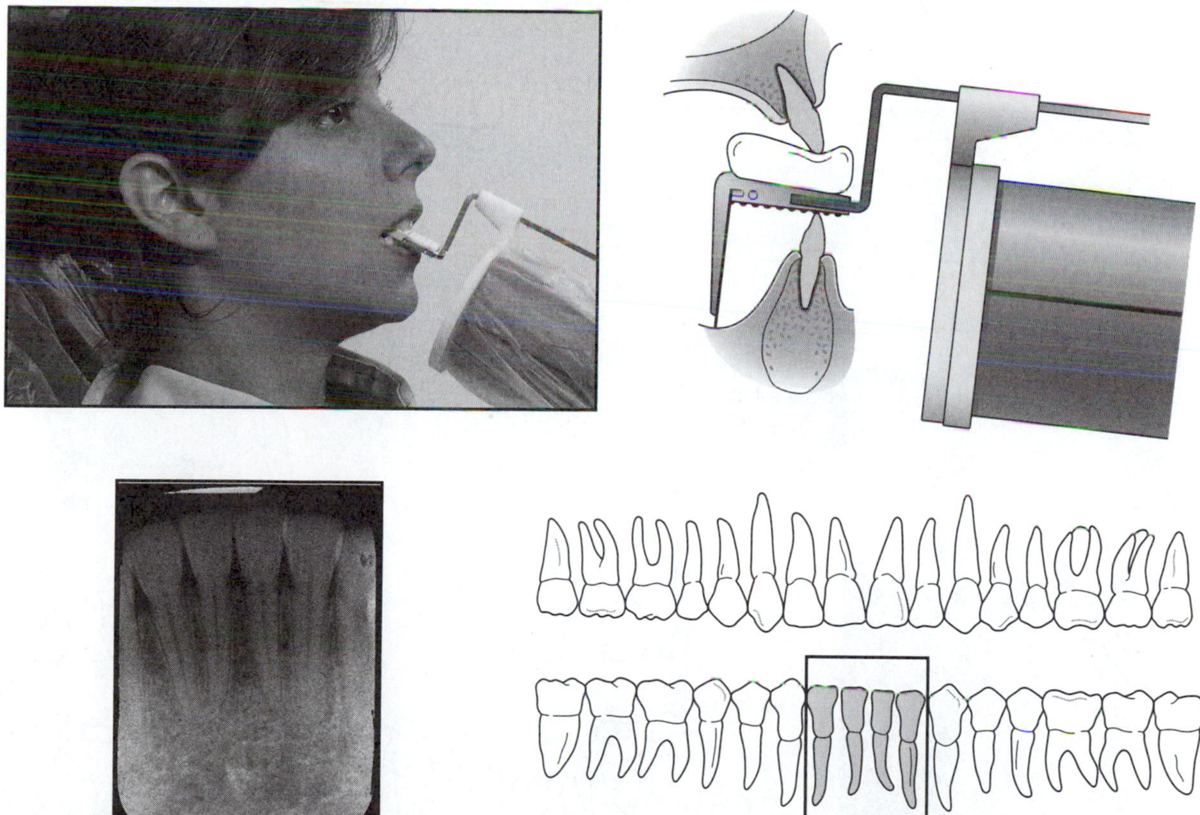

FIGURE 11–8 Mandibular incisors.

5. The mandibular incisors are centered on the bite-block. The incisal edges of the teeth are one-eighth inch from the top of the film.
6. The central ray is directed between the two central incisors to open contact areas. The curve of the arch will cause some overlapping on the distal of the lateral incisors.
7. The drawing illustrates the film placed directly behind the incisors and as far into the mouth as the tongue attachment allows.

Mandibular Cuspids (Figure 11–9)

1. For the mandibular cuspids, tilt the film/film holder, place it in the patient's mouth, and position it away from the lingual surface.
2. Center the bite-block on the cuspid and have the patient slowly close. Move the positioning ring close to the patient's face, bring the cone parallel to the metal rod, and position the open end of the cone flat with the ring.
3. Insert the film toward the floor of the mouth enough to ensure that the film covers the entire length of the cuspid.
4. The film, tooth, and the plane of the open end of the cone are all parallel. The central ray is directed perpendicular to the film plane.

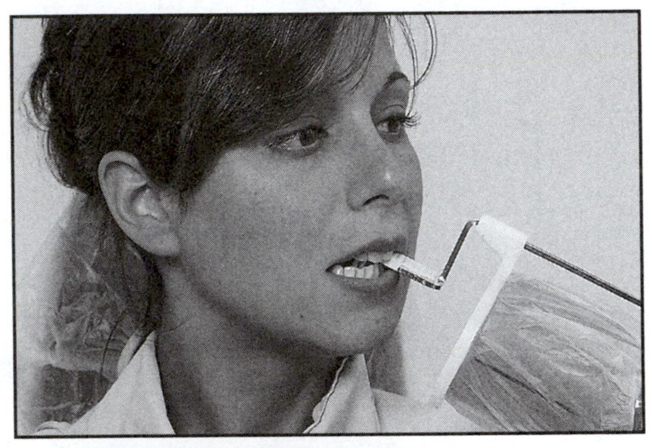

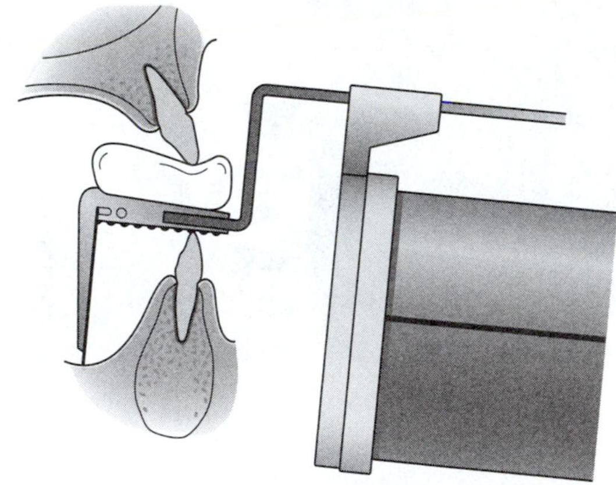

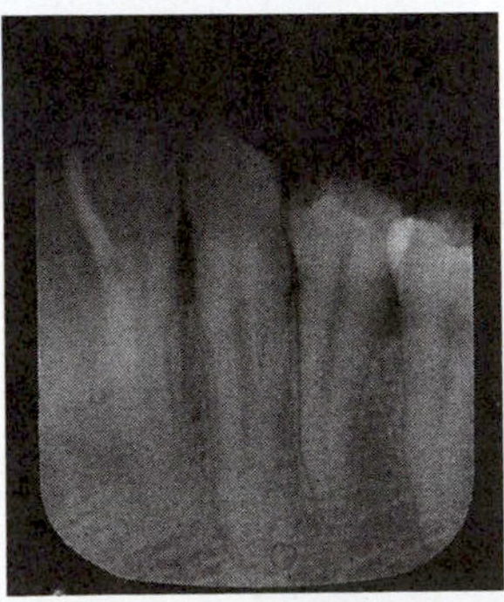

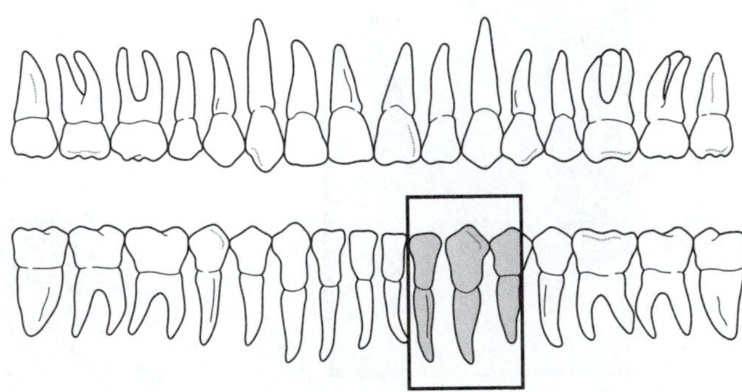

FIGURE 11–9 Mandibular cuspids.

5. In the diagram, the film is angled on the center of the cuspid. As with the incisors, place it toward the base of the tongue, away from the alveolar bone.

Mandibular Premolars (Figure 11–10)

1. For the mandibular premolars, tilt the film/film holder and place the film in the patient's mouth, gently positioning it between the lingual surface of the teeth and the tongue.
2. Place the anterior edge of the film at the middle of the cuspid to ensure that the film covers the area of the two premolars.
3. Have the patient close on the bite-block.
4. Note the position of the film as it is placed in the space between the tongue and the mandibular arch.
5. The film, teeth, and plane of the open end of the cone are all parallel. The first and second premolars are seen on this film with the contact points open.

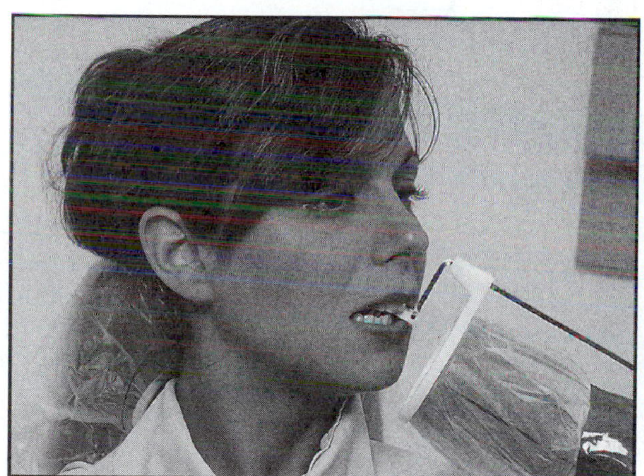

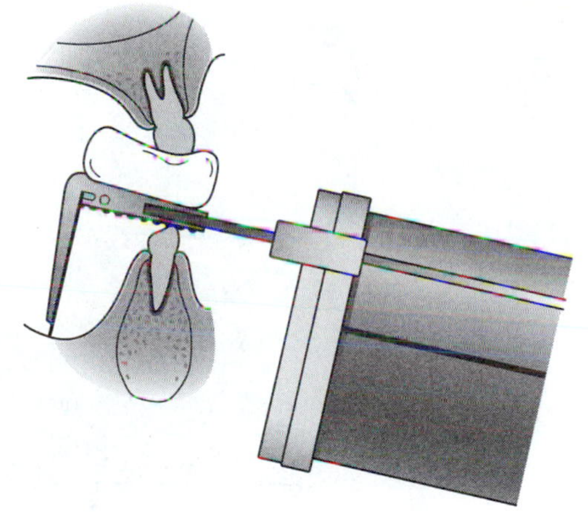

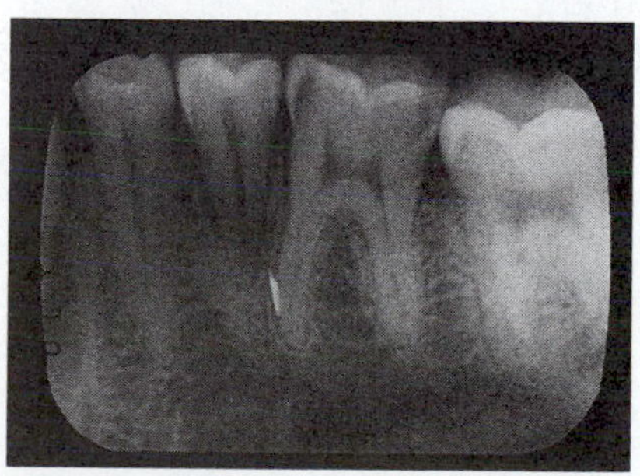

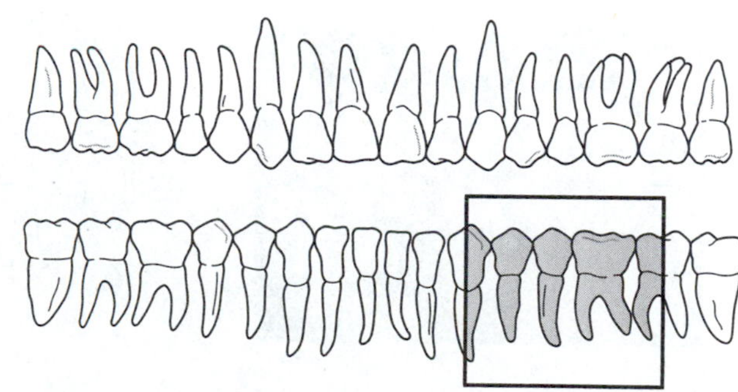

FIGURE 11–10 Mandibular bicuspids (premolars).

◗ **Mandibular Molars** (Figure 11–11)

1. For the mandibular molars, tilt the film/film holder and place the film holder with the film in the patient's mouth, positioning it between the tongue and the lingual surfaces of the teeth.
2. Center the bite-block over the second molar. Hold it in the desired position, and have the patient close to secure it in place.
3. Gently place the patient's cheek over the bite-block, if this is more comfortable for the patient.
4. Align the positioning ring and cone.
5. Note how close the film is to the lingual surface. Move the tongue toward the center of the mouth to make this placement more comfortable for the patient.
6. The edge of the film is positioned only one-eighth inch above the occlusal edge.

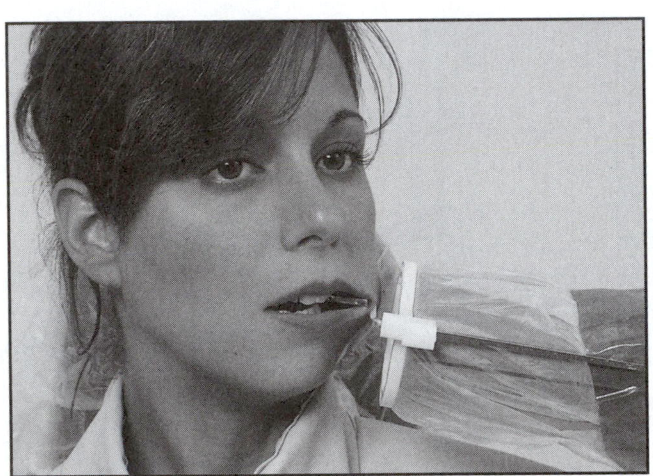

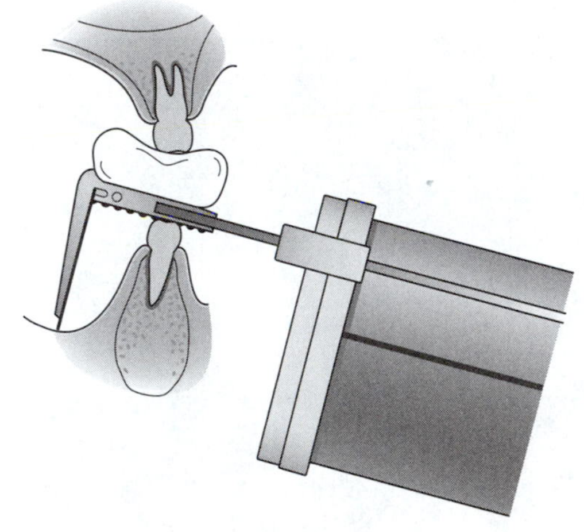

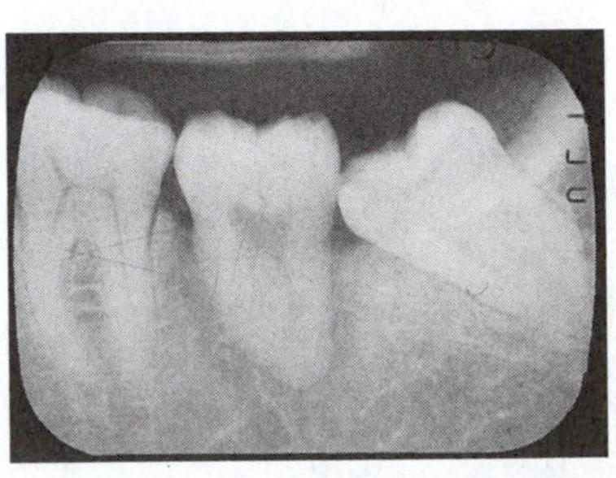

FIGURE 11–11 Mandibular molars.

7. The first, second, and third molars are seen on this film with the contacts open. The third molar may not be erupted into the oral cavity, but it will be seen on the film.
8. During placement, to prevent the film and film holder from moving forward, hold the bite-block in position until the patient closes firmly on it.

Premolar Bite-Wing (Figure 11–12)

1. To position bite-wing radiographs, a tab or positioning instrument is used. Tabs come with adhesive backs or with loops to surround the film. The positioning instrument comes with a bite-wing holder, an indicator rod, and a positioning ring.
2. Holding the film horizontally, place the tab in the center of the film or, if using a positioning instrument, make sure the film is centered on the bite-wing holder with the smooth side of the film directed toward the positioning ring.
3. The drawing/radiograph illustrates the position of the film covering the premolars with the front edge of the film to the middle of the cuspid while the back edge of the film may be to the mesial of the second molar.
4. Hold the tab and place the film near the lingual surface of the teeth in the patient's mouth, positioning the film to cover the mandibular premolars.
5. While holding the tab in place, have the patient close and slowly rotate fingers out of the way.

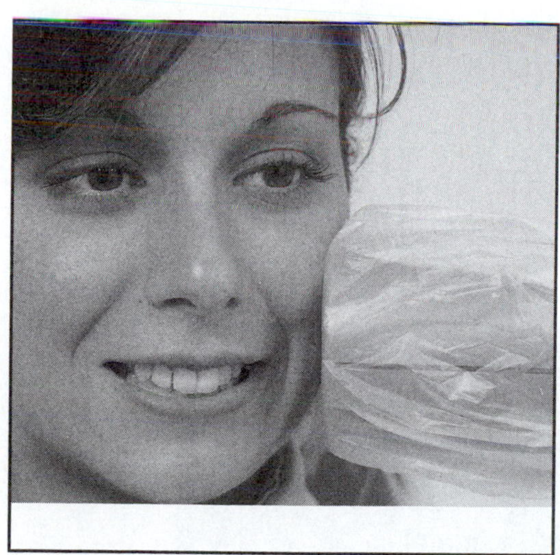

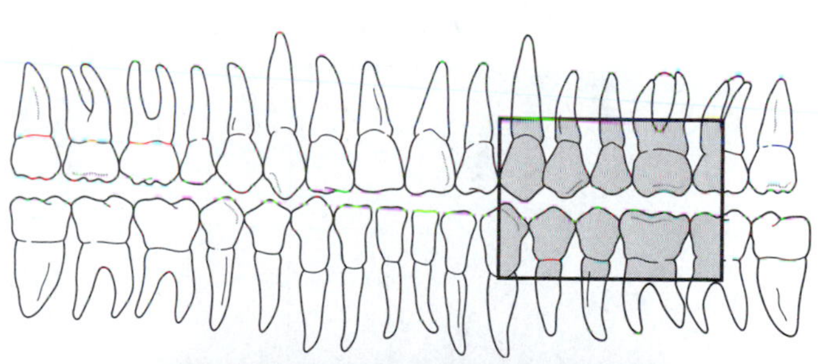

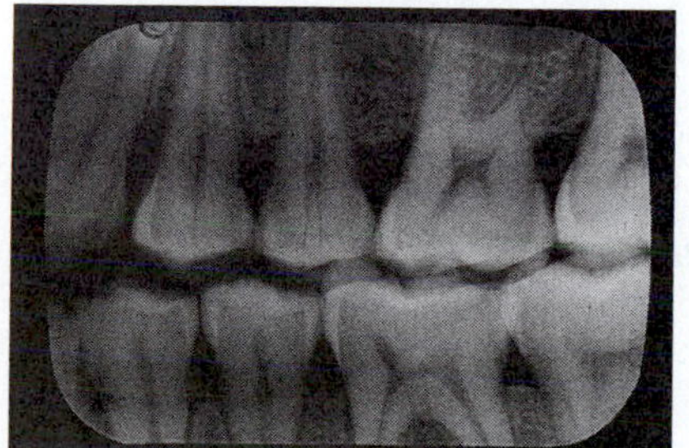

FIGURE 11–12 Premolar bite-wing using bite-wing tab.

6. When using a positioning instrument, place the bite-wing holder in the patient's mouth, away from the lingual surface of the teeth. Position the film to cover the premolars and to be parallel to them. Have the patient close slowly on the bite-wing holder and hold it in place.

7. The cone positioning for the premolar bite-wing begins with the vertical angulation set at 0° so the cone is perpendicular to the film.

8. The horizontal angulation is positioned so that the beam is aimed directly between the contacts of the premolars and the cone is perpendicular to the film. This film placement is sometimes uncomfortable for the patient because of the alveolar ridge curvature near the cuspid. When using the positioning instrument, first hold the indicator rod and then bring the positioning ring close to the patient's face.

◗ **Molar Bite-Wing** (Figure 11–13)

1. Position the film to cover the molars and the distal half of the second premolar. Place the front edge of the film at the distal of the second molar.

2. Holding the tab, place the film in the patient's mouth, away from the lingual surfaces, gently moving the tongue toward the middle of the mouth.

3. When using the positioning instrument, place it in the patient's mouth, pushing the tongue away from the lingual surfaces.

4. The vertical angulation for the molar bite-wing is set at 0° so the cone is perpendicular to the film. The horizontal angulation is directed so that

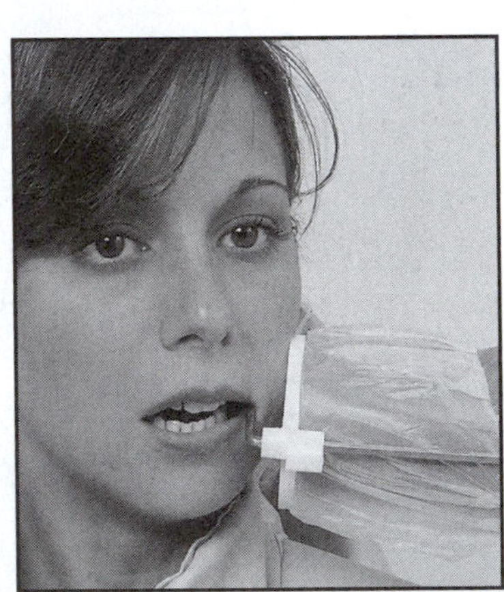

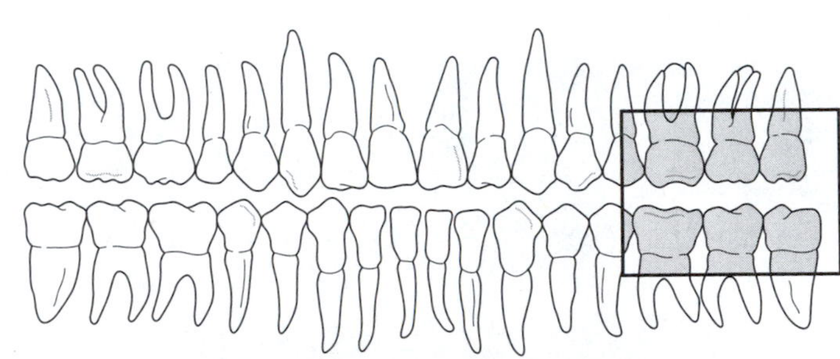

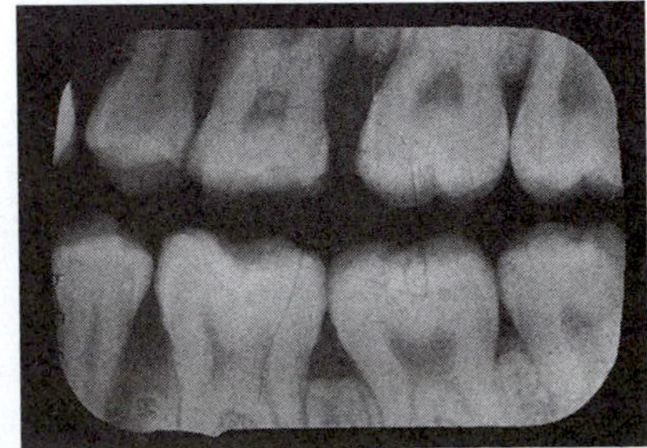

FIGURE 11–13 Molar bite-wing using Rinn XCP.

the beam is between the contacts of the first and second molars. Place the cone near the patient's face, covering the film and perpendicular to the film. Look at the curve of the patient's arch rather than the patient's face to position the cone.

Common Radiographic Errors

Errors during exposing and processing of radiographs are inevitable, especially when learning. Understanding the basic principles helps to produce quality diagnostic x-rays. Perfect x-ray technique skills reduce the number of unnecessary retakes, which expose the patient to more radiation, and require more time for everyone. However, to avoid common radiographic errors, it is necessary to understand what constitutes a quality x-ray.

What is a Quality X-Ray?

- Desired teeth and surrounding area appear on the film.
- Images are dimensionally accurate.
- The contacts between the teeth are open.
- The teeth are not elongated or foreshortened.
- The entire length of the teeth is visible, including 1 to 2 mm beyond the cusps and 4 to 6 mm beyond the apex.
- The film has sufficient contrast and density to show good detail of all anatomy.
- The radiograph is free of spots, stains, handling marks, and other artifacts (black lines).

Correct assembly of the film-holding devices eliminates many errors. Be sure the bite-block is in the correct position for the corresponding arch. Also, be sure the film is centered in the indicating ring. Select the correct size film to cover the area to be exposed. If the film is too small, the apex may be cut off. If the film is too large, it may be difficult for the patient to hold and the x-ray may be distorted. When the film is properly placed in the mouth, a 1 to 3 mm edge of the film should show beyond the occlusal/incisal surface of the tooth.

Distortion. Sometimes the film bends or curves on the palate and in the cuspid area on the mandible; when the film bends, the image distorts. During the film placement, the film may be creased. These crease marks show on the processed film as black lines (artifacts).

Elongation. **Elongation** is a vertical angulation error and is caused by insufficient angulation, meaning there is not enough positive angulation on the maxillary or negative angulation on the mandibular. This error occurs more often when using the bisecting technique.

Foreshortening. **Foreshortening** is also a vertical angulation error. Foreshortening is the opposite of elongation and is caused by too much angulation. This error also occurs more often with the bisecting technique.

Overlapping. **Overlapping** is caused by incorrect horizontal angulation. When the cone is angled toward the mesial or the distal surfaces of the teeth instead of the interproximal areas, overlapping occurs (Figure 11–14).

Cone Cutting. **Cone cutting** means the x-ray beam missed part of the film, causing the film to be only partially exposed. Because the cone is lead lined, the shape of the cone cut on the film will match the shape of the cone (either round or rectangular) (Figure 11–15).

Clear Film. A **clear film** indicates the film was not exposed to any radiation. Check the machine to verify that it was turned on.

Double Exposure. Sometimes, inadvertently, film is exposed twice. A **double exposure** results in blurred images or a dark x-ray. Examine the film closely and two images can be seen.

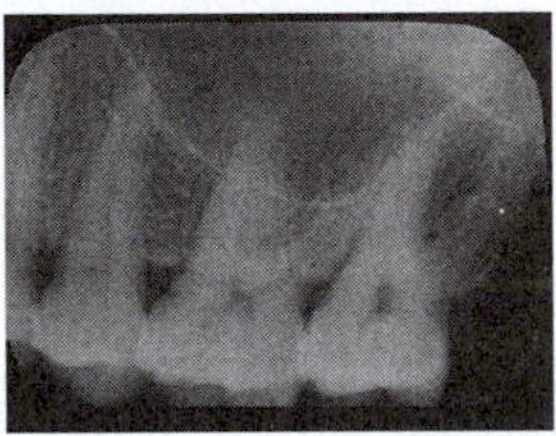

FIGURE 11–14 Overlapping.

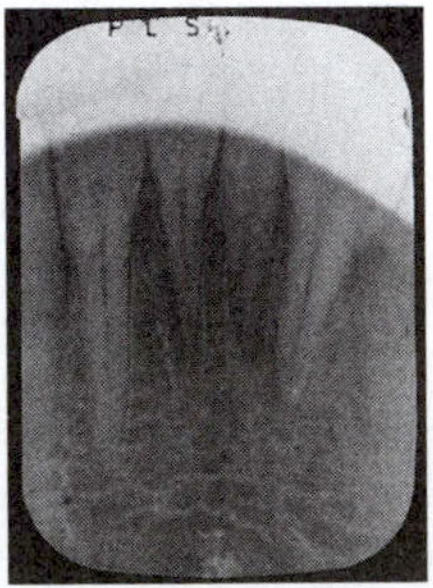

FIGURE 11–15 Cone cut.

Blurred Image. **Blurred images** result from movement of the patient's head or tube head or from the x-ray film moving in the patient's mouth. The images are undefined and unclear.

Underexposed Film. When the film appears light and has a thin image, it may be **underexposed**. Check the mAs, kVs, and the exposure time settings for the type of film being used, the size of the patient, and the x-ray machine.

Overexposed Film. When the film has a dark image, it is overexposed and too dark (dense) to see any structures clearly and accurately for a diagnosis. Use the same checks used for the light film image.

Radiopaque Film Images. Often, metal objects such as eyeglasses, earrings, and partial appliances show as **radiopaque** (not transmitting light) objects on the processed x-ray.

Backward Film. Placing the film in the mouth backward or reversed causes the images on the film to be light and a **herringbone pattern** (tire track). The white, plain side of the film is always placed facing the tube head. If the film is reversed, the amount of x-rays that reach the film are reduced by the lead foil (Figure 11–16).

Film Processing Errors

Light Film Image. Light and dark film images can occur while exposing the film and during processing. A light film is said to be underprocessed. If the film is underprocessed, the developing time was too short, the developer temperature was lower than recommended, or the developing solution was "exhausted" (too weak from over use and needs to be changed).

Dark Film Image. The dark film images can be caused by over-developing, the developing solution temperature being too high, the developing solution being too strong, or the film being left in the developer too long.

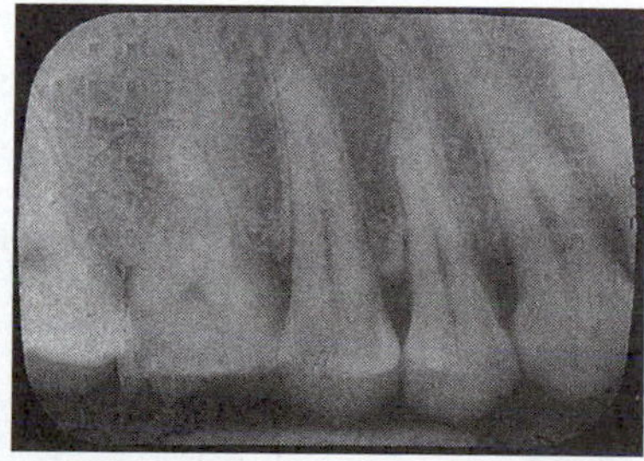

FIGURE 11–16 Film was placed in the patient's mouth backward. Note herringbone pattern on molars.

Fogged Film. **Fogged films** have a gray appearance, film image detail is lost, and contrast is lessened. Fog on films can be caused by improper storage conditions, outdated films, light leaks in the processing room, or light leaks from loose fittings on automatic processors and daylight loaders.

Partial Image. A **partial image** on the film is the result of film placement in the processing tanks when the solution levels are low. The film is not completely immersed and a partial image results.

Film Artifacts. Film artifacts are the result of not handling the films carefully or not keeping the area around the processing tanks clean. Examples of artifacts include water spots on unprocessed film, which leave clear areas on the film; fixer on unprocessed film, which leaves a white area on the film; developer, which leaves black spots. If the film is not washed/rinsed properly, a yellowish brown stain is left on the film. Black film artifacts can occur from a small charge of electricity, such as a lightening streak, when you pull the x-ray film from the packet in a dry climate. Fluoride ions on gloves that are transferred to the film during handling leave dark fingerprint smudge marks. X-rays that overlap (touch) during processing leave an artifact on the films (the artifact is in the shape of the edge or corner of the film).

Torn or Scratched Film. Rough handling of the film can lead to the emulsion on the film being torn or scratched, which leaves a white area or mark on the processed film. Films can be scratched and torn if they are not handled carefully in over-crowded tanks or during retrieval if lost off the film racks (Figure 11–17).

Air Bubbles on Film. Air bubbles are trapped on the film if it is not agitated when placed in the processing solutions. The air bubbles leave round, white spots where they were attached to the film.

Reticulation. **Reticulation** is when a film has been exposed to a high temperature followed by a low temperature. The film emulsion swells and then shrinks.

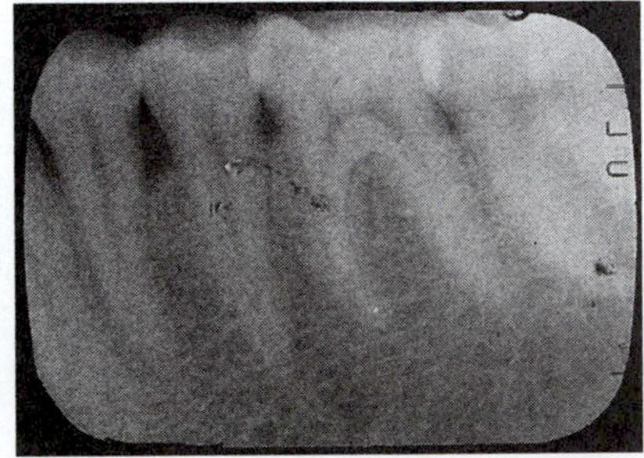

FIGURE 11–17 A radiograph with torn or scratched emulsion.

Streaks. Streaks on films can be caused by rollers not being clean when using automatic processors or from unclean x-ray racks. Debris is picked up as the films pass though the rollers, leaving a streaked appearance on the film. Streaks from unclean x-ray racks occur during the processing procedure; debris, including processing solutions, runs from the racks onto the film.

PROCESSING QUALITY RADIOGRAPHS

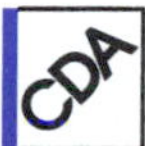

Dental radiographs are processed either in manual tanks or in the automatic processor. The manual tank (Procedure 11–2) utilizes more of the assistant's time. The added time is due to the required movement of the x-rays from the developer tank after a specified time, which the assistant must monitor, to the water bath. Then the x-rays go from the water bath to the fixer tank, and then again from the fixer tank back into the water (Figure 11–18). The x-rays must be again removed from the second water wash and placed in a dryer or left to dry on a rack. By comparison, the dental assistant can place the x-rays into the automatic processor and when they come out they are dry and ready for mounting. The automatic processor does not need to be timed. Both techniques produce quality radiographs.

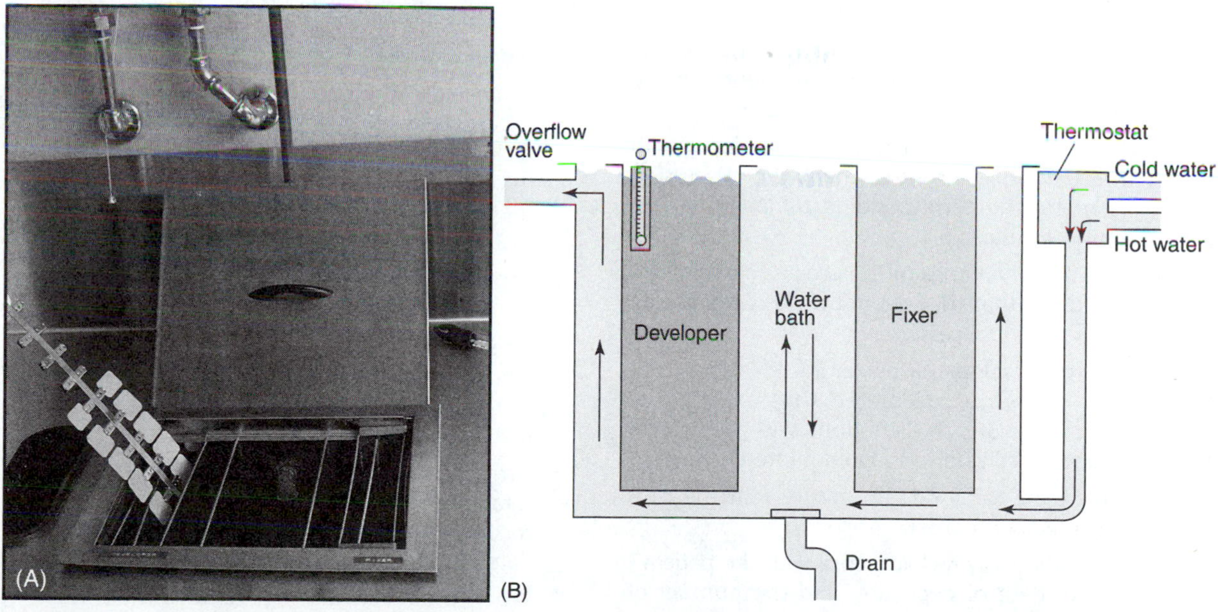

FIGURE 11–18 (A) Typical manual processing tank showing developer and fixer insert tanks in the water bath. (B) Line drawing of manual processing tank.

PROCEDURE

11-2 Processing Radiographs Using a Manual Tank

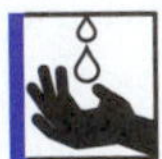
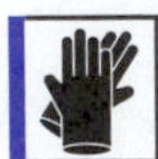

This procedure is performed by the dental assistant, who prepares the equipment, supplies, and the area. The exposed radiographs are taken to the darkroom by the dental assistant to process.

EQUIPMENT AND SUPPLIES

- Barriers for the darkroom counter
- Exposed radiographs
- X-ray rack
- Processing tank
- Safety light
- Timer
- Thermometer
- Stirring rods
- Pencil
- Electric film dryer

PROCEDURE STEPS *(Follow aseptic procedures)*

1. Wash and dry hands (gloves must be worn if the x-rays are contaminated).
2. Make sure the area is clean and free of splashes. Place barriers on the counter in the darkroom.
3. Check the temperature of the developer with the thermometer. Also, check the processing chart for the corresponding temperature and time information.
4. Check the volumes of the processing solutions to ensure that they do not need replenishing. (Replenish if necessary.)
5. Stir the developer and fixer if it is the first processing being completed that morning or afternoon. Stir the solutions with the corresponding stirring rods. Do not interchange.
6. Check the x-ray rack to ensure that the clips are in working order.
7. Label the x-ray rack in pencil with the patient's name, date of exposure, and the number of x-rays taken.
8. Turn on the safelights and turn off the white lights.
9. Remove the films from their wrappers and place on the x-ray racks. (Use gloves if the x-rays are contaminated.)
10. Check each film to make sure it is attached securely and placed in a parallel manner so it does not touch the adjacent film.
11. Submerge in the developer tank and agitate the rack slightly in the developing solution to eliminate bubbles on the surface of the emulsion.
12. Place the tank cover on the processing tank. Set the timer for four and one-half minutes if the temperature of the developer is at 68°. Clean the area and dispose of the barrier and x-ray wrappers.
13. When the timer goes off, remove the x-ray rack from the developer, letting the excess solution drip into the developer prior to placing the rack in the running water (the middle area in the processing tank). Rinse for thirty seconds.
14. Remove the x-ray rack from the rinsing, let the excess water drip off, and then immerse the rack in the fixing solution for ten minutes. If the dentist needs to view the patient's x-rays, they can be removed after three minutes and then returned to the fixer for the remaining time.
15. Replace the processing lid and set the timer for ten minutes.
16. After the ten minutes, remove the x-ray rack from the fixer and place it in the running water at the center of the processing tank. The final wash takes twenty minutes.
17. After twenty minutes remove the rack of x-rays from the water and place it in the dryer for fifteen to twenty minutes or until drying is completed.
18. When the x-rays are dry, remove them from the rack and place them in a labeled x-ray mount.

Preparation for Film Processing

Dental developer and fixer are prepared from liquid concentrates, following the manufacturer's instructions. These solutions are supplied in two packs with color-coded lists and labels. Before using these chemicals, the dental assistant must verify that the correct solution is placed in the proper tank to prevent cross-contamination. After checking the date on the solution, the dental assistant carefully opens the top and pours the developer into the developing tank. The dental assistant then adds the proper amount of water at approximately 68°F to the indicator line at the top of the tank. The dental assistant prepares the developer in the same manner.

After the insert tanks are in the processing tank, the dental assistant starts the water at the inlet valve to the proper height in the tank. The dental assistant then stirs the solution in each insert tank using a special paddle to mix the chemicals thoroughly. The dental assistant checks the temperature of the developing solution; when it is at 68°F it is ready to process dental x-rays. A time/temperature chart is included on each of the developer/fixer solution bottles. The dental assistant should keep this chart available in the dark room for ready reference.

The dental assistant should discard and change the processing solutions every three to four weeks, depending upon the number of films processed, to maintain optimal processing. With heavy use, the solutions should be changed more frequently.

Temperature	Duration in the Developer
80°F	2 1/2 minutes
75°F	3 minutes
70°F	4 minutes
68°F	4 1/2 minutes
60°F	6 minutes

Manual Film Processing

After the solutions are stirred thoroughly and proper temperature has been attained, the dental assistant is ready to process the films (Figure 11–18). The work area must be clean and dry. The dental assistant obtains the correct processing rack and indicates the patient's name, the date, and number of x-rays on the identification tab at the top of the rack using a pencil (Procedure 11–2).

The dental assistant dons gloves, remembering to avoid touching any portion of the film directly (Figure 11–18). Films should be handled carefully, by the edges only.

The dental assistant turns off the white light, closes and locks the darkroom door, and turns on the safety light. The dental assistant then carefully unwraps each film and retracts the plastic coating, the black paper, and the lead foil; then the dental assistant attaches each film to the hanger. The dental assistant holds the film by the edges to confirm that it is securely clipped onto the hanger and places each individual film on the rack in the same manner. When all the films have been clipped to the rack, the dental assistant lifts the lid off the processor and submerges the rack into the developer. The assistant gently agitates the rack in the solution by raising and lowering it several times before hanging it on to the side of the rack to ensure that the films are completely bathed in the developer and that no bubbles are present on the surfaces of the individual films.

The dental assistant returns the lid to the processing tank and sets the time at 4½ minutes. The dental assistant may wait in the dark room with the safety light on while developing takes place, or he or she may open the door and resume other necessary clinical functions during the developing time.

When the x-ray timer rings, the dental assistant, working with the door closed and locked and the safety light on, removes the lid from the processor and rinses the film rack in the water bath for a minimum of 30 seconds to curtail the developing phase and to remove excess solution from the films. Next, the dental assistant submerges the rack of films into the fixer insert tank. The dental assistant replaces the processor lid and resets the timer for twice the developing time, or at 9 minutes when the temperature is at 68°F.

When the timer rings and fixing time is complete, the dental assistant removes the films from the fixer and places them back into the water bath in the center of the tank for the final rinse. (The safety light is no longer required, as the light-sensitive phase is over.) The x-rays should be rinsed with clean running water for 20 minutes. When rinsing is complete, the dental assistant removes the tank with the films still attached and hangs it from a towel rack or places it in an electronic dryer for 15 minutes. When drying time is complete, the dental assistant removes the film from the dryer. The films are then ready for mounting and filing in the patient's chart (Procedure 11–5).

Automatic Processor

Automatic processors are used in most dental offices (Figure 11–19) because they are easy to use and reduce processing time. The x-rays are consistently of good quality. Most processors are compact and require minimum space in the darkroom. If space in the darkroom is a concern, some processors have daylight loading units that can be added. With the daylight loading units, the processors can be placed wherever they are convenient to use. One important factor to consider when using automatic processors is that maintenance of the units and daily chemical control is essential.

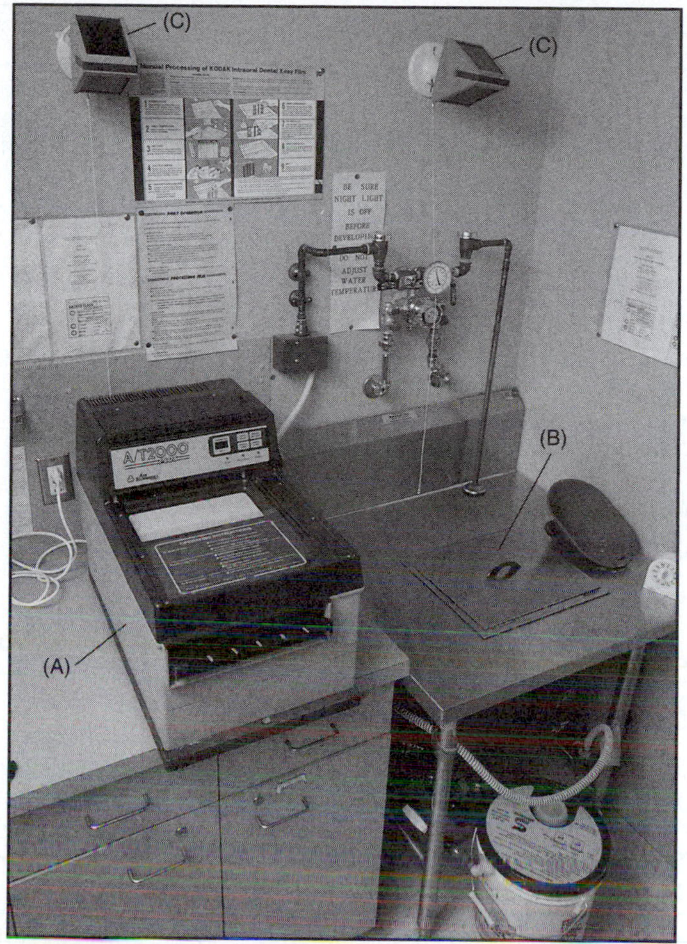

FIGURE 11–19 (A) Automatic film processor. (B) Manual processing tank in darkroom. (C) Safelights.

Although **automatic processing** follows the same basic steps as manual processing, the order in which the film is soaked in solutions is different. With automatic processors, a series of rollers moves the x-ray film through the developing compartment, the fixing compartment, the water compartment, and, last, through the drying compartment before depositing it onto a tray (Procedure 11–3).

The rollers are moved by gears, belts, or chains that must be lubricated and maintained according to manufacturer's instructions. The x-ray film is processed in four to seven minutes, depending on the temperature of the developing solution. The temperature also determines the speed at which the rollers are set. Automatic processing is done at temperatures between 85°F and 95°F

PROCEDURE

11-3 Processing Radiographs Using an Automatic Processor

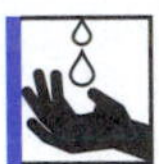
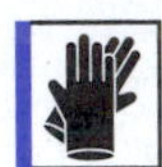

This procedure is performed by the dental assistant who prepares the equipment, the supplies, and the area. The exposed radiographs are taken to the automatic processor by the dental assistant to process.

EQUIPMENT AND SUPPLIES

- Exposed radiographs
- Gloves
- Automatic x-ray processor with daylight loader

PROCEDURE STEPS *(Follow aseptic procedures)*

1. Turn on the automatic x-ray processor at the beginning of each day. This ensures that it is warmed up and ready to process after the x-rays are exposed. (The chemicals must be heated to the correct temperatures or the x-rays will appear light and the diagnostic quality will be diminished.)
2. Wash and dry hands.
3. Place exposed radiographs in the daylight loader with two additional containers.
4. Put on gloves and position gloved hands through the sleeves of the daylight loader.
5. Remove each radiograph from its packet and place the film in the container that is not contaminated. Be careful not to touch and contaminate the film as the packet is removed.
6. Place the empty packets in a contaminated cup.
7. After all x-rays are unwrapped, remove the gloves and place them in a contaminated container.
8. With clean hands, feed the unwrapped films into the machine *slowly.* Start on one side of the processor and rotate to the other side. Repeat. If using a film holder, place all films in the holder and release for processing. Continue until all films are placed in the processor.
9. Remove processed films from the outlet area and place in a labeled x-ray mount.

This increase in temperature significantly reduces the total processing time. The rollers move the film through each compartment and also "squeeze" off the excess solution between compartments. This prevents processing chemicals from being carried into the next stage of processing.

Care of the Automatic Processor. Proper care of automatic processors is crucial. To ensure quality x-ray film processing, daily and weekly maintenance must be followed. The dental assistant must read the manufacturer's instructions and set a schedule for maintenance.

PROCEDURE

11-4 Processing Duplicating Technique

This procedure is performed by the dental assistant who prepares the equipment, the supplies, and the area. The radiographs to be duplicated are taken to the darkroom by the dental assistant to duplicate.

EQUIPMENT AND SUPPLIES

- Duplicating film and radiographs to be duplicated
- X-ray duplicating machine
- Automatic x-ray processor with daylight loader

PROCEDURE STEPS *(Follow aseptic procedures)*

1. Place the x-rays in the desired position on the duplicator (Figure 11–20). Make sure the dot on the film is upward (convex).
2. If the machine has a viewing light, turn it on to assist during placement of the x-rays.
3. Turn off the viewing light and under safelight conditions, place the duplicating film over the x-rays with the emulsion side facing downward so that it is contacting the x-rays (the notch will be in the upper left corner).
4. Cover with the lid and latch tightly. Set the timer to four to five seconds (this may vary with machines).

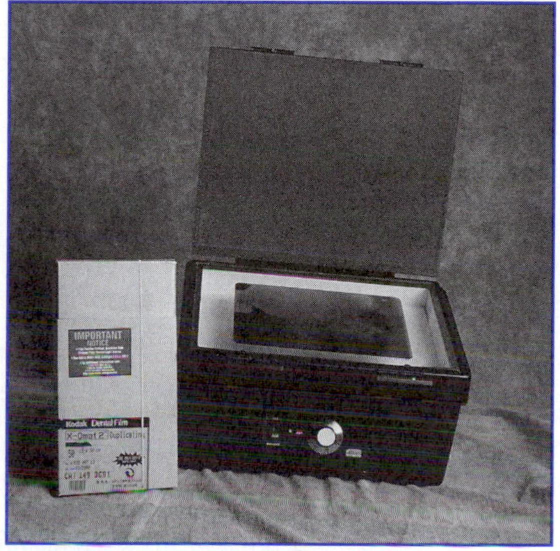

FIGURE 11–20 Example of a radiographic duplicator and film.

5. Activate the machine to expose the film.
6. When completed, remove the duplicating film under safelight conditions and process the film.

Duplicating Radiographs

Dental x-rays can be duplicated (Procedure 11–4) so the originals never have to leave the office. The need for duplication is increasing because more patients have dental insurance, patients request that x-rays be sent to specialists, and requests are made to forward x-rays when patients move. Also, malpractice suits have increased, which require radiographs for defense support. Copies of x-rays can be made by a duplication process in the darkroom. These copies offer protection for the dentist as well as reference sources for the patient.

The **duplication technique** requires the purchase of duplicating film and a duplication machine. The film is supplied in a variety of sizes and can be processed either manually or with an automatic processor. Duplicating film has emulsion on one side only and is coded with a notch in the upper right corner, when the emulsion side is facing you. Duplicating film is a direct positive film; thus, if an increase in film darkness (density) is desired, the exposure time is reduced.

Duplicating machines have light sources with glass over them. The lid closes with a latch to prevent light leaks. There is a setting for viewing the x-rays and a timing selector. These machines fit conveniently on a counter top.

Mounting Radiographs

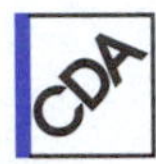

Each radiograph has a raised dot to aid in the mounting process (Procedure 11–5). The film pack is placed in the patient's mouth so the raised dot, or convex side, is toward the x-ray cone. Mounting the radiographs so that the dot is toward the operator means that the operator looks at the film as if the operator were facing the patient. The patient's left side is on the operator's right side when the operator is facing the film mount. This type of mounting is called labial mounting. The ADA recommends that dental offices use the labial mounting. An x-ray viewbox may be used to mount dental radiographs. A viewbox is a lighted box that has a white, frosted surface so that x-rays can be viewed easily for diagnostic purposes.

A number of different mounts are available. They range in size from 1, 2, 4, 7, 14, 16, 18, 20, and 28 windows. Bite-wing x-ray mounts come in either 2 or 4 windows. The 14 or 16 window mounts are used most commonly for periapical mounts. The 18 or 20 windows are used for full-mouth (both periapical and bite-wing) mounting.

After selecting the correct mount, the dental assistant places the x-rays on a clean counter in front of a viewbox. If mounting a full mouth set of x-rays (Procedure 11–4), divide the x-rays into three groups: bite-wings, anterior periapicals, and posterior periapicals. It is easy to identify the bite-wing x-rays because they have both the crowns of the mandibular and the maxillary teeth on them.

The four bite-wing x-rays are mounted so that the molar x-rays are on the outside and the corresponding bicuspid x-rays are on the inside, just as if looking directly at the patient (Figure 11–21). Notice the curve of spee (or formation of a smile pattern), which comes from the curvature of the mandible on correctly mounted x-rays. The dental assistant checks carefully that the dots are convex, the molars are on the outside, the bicuspids are on the inside, and the occlusal plane is curved in a smile pattern.

Next, the anterior periapical x-rays are mounted. The maxillary anterior teeth are always larger and wider than the mandibular anterior teeth. The maxillary central teeth are the easiest to identify. They are placed in the full-mouth mount in the center upper portion as they appear in the mouth, with the incisal edge in the middle of the mount and the roots toward the outside of the mount.

PROCEDURE

11-5 Mounting Radiographs

This procedure is performed by the dental assistant. A viewbox may be utilized when mounting the radiographs.

EQUIPMENT AND SUPPLIES

- Radiographs
- Lighted viewbox
- X-ray mount (using full-mouth, 18 x-ray mount)
- Clean, dry surface

PROCEDURE STEPS *(Follow aseptic procedures)*

1. Wash and dry hands.
2. Label the x-ray mount with the patient's name and the date of the exposure (in pencil).
3. Turn on the viewbox (optional).
4. Place the radiographs on a clean surface with all dots outward (or convex) to viewing.
5. Categorize all x-rays into three groups: bite-wings (four in number), anterior (six in number), and posterior (eight in number).
6. Place the bite-wing x-rays in the mount, making sure the dots remain convex, the molars are toward the outside, and the bicuspids (premolars) are toward the inside. Make sure that the x-rays are mounted according to the curve of the spee.
7. Put the anterior x-rays in place, with the maxillary on the upper and the mandibular on the lower. The incisal edges should be closest to each other in the mount and the roots positioned as they grow. The centrals are placed in the middle with the cuspids on the outer sides. (The maxillary centrals are much larger than the mandibular centrals.)
8. Place the remaining posterior x-rays. The molars should be toward the outside and the bicuspids (premolars) toward the inside. (The maxillary molars have three roots and the mandibular molars have two roots.) Both should be placed according to how they are in the mouth, with the roots opposite each other and the biting surfaces more closely positioned.
9. Review the mounted x-rays to verify they have been placed properly.

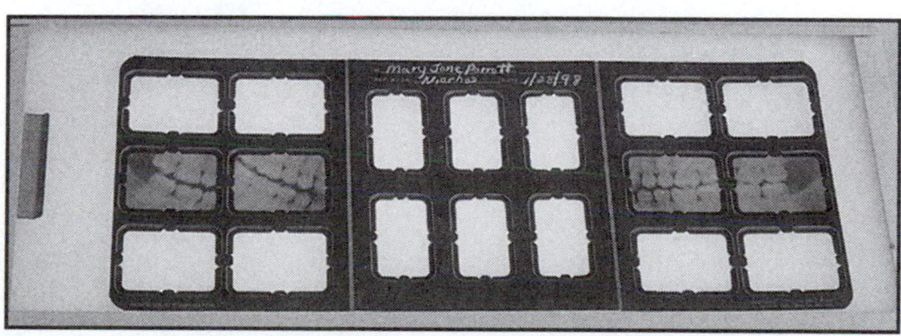

FIGURE 11–21 Full-mouth mount with bite-wing x-rays in place.

The mandibular central x-rays appear to have the smallest teeth on them. Place them directly below the maxillary teeth with the incisal edges toward each other. There are four cuspid x-rays (two maxillary and two mandibular) left to mount. The maxillary cuspids appear larger and may show the maxillary sinuses near the distal side of the apex of the roots. The roots always tend to curve distally. The dental assistant mounts both the maxillary and the mandibular cuspid x-rays with the lateral incisor sides toward the center and the bicuspids side outward. All the incisal edges come together in the center of the mount.

The mandibular and maxillary posterior films are differentiated from each other on the basis of root and crown shape, along with anatomic landmarks. The maxillary posterior x-rays may show the nasal cavity or sinuses. The maxillary premolars usually have two roots and the molars have three roots. The roots of the maxillary molars may look unclear because of the lingual root showing through the mesial and distal roots. The dental assistant mounts the maxillary molars on the upper part of the mount toward the outside. The bicuspids are placed between the molars and the anterior cuspids. The bicuspid and molar x-rays must match each other as well as the corresponding crowns of the bite-wing x-rays. The mandibular periapical x-rays should be mounted in much the same manner as the maxillary. The molars have two roots that are more clearly defined than the maxillary; the bicuspids will have one root. After all the x-rays are in the mount, perform a quick check to see whether all the x-rays are mounted similar to the position of the teeth in the mouth.

Legal Implications of Radiographs

X-rays are legal records and should not be destroyed. They belong to the dentist and should not be given to the patients. If a patient switches to another dentist, send a duplicate of the x-rays to the new dentist; keep the original for the office files.

CHAPTER 12

Topical and Local Anesthesia

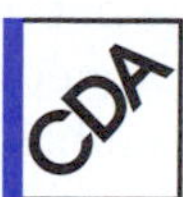

OBJECTIVES

The student should strive to meet the following objectives and demonstrate an understanding of the facts and principles presented in this chapter:

1. List the steps for preparing for the administration of topical and local anesthetic.
2. Describe the equipment and materials required to administer local anesthetic.

KEY TERMS

local anesthesia (p. 192)
topical anesthetic (p. 192)

INTRODUCTION

One of the biggest fears for patients visiting the dentist is the injection. Over the years many advances have been made to control patients' pain and anxiety. Improved administration techniques and equipment for management of pain and anxiety for the patient continues to be a focus of research.

Because most procedures require some form of anesthesia, the dentist may select one or a combination of methods to control pain, depending on the patient and the procedure.

Local Anesthesia

Local anesthesia produces a deadened or pain-free area while the dentist performs a procedure.

Topical Anesthesia

Before the local anesthesia is injected, the area may be numbed with **topical anesthetic**. This material desensitizes the oral mucosa for a brief period so the patient will not feel the "pinch" of the needle. Topical anesthetics affect the small nerve endings located in the surface of the skin and oral mucosa.

ANESTHETICS, SYRINGES, AND NEEDLES

The equipment necessary for the administration of local anesthetic includes a syringe, a needle, and an anesthetic carpule.

The Syringe

There are various types of syringes used for dental procedures, however the most common is the **aspirating syringe.** The aspirating syringe, recommended by the ADA, is designed to allow the operator to check the position of the needle before depositing the anesthetic solution. The aspiratory syringe has a harpoon on the end of the piston. The harpoon penetrates the rubber end of the anesthetic cartridge. Once the needle is placed in the tissues, the operator retracts the thumb ring, creating negative pressure. If the needle has penetrated a blood vessel, a thin line of blood is drawn into the cartridge. The operator then repositions the needle to avoid injecting the anesthetic into the blood vessel and retests until there is evidence that the needle is not placed in a blood vessel. Use of an aspirating syringe allows the operator to place the anesthetic for maximum benefit.

Syringes may be metal (stainless steel) or non-metal (plastic). The metal syringes are autoclavable while the non-metal syringes may be disposable or autoclavable (Procedure 12–1 and 12–2).

PROCEDURE

12-1 Preparing the Anesthetic Syringe

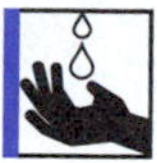 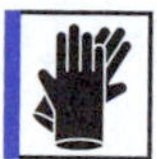 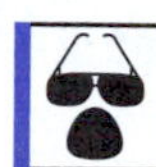

The dental assistant prepares the syringe out of the view of the patient. A topical anesthetic is applied by either the dentist or the dental assistant. The equipment and materials are on the procedure tray or stored at the dental unit.

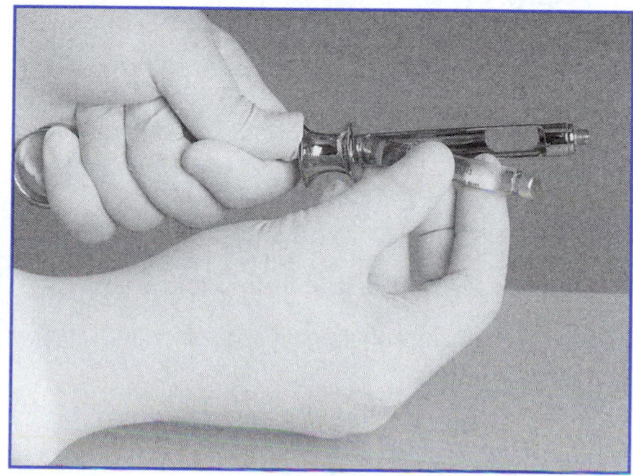

FIGURE 12–1 Technique to place a cartridge in an aspirating syringe.

EQUIPMENT AND SUPPLIES

- Sterile syringe
- Selected disposable needle
- Selected anesthetic cartridge
- 2 × 2 gauze sponge moistened with 91 percent isopropyl alcohol or 70 percent ethyl alcohol

PROCEDURE STEPS *(Follow aseptic procedures)*

This procedure is described for a right-handed person.

1. Following aseptic procedures, select the disposable needle and the anesthetic the dentist has specified for this procedure.
2. Remove the sterilized syringe from its autoclave bag or pouch. Inspect the syringe to be sure it is ready for use.
3. Hold the syringe in the left hand and use the thumb ring to fully retract the piston rod.
4. With the piston rod retracted, place the cartridge in the barrel of the syringe. The plunger end (rubber stopper end) goes in first (Figure 12–1). To prevent contamination, do not place a finger over the diaphragm while placing the cartridge in the syringe. Once the cartridge is in place, release the piston rod.
5. With moderate pressure, push the piston rod into the rubber stopper until it is fully engaged. Do not hit the piston rod to engage the harpoon, and do not hold your hand over the cartridge while engaging the harpoon.
6. Remove the protective plastic cap from the syringe end of the needle, and then screw or press the needle onto the syringe, depending on the type of needle hub. Make sure the needle is secure but not too tight. A disposable needle guard is often placed on the protective cap covering the needle.
7. Carefully remove the protective cover from the needle. Holding the syringe upright, expel a few drops to ensure that the syringe is working properly. Replace the cap and place on the tray, ready for use.

Note: The needle may be placed on the syringe before the cartridge. This technique also requires pressure on the thumb ring to engage the harpoon into the rubber plunger.

PROCEDURE

12-2 Assisting with the Administration of Topical and Local Anesthetics

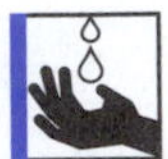
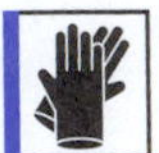
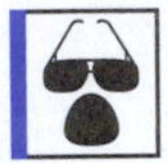
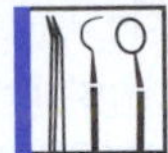
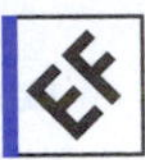

The dental assistant checks with the dentist for instructions on the type of anesthetic and needle for the procedure. The equipment and materials are either on the procedure tray or stored at the dental unit.

EQUIPMENT AND SUPPLIES *(Figure 12–2)*

- Patient's medical/dental history and chart
- Basic setup: mouth mirror, explorer, and cotton pliers
- Air-water syringe tip and evacuator tip (HVE)
- Cotton rolls, cotton-tip applicator, and 2 × 2 gauze sponges
- Topical anesthetic
- Aspirating syringe
- Anesthetic cartridge
- Selection of needles

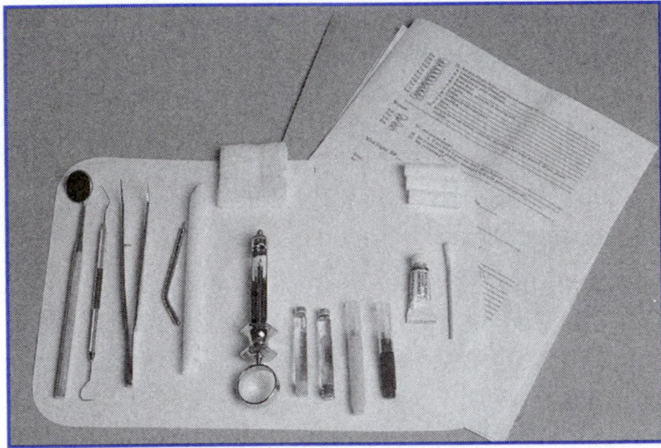

FIGURE 12–2 Equipment and supplies needed to place the topical anesthetic and to pass the prepared syringe.

PROCEDURE STEPS *(Follow aseptic procedures)*

Placing Topical Anesthetic (by the dentist or the assistant)

1. After seating the patient, review and update the medical/dental history.
2. Prepare the patient for the procedure and explain what tastes and sensations he or she may experience. (The explanations should be brief and avoid such words as "pain," "shot," and "injection.") Explain that the topical anesthetic is being applied to make him or her more comfortable during the procedure.
3. Place a small amount of topical anesthetic on a cotton-tip applicator.
4. Prepare the oral mucosa by drying with a sterile 2 × 2 gauze sponge. Keep the tissue retracted.
5. Place the topical anesthetic on the site of the injection and leave in place for one minute (Figure 12–3).

Administering the Local Anesthetic

6. While waiting for the topical anesthetic to take effect, prepare the syringe if this has not been completed. Assemble the syringe, cartridge, and needle as described previously.
7. When the operator indicates, remove the cotton-tip applicator and prepare to pass the syringe.

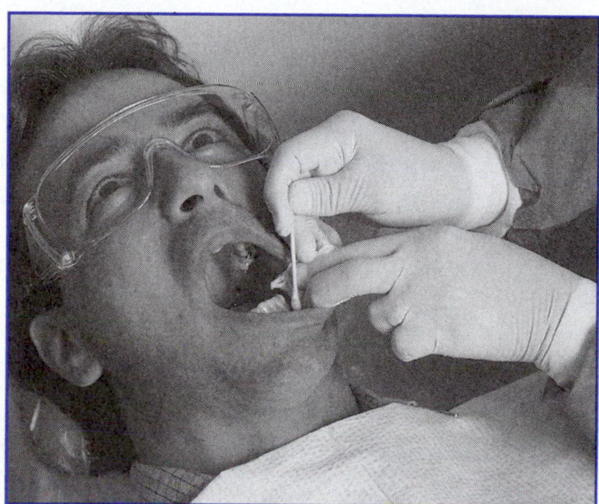

FIGURE 12–3 Placing the topical anesthetic on the mandibular injection site.

8. Check the needle bevel (slanted tip of the needle that penetrates the soft tissue) so it is directed toward the alveolar bone, and then loosely replace the cap on the needle. The protective cap is placed on the hub of the needle so that it is secure but can be removed easily.
9. Pass the syringe below the patient's chin (or behind the patient's head), placing the thumb ring over the dentist's thumb (the dentist grasps the syringe at the finger rest and takes the syringe). As the dentist takes the syringe, remove the protective guard. During the injection, watch the patient for any adverse signs or reactions.

Note: There are different methods to safely remove the cap and complete the transfer. It is important for the dentist and the assistant to establish a routine.

10. The operator recaps the syringe by sliding (scooping) the needle into the protective guard or placing the needle of the syringe in a mechanical recapping device. If a second injection is given, remove the cartridge, insert a new cartridge, test the syringe by expelling a few drops, check the bevel, and position the needle for the dentist to retrieve.

Note: At this time, the syringe is contaminated. It is during recapping that most needle sticks occur. To prevent this, the dentist should recap the needle and retrieve it after the assistant has replaced the cartridge and has repositioned the syringe on the tray or counter. There are a variety of needle holders available, which hold the needle cap so that the needle can be recapped while protecting the hand.

11. The recapped syringe is placed on the tray out of the way for the rest of the procedure but close in case more anesthetic is needed.
12. Rinse the patient's mouth with the air-water syringe and evacuate to remove the water, saliva, and taste of the anesthetic solution.

Unloading the Anesthetic Syringe

1. After the procedure is completed and the patient is dismissed, don utility gloves, take the syringe apart, and prepare it for sterilization.
2. Carefully remove the needle with the protective cap in place. Carefully unscrew the needle. A hemostat can be used to hold the needle while it is being removed from the syringe. The needle is discarded in the sharps container.

Note: The needle can also be removed after the cartridge.

3. Retract the piston to release the harpoon from the cartridge.
4. Remove the cartridge from the syringe by retracting the thumb ring enough to release the cartridge. Turn the syringe until the cartridge is free.
5. Prepare the syringe for sterilization.

The Needle

The needle is used to penetrate the tissue and to direct the local anesthetic solution from the carpule into the surrounding tissues. Most needles are made of stainless steel and are disposable.

One factor to consider when selecting a needle for a dental procedure is the length of the needle. Dental needles are available in two lengths: short (one inch) and long (one and five-eighths inch). The selection usually depends on the operator's preference, the approximate depth of the soft tissues to be penetrated, and the aspiration potential.

The Anesthetic Cartridge

The anesthetic cartridge, also called the carpule, is a glass cylinder that contains the anesthetic solution.

CHAPTER 13

Dental Cements and Restorative Materials and Techniques

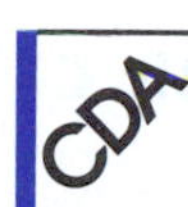

OBJECTIVES

The student should strive to meet the following objectives and demonstrate an understanding of the facts and principles presented in this chapter:

1. Explain the types of dental restorative materials.
2. List the types of materials used to restore cavity preparations.
3. Identify the types of dental cements. Explain their properties, composition, uses, and manipulation.
4. Describe bonding agents and their manipulation.
5. Identify the types of direct restorative materials and where they are used.
6. Explain dental amalgam restorative material.
7. Identify the armamentarium and steps of an amalgam procedure.
8. Explain the composition of composite resins.
9. Explain the properties and manipulation of various composite restorations.
10. Identify the armamentarium and steps of a composite restoration.
11. Explain the use of glass ionomer/resin restorative materials.

KEY TERMS

acid etchant (p. 208)
adhesives (p. 209)
alloy (p. 213)
amalgam (p. 212)
base (p. 199)
bonding agents (p. 209)
compules (p. 218)
dual-cured materials (p. 209)
light-cured (p. 199)
liner (p. 199)
luting (p. 199)
primer (p. 220)
sedative or pallative effect (p. 199)
self-curing (p. 199)
varnish (p. 199)

INTRODUCTION

A wide variety of material is used in dentistry. Although some materials have been around for a long time, new products are always being introduced.

Generally, the materials are divided and categorized according to their functions. Some materials have a wide range of uses. After the tooth has been prepared and the decay removed, certain materials are utilized to restore the tooth.

The Role of the Dental Assistant

The general chairside dental assistant prepares and mixes the material and the dentist places the material in the oral cavity.

Knowledge of the properties of the dental material is necessary for the dental assistant to properly prepare and manipulate restorative materials.

TYPES OF RESTORATIVE DENTAL MATERIALS

Dental materials used to restore the teeth can be divided into two classifications:

1. Liners, bases, cements and bonding agents—Materials to prepare the teeth for the actual restorative materials
2. Amalgam and composite restorative materials

These materials are mixed at chairside by the dental assistant as indicated by the dentist, following manufacturer's instructions and the dentist's preferences. It is the dental assistant's responsibility to maintain the materials and mixing equipment and supplies.

Dental Cements

Dental cements are usually supplied in a powder/liquid form, a two-paste system, a capsule, or a dispensing syringe. Most of these materials are mixed manually, however a few of the powder/liquid cements are in capsules that are mixed mechanically. Cements are mixed in a precise ratio to attain a specific consistency, ranging from a liquid solution to a putty consistency.

Dental cements set or cure by either **self-curing** (chemical reaction between two materials) or with a curing light (**light-cured**). The light-cured materials are becoming very popular because the operator has more time to place and manipulate the materials before curing them. These materials are sensitive to overhead lights, however, and must be protected from light if dispensed ahead of time.

There are several terms used in conjunction with dental materials. Knowing these terms helps the dental assistant to understand the uses and functions.

- **Luting**—Bonding or cementing together. Dental cements may be used as luting agents to bond inlays, bridges, and so on to teeth.
- **Permanent luting cement**—A long-term cementing agent.
- **Temporary luting cement**—A short-term cementing agent.
- **Intermediate luting cement**—A material that lasts six months to a year.
- **Liner**—A material placed in a thin layer on the walls and floor of the cavity preparation. The liner protects the pulp from bacteria and irritants.
- **Base**—Applied in a putty or thick layer between the tooth and the restoration to protect the pulp from chemical irritation, temperature changes, electrical protection, and mechanical injury. Bases are strong enough to be placed under restorative materials and to support the materials from occlusal stresses.
- **Sedative** or **palliative effect**—Soothing effect a material may have on a tooth. The sedative or palliative material may relieve pain but does not provide a cure for the problem.
- **Varnish**—A thin layer of material that is placed to seal the walls and floor of the cavity preparation.

Uses of Dental Cements

There are many types of dental cements; each type of cement can have several uses. Some cements are combined with other materials to modify or expand their functions. Examples include reinforced zinc oxide eugenol cements and glass ionomers.

Zinc Phosphate Cement

Zinc phosphate cement is one of the oldest cements, and although it has some disadvantages, it is still a reliable choice for a luting and as a base cement. It is supplied in a powder/liquid form.

Manipulation Considerations. When the zinc phosphate powder is mixed with the liquid, an exothermic reaction occurs. Zinc phosphate cement is mixed on a cool glass slab to dissipate (spread) the heat of the mix. The slab is first cooled in cold water and then dried completely. (Any moisture left on the slab affects the properties of the cement.) The glass slab should be clean and free of scratches and dried cement. A stainless steel cement spatula is used to mix the powder into the liquid. The spatula also should be cool (Procedure 13–1).

PROCEDURE

13-1 Mixing Zinc Phosphate Cement

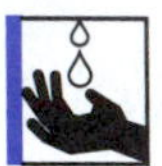 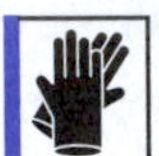 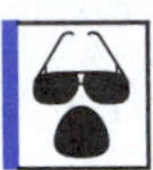

This procedure is completed by the dental assistant for the dentist. The equipment and materials are prepared and the material is mixed and passed to the dentist. Sometimes the dental assistant places the cement in the cast restoration while the dentist places material on the prepared tooth.

EQUIPMENT AND SUPPLIES

- Zinc phosphate powder and liquid (dispensers, if needed)
- Cooled glass slab
- Flexible stainless steel cement spatula
- 2 × 2 gauze sponge
- Timer
- Plastic filling instrument

PROCEDURE STEPS *(Follow aseptic procedures)*

1. Shake the powder to fluff it before removing the cap.
2. Place an appropriate amount of powder on one end of the slab. The amount of powder to be used is determined by the powder-liquid ratio and the amount of cement required for the procedure. For example, it would take less cement to cement a crown than a bridge.
3. Level the powder with the flat side of the spatula blade into a layer about 1 mm thick.
4. Divide the powder, according to the manufacturer's instructions, into two equal portions with the edge of the spatula; divide each of these portions into quarters, then two sections into eighths and one of the eighths into sixteenths.
5. Gently shake the liquid. Dispense the liquid from a dropper bottle onto the opposite side of the glass slab. Hold the liquid vertical while dispensing to produce uniform drops. Recap to avoid spilling and evaporating the liquid.
6. Incorporate one small portion of powder into the liquid, following specific manufacturer's directions on mixing times. Use the flat side of

the spatula blade to wet the powder particles (for about fifteen seconds).

7. Hold the spatula blade flat against the glass slab. Using a *wide sweeping motion,* spatulate the powder and liquid over a *large area of the glass slab.*
8. Adding small amounts of powder helps neutralize the acid, control the setting time, and achieve a smooth consistency of the mix. Incorporate each increment of powder thoroughly into the mix before adding more powder.
9. The mix appears watery at first and then, as more powder is incorporated, the mix will become creamy. Gather all particles of powder and liquid from around the edges of the mix from time to time.
10. Turn the spatula blade on edge and gather the mass to check the consistency.
11. Continue to add additional increments to the mix until the desired consistency is reached and within the prescribed time.
12. Gather the entire mass into one unit on the glass slab.
13. The consistency for luting (cementing) is creamy. It will follow the spatula for about one inch as it is lifted off the glass slab before breaking into a thin thread and flowing back into the mass.
14. The consistency of the base should be putty-like, and the base should be able to be rolled into a ball or cylinder with the flat side of the spatula.
15. Once the cement has been mixed to the desired consistency, wipe off the spatula with a 2 × 2 gauze. Hold the glass slab under the patient's chin, and pass the plastic filling instrument.
16. Wipe the spatula and the glass slab off with a moistened 2 × 2 gauze.
17. To clean the glass slab and spatula, soak them in water or a solution of bicarbonate of soda to loosen the hardened cement and then sterilize/disinfect accordingly.

Zinc Oxide Eugenol Cement

Zinc oxide eugenol cement, often referred to as ZOE, is another cement that has been used for many years. It is noted for its sedative or soothing effect on the dental pulp. The functions of this cement are diverse because of additives that enhance its properties. There are two types: **type I** is not as strong and is used for temporary restorations and cementation; **type II** has been reinforced and is stronger and can be used for permanent cementation (Procedure 13–2).

One of the type II zinc oxide eugenol cements is different from the rest in function. It is called an **intermediate restorative material (IRM).** This material is placed in the patient's mouth and lasts up to one year. This material is supplied in a powder/liquid form and in capsules. It is used when a tooth cannot be restored immediately, during illness, when the patient is moving, and because of economic reasons (Procedure 13–3).

Manipulation Considerations. Most zinc oxide eugenol materials are mixed on a paper pad with a stainless steel cement spatula. A glass slab may be used to control the setting time. Gently shake the powder before dispensing and swirl the liquid. These materials have specific powder dispensers and

13-2 Mixing Zinc Oxide Eugenol Cement: Powder/Liquid Form

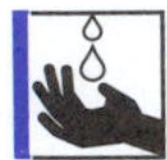 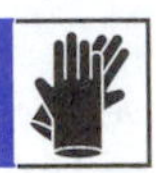 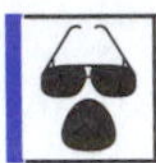

This procedure is completed by the dental assistant when the dentist signals. The equipment and materials are prepared and the material is mixed and passed to the dentist. The dental assistant follows the manufacturer's directions for specific information on proportions, incorporation technique, and the mixing and setting times.

EQUIPMENT AND SUPPLIES

- Zinc oxide eugenol cement
- Dispensers that go with the specific material
- Paper pad or glass slab
- Cement spatula
- Timer
- Plastic filling instrument
- 2 × 2 gauze sponges
- Alcohol or orange solvent

PROCEDURE STEPS *(Follow aseptic procedures)*

1. Fluff the powder before removing the cap.
2. Place the powder on the mixing pad according to manufacturer's directions. Replace the cap to avoid spilling and contamination.
3. After swirling, place the liquid on the paper pad. Hold the dispensing dropper perpendicular to the mixing pad and dispense the drops. Dispense near the powder but not touching it.
4. Incorporate the powder into the liquid in divided increments or all at once, according to manufacturer's directions.
5. Spatulate with the flat part of the blade and with an even pressure to wet all the particles of the powder. With some cements, a firm pressure is required to accomplish this.

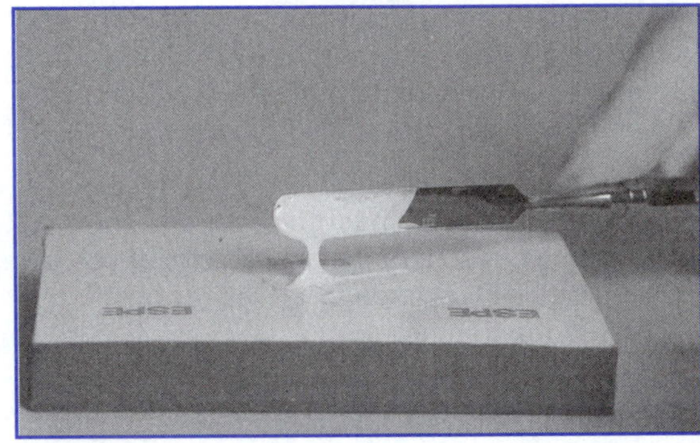

FIGURE 13–1 ZOE temporary luting cement's consistency.

6. Gather up the powder and liquid from the edges of the mix.
7. Gather up the entire mass into one unit on the slab to test the consistency.
8. The consistency for temporary luting will be creamy, like frosting (Figure 13–1).
9. The consistency for an insulating base or IRM will be putty-like and can be rolled into a ball or cylinder.
10. Once the material has been mixed to the desired consistency, wipe the spatula with a 2 × 2 gauze. Hold the pad under the patient's chin and pass the plastic filling instrument.
11. Receive the plastic filling instrument and wipe it off. The top page of the paper pad is removed and folded to prevent accidental contact with the cement.
12. To clean material that has hardened on the spatula or glass slab, wipe it with alcohol or orange solvent.

PROCEDURE

13-3 Mixing Zinc Oxide Eugenol Cement: Two-Paste System

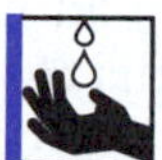
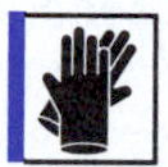
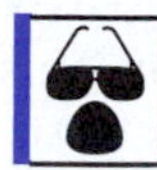

This material is often used for temporary luting of provisional coverage. The dental assistant dispenses and mixes the material according to manufacturer's directions. The dental assistant assists the dentist during the placement of the temporary. Sometimes the dental assistant places the cement in the provisional coverage of the tooth, if this procedure is included in expanded function regulations.

EQUIPMENT AND SUPPLIES

- Two-paste zinc oxide eugenol (accelerator and base)
- Paper pad
- Cement spatula
- 2 × 2 gauze sponge (moistened)
- Plastic filling instrument

PROCEDURE STEPS *(Follow aseptic procedures)*

1. Dispense the amount of material required for the procedure. This is equal lengths of the accelerator and the base. They usually are placed parallel to each other on the paper pad.
2. Gather the materials and mix into a homogenous mass. Spread over a small area, then gather. Repeat the process. The material should be a creamy mix that follows the spatula up for an inch (luting consistency).
3. Wipe both sides of the spatula and then gather all the material into one area.
4. Wipe off the cement spatula with the moist 2 × 2 gauze sponge.

liquid droppers. Care should be taken not to allow the eugenol into the rubber bulb of the dropper. The eugenol breaks down the rubber, thereby contaminating the liquid (Procedure 13–2 and 13–3).

The setting time ranges from three to five minutes in the oral cavity for most zinc oxide eugenol materials. They are mixed to either a luting or base consistency depending on the use and the specific material.

Polycarboxylate Cement

Polycarboxylate cement, also known as zinc polycarboxylate, is used for permanent cementation and as an insulating base. This cement is said to be "kind" to the pulp and was the first cement that had the ability to chemically bond to the tooth structure. There are several brands of polycarboxylate cement, and the cement is supplied in a powder/liquid form.

Manipulation Properties. Polycarboxylate cement is mixed on a paper pad or a glass slab with a stainless steel cement spatula. The powder is fluffed before the dispenser is used. The viscous liquid is dispensed from a squeeze bottle or a calibrated syringe. The liquid bottle is held perpendicular and squeezed until a drop begins to fall. The size of the drop varies because of this dispensing technique and the viscosity of the liquid. The syringe improves the accuracy of dispensing the liquid.

Polycarboxylate cements are mixed in thirty to sixty seconds and have a short working time of about three minutes. After this, the material loses its shine and becomes stringy or forms "cobwebs." At this point, the cement should not be used (Procedure 13–4).

3 PROCEDURE

13-4 Mixing Polycarboxylate Cement

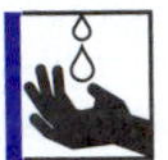
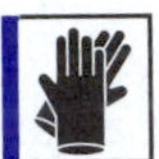
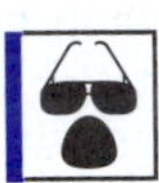

The dental assistant prepares and mixes the polycarboxylate materials to the desired consistency. The amount of material dispensed depends on the size of restoration and the number of units involved.

EQUIPMENT AND SUPPLIES

- Polycarboxylate powder and liquid and a dispenser for the powder
- Paper pad or glass slab
- Flexible stainless steel spatula
- 2 × 2 gauze sponge (moistened)
- Timer
- Plastic filling instrument

PROCEDURE STEPS *(Follow aseptic procedures)*

1. The powder is fluffed before dispensing with the dispensing scoop.
2. The powder is measured and dispensed on one side of a paper pad or a glass slab.
3. Uniform drops of liquid are placed toward the opposite side of the powder. Follow manufacturer's directions for the appropriate number of drops per scoop of powder.
4. Incorporate from three-fourths to all of the powder into the liquid and use a folding motion while applying some pressure to wet all the powder. Mix quickly until all the powder is incorporated. (Because the liquid is thick, it is harder to incorporate the powder.)
5. The mix will be slightly more viscous (sticky) than zinc phosphate cement and is glossy. Gather all the cement, wiping both sides of the spatula.
6. For luting consistency, the mix will follow the spatula up one inch.
7. For a base consistency, the same amount of powder is used, but the liquid ratio is decreased. The mix for the base should be glossy, but the consistency is tacky and stiff.
8. The mix must be used immediately before it becomes dull and stringy.
9. The cleanup is done immediately by wiping the spatula with a wet 2 × 2 gauze or by soaking the spatula with the dried cement in a 10 percent sodium hydroxide solution. The paper pad sheet is removed, folded, and disposed of. (Fold the paper pad to prevent touching the cement and spreading it onto instruments and the patient's face.)

Glass Ionomer Cement

Glass ionomer cement is one of the newer cement systems. This cement is diverse in its applications.

- **Type I**—A finer grain glass ionomer used for cementation of crowns and bridges because it chemically bonds to the tooth structure. Type I is also used for orthodontic bonding and pit and fissure sealant.
- **Type II**—A coarser grain glass ionomer that comes in various shades for use in selected restorations, such as Class III and V and pediatric restorations.
- **Type III**—Glass ionomer used as a liner and dentin bonding agent.
- **Type IV**—Reinforced or admixtures of glass ionomers. Silver or amalgam filings are combined with the glass ionomer material to be used for crown and core buildups.

Glass ionomer cements are supplied in numerous brands. Forms include powder/liquid, paste systems, syringes, and capsule forms, in both self-curing and light-curing materials.

Manipulation Considerations. Glass ionomer cements are mixed on a paper pad or a cool glass slab. Paper pads are preferred for easy cleanup; however glass slabs may be used to retard the setting action. The materials should be mixed quickly following manufacturer's directions because of the water content of the liquid. Water evaporation affects the properties of the cement.

Although many properties are the same as those of the polycarboxylate cements, the liquid of the glass ionomers is not as viscous and is therefore easier to dispense and mix. The powder is dispensed first, using the scoop and the amount indicated in the manufacturer's instructions. The liquid is dispensed just prior to manipulation. The mixing time is usually thirty to sixty seconds. The working time for the material is about two minutes.

The tooth must be completely isolated, cleaned, and dried before the cement is placed. The glass ionomer cement sets in the mouth in about five minutes (Procedure 13–5).

Calcium Hydroxide Material

Calcium hydroxide is a cement that is used as a low-strength base under any restoration. It is used for indirect or direct pulp capping procedures (near or direct pulp exposures). This material has a therapeutic effect on the pulp. The area is sealed with the calcium hydroxide so that secondary dentin may form.

Calcium hydroxide comes in powder/liquid, a two-paste system, or a one-paste system. The form many offices use is the two-paste system: catalyst and base. Calcium hydroxide comes in a self-curing and a light-curing formula.

PROCEDURE

13-5 Mixing Glass Ionomer Cement

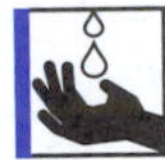 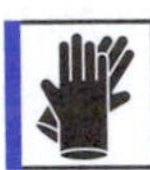 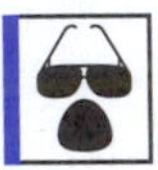

This procedure is completed by the dental assistant. The equipment and materials are prepared and mixed when the dentist indicates. The material must be used immediately after it is mixed. This material requires that the tooth be clean of debris and dry, so the dental assistant should rinse and evacuate and then isolate the area before beginning to mix the cement.

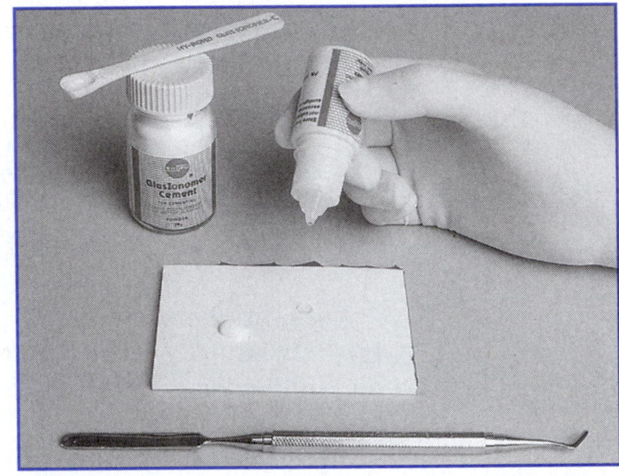

FIGURE 13–2 Dispensed glass ionomer powder and liquid.

EQUIPMENT AND SUPPLIES

- Glass ionomer materials and appropriate dispensers
- Paper pad or cool glass slab
- Flexible stainless steel spatula
- 2 × 2 gauze sponges (moistened)
- Timer
- Plastic filling instrument

PROCEDURE STEPS *(Follow aseptic procedures)*

1. Fluff the powder and, using the recommended scoops, place the appropriate number of scoops on the paper pad or glass slab.
2. Swirl the liquid and then place the specified number of drops on the pad near the powder. Replace the cap on the liquid immediately to prevent evaporation (Figure 13–2).
3. Divide the powder into halves or thirds and then draw the sections into the liquid one at a time.
4. Mix over a small area until all the powder is incorporated. The cement should be creamy and glossy for the luting consistency and tacky and stiff for the base consistency.
5. Once the cement has obtained the final consistency, wipe off the spatula with a 2 × 2 gauze. Hold the paper or glass slab under the patient's chin and pass the plastic filling instrument to the dentist.
6. To clean up, remove the top paper, fold it, and dispose of it. The instruments are wiped after use for easier cleanup.
7. Glass ionomer capsules are also available for use. They are activated by placement in an "activator" or dispenser to break the seal between the powder and liquid in the capsule.
8. The capsules are then placed in an amalgamator to be mixed (triturated) for a specific amount of time, usually ten seconds. Follow manufacturer's directions.
9. Insert the capsule in the appropriate dispenser and pass it to the dentist for dispensing the material needed.
10. To clean up, the capsule is discarded and the activator and the dispenser are disinfected.

PROCEDURE

13-6 Mixing Calcium Hydroxide: Two-Paste System

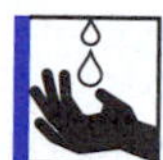
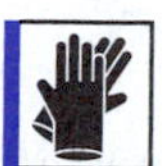
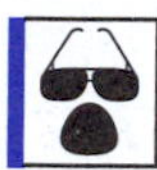

This material is dispensed and mixed by the dental assistant. It is often the first step in restoring the cavity preparation.

EQUIPMENT AND SUPPLIES

- Calcium hydroxide two-paste system
- Small paper pad
- Small ball-ended instrument or explorer
- 2 × 2 gauze sponge

PROCEDURE STEPS *(Follow aseptic procedures)*

1. Dispense small and equal amounts of both the catalyst and base onto the paper pad.
2. Wipe off the ends of the tubes and replace the caps.
3. Mix the two materials together using a circular motion.
4. Mix until the materials are a uniform color within the ten to fifteen second mixing time.
5. Use a 2 × 2 gauze to remove excess material from the mixing instrument.
6. Pass the instrument to the dentist and hold the paper pad close to the patient's chin.
7. Wipe off the instrument with a gauze for the dentist between applications.
8. Receive the instrument, wipe it off, tear and fold the top page of the paper pad, and dispose of it.

Manipulation Considerations. The two-paste system is mixed on a small paper pad with a metal spatula, an explorer, or a small ball-ended instrument. The base and the catalyst of the two-paste system come as a set and cannot be interchanged with those of other calcium hydroxide paste systems.

This material is dispensed in equal portions and mixed for ten to fifteen seconds. The setting times vary from two to seven minutes (Procedure 13–6).

Cavity Varnish

Cavity varnish is a material used to seal the dentinal tubules that are exposed during an amalgam cavity preparation. This thin liquid is placed on the surface of the dentin only. There are various types of varnish, and some come with solvents.

Manipulation Properties. Cavity varnishes are often placed in two layers for greater protection and to prevent voids. (Recap the varnish immediately to

PROCEDURE

13-7 Preparing Cavity Varnish

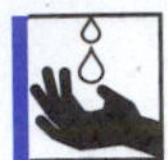 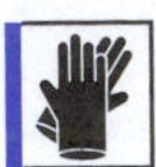 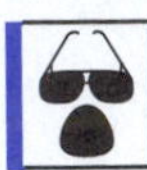

The materials needed for application of cavity varnish are prepared by the dental assistant. Depending on expanded function laws, the dental assistant applies the varnish or assists the dentist during placement.

EQUIPMENT AND SUPPLIES

- Cavity varnish and solvent
- Two cotton pliers
- Cotton pellets or pieces of cotton rolled into small, football-shaped balls, or a small brush
- Cotton roll

PROCEDURE STEPS *(Follow aseptic procedures)*

1. Clean and dry the cavity preparation.
2. Prepare cotton pellets for application of two layers of varnish. The pellets must be small to apply the varnish to the cavity preparation.
3. Remove the cap from the varnish bottle. Holding the two cotton pellets in the pliers, dip them into the varnish until they are moistened. Then, replace the cap on the varnish to prevent evaporation.
4. Place the cotton pellets on a 2 × 2 gauze and dab off the excess varnish.
5. Using one pellet, apply the varnish to the cavity preparation. Coat the surface of the preparation.
6. Allow the first coat to dry, and then apply a second coat in the same manner.
7. Dispose of the cotton pellets and clean the cotton pliers with solvent before sterilizing them.
8. To prepare the cotton pellets one at a time, two separate cotton pliers must be used to avoid contamination.

minimize evaporation of the varnish.) The cavity varnish comes with a separate bottle of solvent. If the varnish becomes too thick, solvent can be added. The solvent also can be used to clean the applicator and to remove any varnish on the external tooth surfaces.

Cavity varnish is not mixed; it is placed directly into the tooth preparation with one of various types of applicators such as small cotton pellets or brushes (Procedure 13–7).

Resin Cement

Resin cements have multiple uses with a wide variety of procedures, including permanent cementation of cast metal restorations and porcelain/resin restorations and veneers, orthodontic brackets, and endodontic posts. Resin cements may be supplied in a two-paste system, powder/liquid set, or syringe. The manufacturer may supply the **acid etchant** gel or liquid with the material. Some of these materials may be shaded to complement the translucency of the crown or inlay.

There are three types of resin cements: self-curing (chemical), light cured, and dual cured. **Dual-cured materials** contain chemicals for a self-curing as well as a light-curing reaction. Self-cured materials are used with metal or metal combination materials and endodontic posts; light-curing materials are used with porcelain/resin restorations, veneers, and orthodontic brackets.

Manipulation Considerations. Resin cements do not adhere to metal or ceramic materials; these materials must be roughened with etchants to produce mechanical bonding or the tissue surfaces of ceramics are treated with a silane coupling agent to produce a chemical bond with the resin cements. Sometimes, a wire mesh or undercuts may be added to the tissue side of the prosthesis to aid in retention.

Self-cured materials are supplied with an initiator and an activator. These are mixed on a paper pad for twenty to thirty seconds. Excess cement must be removed before the material is set completely to prevent any marginal leakage. Light-cured materials are supplied in syringes and must be cured for at least forty seconds. Dual-cured materials are supplied in two component systems that are mixed together for twenty to thirty seconds. Once mixed, these materials begin to set slowly, allowing for placement of the cement on the prosthesis and the prosthesis to be seated in the oral cavity. Once in position, the visible light unit is activated to harden the cement (Procedure 13–8).

Bonding Agents

Bonding agents are also known as **adhesives** and **bonding resins.** These materials are used to improve the retention between the tooth structure (enamel and dentin) and the restoration. These materials are supplied in many forms and are often complete systems (Figure 13–3). These materials bond enamel and dentin to porcelain, resins, precious and non-precious metals, composites, and amalgam.

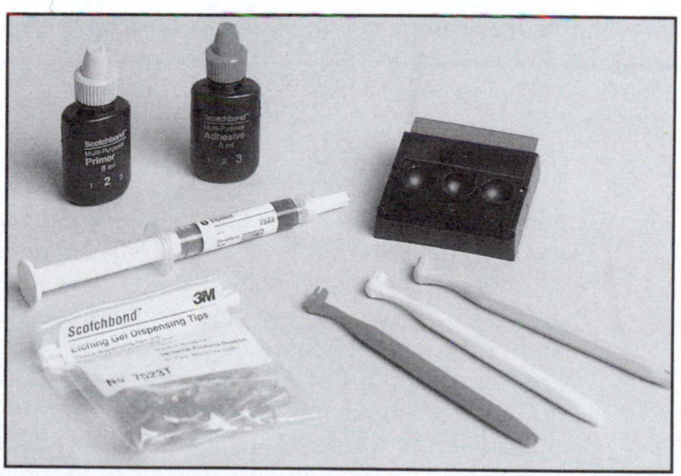

FIGURE 13–3 Bonding agents and systems.

PROCEDURE

13-8 Placing Resin Cement: Dual-Curing Technique

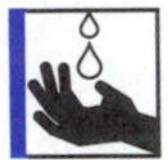 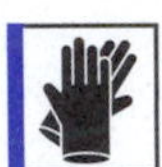 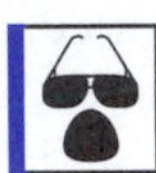

This procedure is done by the dental assistant for the dentist. The equipment and materials are prepared, and the material is mixed and passed to the dentist. Because this material is dual-curing, a curing light and eye protection are needed.

EQUIPMENT AND SUPPLIES

- Resin cement system
- Paper pad
- Stainless steel spatula
- Plastic filling instrument
- Curing light and protective shield or glasses
- 2 × 2 gauze sponges

PROCEDURE STEPS *(Follow aseptic procedures)*

1. Clean and dry the tooth and isolate the area with cotton rolls.
2. Pass the etchant to the dentist.
3. Wait the required time for the etchant and rinse the tooth thoroughly.
4. Lightly air dry the tooth and apply the adhesive.
5. Dispense and mix the two components together to a homogeneous, creamy mixture.
6. Hold the pad close to the patient and pass the placement instrument. The dentist places the material on the tooth and restoration.
7. Hold a 2 × 2 gauze to remove any excess materials.
8. Receive the placement instrument and prepare the curing light.
9. Either the dental assistant or the dentist holds the curing light and uses the protective shield when the light is activated.
10. Clean up immediately. Wipe any excess cement off the instruments and discard disposable items.

Bonding materials are low-viscosity resins that may or may not contain fillers. Some of the bonding agents contain additives with adhesive enhancers, and some contain fluoride. These materials are mainly light-cured or dual-cured.

Adhesion of dental materials to enamel and dentin is accomplished by acid etching with phosphoric acid. This solution alters the surface of the enamel and creates microscopic undercuts between the enamel rods and the dentin. Low-viscosity, unfilled resin bonding agents then penetrate into these undercuts and mechanically lock into them. The restorative material then bonds to this layer and becomes a solid unit (Procedure 13–9).

The acid etching process uses phosphoric acid solution. The etchant is supplied in liquid or gel form and is supplied in bottles or syringes. The liquids are

PROCEDURE

13-9 Placing Bonding Agent

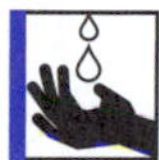 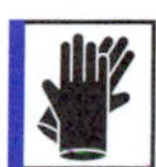 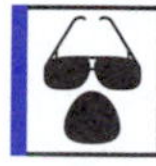

Steps in the application of bonding agents vary with manufacturers. The dental assistant prepares the materials for each step and keeps the area dry and free of debris.

EQUIPMENT AND SUPPLIES

- Bonding system that contains acid etchant, primer or conditioner, adhesive material
- Applicators (disposable tips or brushes)
- Dappen dish
- Isolation means
- Air-water syringe
- Curing light and shield
- Timer

PROCEDURE STEPS *(Follow aseptic procedures)*

1. If the cavity preparation is near the pulp, place calcium hydroxide or glass ionomer lining cement over the area.
2. The etchant is placed on the enamel and the dentin for the specified time, usually fifteen to twenty seconds. Usually, the etchant is placed on the enamel first and then the dentin, because the dentin is more sensitive to the etchant.
3. Rinse the tooth as soon as the time has lapsed. Continue to rinse for at least five to ten seconds. Move quickly to prevent bacterial contamination of the dentin.
4. If the bonding involves both the enamel and dentin, a primer step is included. The primer or conditioner is placed with a brush or an applicator. This material wets the dentin and penetrates the dentinal tubules.
5. The bonding resin is then applied, and the curing light is used to harden the material.
6. Cleanup involves disposing of applicator tips or brushes.

placed with small cotton pellets, sponges, brushes, or disposable applicators (Procedure 13–10).

RESTORATIVE DENTISTRY

Restorative dentistry, also known as operative dentistry, employs a variety of materials and techniques. There are many reasons why a tooth needs to be restored, including decay, fracture, abrasion, esthetics, and attrition. Restorative materials such as amalgam and composite are used to restore the tooth. These materials are called direct restorative materials because they are mixed and placed directly in the cavity preparation in one appointment.

PROCEDURE

13-10 Placing Etchant

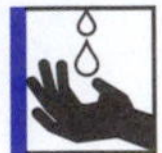
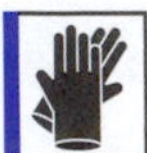
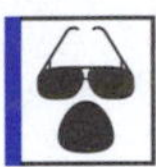

The dental assistant prepares the materials and isolates the area. The dentist places the etchant. When the allotted time has passed, the dental assistant thoroughly rinses the tooth.

EQUIPMENT AND SUPPLIES

- Acid etchant, usually a thirty to forty percent solution
- Isolation materials (dental dam or cotton rolls)
- Applicator (syringe, cotton pellets, or small applicator tips)
- Dappen dish
- Air-water syringe
- Timer

PROCEDURE STEPS *(Follow aseptic procedures)*

1. Isolate the area.
2. Clean the surface thoroughly.
3. Prepare the etchant applicator or syringe.
4. Place the etchant on the surface for fifteen to thirty seconds, following the manufacturer's directions.
5. Rinse the tooth after the designated time for fifteen to twenty seconds with the air-water syringe and evacuate thoroughly for ten to twenty seconds.

Note: The etched surface will have a frosty appearance. This surface needs to be isolated until the cementation is complete. If saliva or other fluids contact the surface, the etching process must be repeated.

Cavity Detection

Cavities can be detected with radiographs, probing with an explorer, or the use of a special dye. This dye detects caries by distinguishing between good, sound dentin and dentin that is infected with bacteria and softened. The dye is placed in the preparation early in the procedure to keep from removing too much tooth structure. The dye is applied for about ten seconds and then rinsed off. Burs and spoon excavators usually remove all the stained dentin. This process is repeated until no caries remain. This material also can be used to identify cracks and root canals.

Amalgam Restorative Materials

After the cavity has been prepared and the liners and bases have been placed, the tooth is ready to be restored. One of the most common restorative materials is dental **amalgam**, which has been used for many years. Dental amalgam is an effective, long-lasting, and comparatively inexpensive restorative material. Amalgam is a combination of an alloy with mercury. An **alloy** is the combination of two or more metals.

Dental amalgam is pliable when first mixed, so it is easily placed in the cavity preparation. It is carved before hardening to resemble tooth structure. This material is used on the posterior teeth because of its strength.

Mercury

Dental **mercury** is a very toxic chemical and must meet the specifications of the ADA. Dental professionals are aware of the hazards and safety measures when working with dental mercury to prevent problems from occurring.

Potential office hazards involving mercury can be eliminated by practicing appropriate mercury hygiene. The guidelines should include:

1. Wear disposable gloves, a face mask, and glasses when working with amalgam.
2. Educate all personnel regarding the potential hazards of mercury and good mercury hygiene practices.
3. A no-touch technique should be used when handling mercury. If the skin is exposed, wash with soap and water, and rinse under running water.
4. Use capsules containing a measured amount of mercury and alloy.
5. Use an amalgamator with a protective cover to reduce the likelihood of mercury vapor being released and to confine mercury that might be sprayed from an ill-fitting capsule.
6. Store mercury and amalgam scraps in capped, unbreakable jars containing used x-ray fixer, finely divided sulfur, glycerin, or mineral oil.
7. Carpeting in the dental treatment rooms is not recommended. Carpeting retains mercury, which is difficult to retrieve.
8. Use water spray and high-volume evacuation when cutting old amalgams or polishing new restorations. Wear PPE during these procedures.
9. Avoid working with mercury or amalgam near a heat source, such as the autoclave.
10. Handle mercury only over impervious surfaces. The area should have a continuous lip to retain any spillage.
11. The office should have proper ventilation to reduce the possibility of mercury vapor inhalation.
12. Office personnel should have periodic urinalyses to detect mercury in the body.
13. Monitor the dental office to determine mercury levels.
14. Keep a mercury spill kit if the office uses large quantities of mercury in the case of a spill. Clean up any mercury scraps or spills immediately, following OSHA recommendations.

Forms of Dental Alloy

Dental alloy is purchased in disposable capsule form. The **capsule** contains a premeasured amount of alloy and mercury and sometimes a **pestle.** The pestle, a small pellet, is made of metal or plastic and aids in the mixing of the alloy and mercury. In the capsule, a thin membrane separates the alloy and the mercury until they are mixed. Some capsules are supplied with activators to break the membrane or the capsules are twisted or compressed before being mixed.

Manipulation

Trituration is the mechanical method of combining (mixing) the dental alloy and mercury. **Amalgamation** is the actual chemical reaction that occurs between the alloy and the mercury to form the silver amalgam. Specially designed machines used to triturate (amalgamate) the alloy and mercury are called dental **amalgamators** or **triturators.** These machines have cradles to hold the capsules, cradle covers, timers, and variable speed controls. Trituration of the alloy and mercury is ten to fifteen seconds. This produces a homogeneous and uniform mix (Procedure 13–11).

PROCEDURE

13-11 Using the Dental Amalgamator (Triturator)

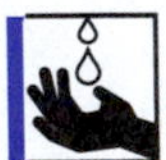
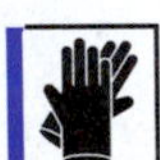
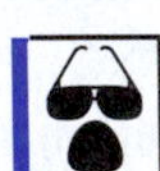

This procedure is completed by the dental assistant. The materials and equipment are prepared before the procedure begins.

EQUIPMENT AND SUPPLIES

- Amalgamator (triturator)
- Premeasured capsule of dental alloy and mercury
- Amalgam well, dappen dish, or squeeze cloth
- Amalgam carrier/condenser
- Scrap container for excess amalgam

PROCEDURE STEPS *(Follow aseptic procedures)*

1. Assemble materials for the procedure. Select trituration time and speed for the type of alloy and amalgamator.
2. Prepare the capsule by twisting the cap, squeezing the capsule, or using an activator.
3. Insert the capsule into the cradle (prongs) of the amalgamator. Place one end first, then slide the other end down into place. Practice placing the capsules into the cradle with one hand (Figure 13–4).
4. Close the cover of the amalgamator.

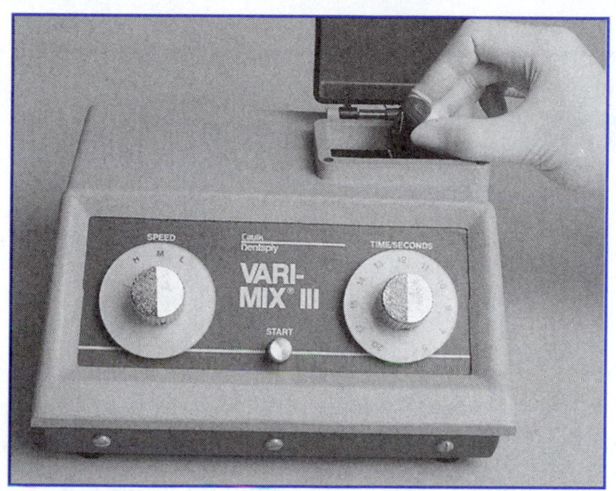

FIGURE 13–4 Placing capsule in the amalgamator.

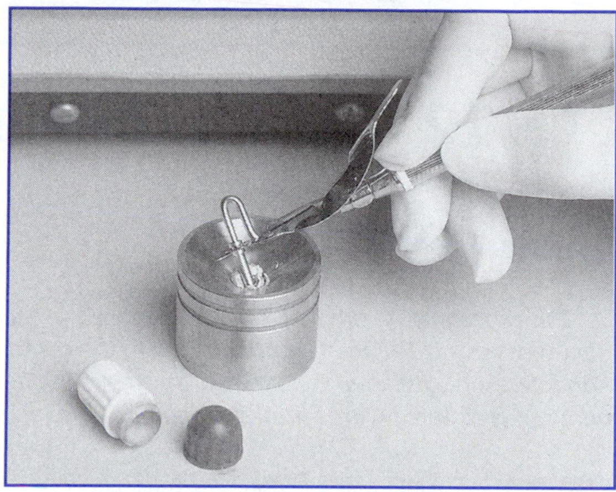

FIGURE 13–5 Loading an amalgam carrier.

5. Activate the amalgamator for the prescribed time and speed. (The timer will automatically switch off after the prescribed trituration time.)
6. Lift the cover and remove the capsule.
7. Open the capsule and empty the amalgam into an amalgam well. Avoid touching the amalgam with gloved hands. Use cotton pliers, if necessary. A well-mixed amalgam will have a glossy appearance with a smooth, velvety consistency.
8. Reassemble the capsule and place it to the side.
9. Hold the carrier and load the amalgam (Figure 13–5).
10. Pack the carrier, applying pressure so the cylinder is packed tightly. Wipe excess material from the end of the carrier on the sides of the amalgam well.
11. Pass the amalgam carrier to the dentist and prepare to exchange a condenser for the carrier. When practicing, dispense the amalgam from the carrier into a dappen dish and evaluate the mix. The cylinders of amalgam should be smooth and shiny.
12. Repeat loading and dispensing of all the material. Toward the end of the manipulation, the amalgam becomes harder to load into the carrier because it begins to set. This is the stage that takes practice to become proficient.
13. To clean up, expel any excess amalgam into the appropriate container. The instruments are cleaned and sterilized.

Complete Amalgam Procedure

The sequence of the procedure is for a complete amalgam restoration (Procedure 13–12). The steps include administrating anesthetic; placing the dental dam; placing liners and bases; assembling the matrix and wedge; and mixing, placing, condensing, and finishing the amalgam restoration. This gives the dental assistant an overall view of assisting during an amalgam procedure. Many of these steps, such as placing dental dam, are discussed in detail in other chapters because they can be performed by an expanded function dental assistant. (These steps are indicated with EF after the procedure.)

PROCEDURE

13-12 Amalgam Restoration: Class II

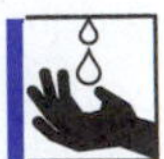
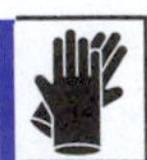
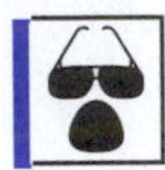

This procedure is completed by the dentist and the dental assistant. The tooth is prepared with the dental handpiece and assorted burs. Once the tooth is prepared, it is restored with dental amalgam.

EQUIPMENT AND SUPPLIES *(Figure 13–6)*

- Basic setup: mouth mirror, explorer, cotton pliers
- Air-water syringe tip, HVE tip, and saliva ejector
- Cotton rolls, gauze sponges, pellets, cotton tip applicators, and floss
- Topical and local anesthetic setup
- Dental dam setup
- High- and low-speed handpieces
- Assortment of dental burs
- Spoon excavator
- Hand cutting instruments (hatchets, chisels, hoes, and gingival margin trimmers)
- Base, liner, varnish
- Paper pad, cement spatula, and placement instrument
- Matrix retainer, matrix bands, and wedges
- Locking pliers or hemostat
- Amalgam capsules
- Amalgam well
- Amalgam carrier and condensers
- Amalgamator
- Carving instruments
- Articulating paper and forceps

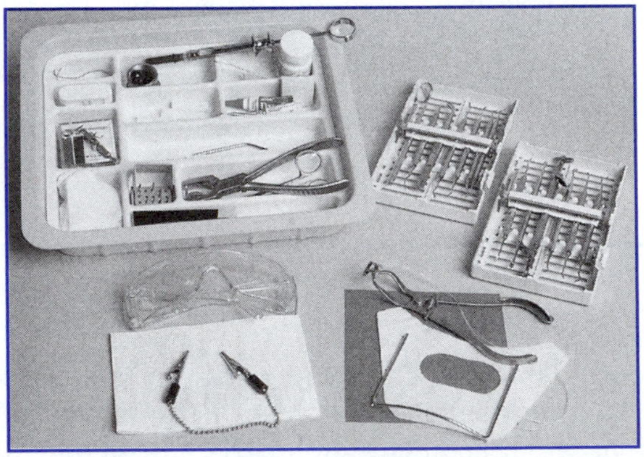

FIGURE 13–6 Amalgam procedure tray setup and armamentarium.

PROCEDURE STEPS *(Follow aseptic procedures)*

1. Greet and prepare the patient for the procedure. Review the medical history.
2. Prepare for the administration of the topical and local anesthetic. Dry the injection site and apply topical anesthetic (Expanded Function—EF). Prepare the syringe and summon the dentist. Transfer the mirror and explorer for the dentist to examine the tooth before beginning the procedure. When the dentist is ready, transfer a 2 × 2 gauze in one hand and the syringe in the other. The dentist replaces the needle cap and places the syringe on the tray. After the injection, rinse and evacuate the patient's mouth.
3. Prepare dental dam materials and equipment to assist the dentist in the placement (EF).

4. Transfer the mouth mirror and the high-speed handpiece with a bur. Position the HVE tip and maintain visibility throughout the procedure by retracting the cheek and tongue, keeping the mirror clear with the air-water syringe, and evacuating the site. Transfer and receive instruments at the dentist's signals. Instruments used at this point may include the explorer, the excavator, hatchets, hoes, angle formers, gingival margin trimmers, and chisels.
5. When the preparation is finished, transfer a cotton pellet with a cavity cleaning preparation to clean the inside of the tooth (EF). The area is then rinsed and dried. At the dentist's direction, mix the cavity liner (calcium hydroxide or glass ionomer), prepare the varnish and the base (glass ionomer, polycarboxylate, zinc phosphate, or modified ZOE), and transfer them to the dentist for placement. If the materials are light-cured, hold the light tip near the material to be cured and, with the protective shield in place, activate the light to cure the material.
6. Assemble the matrix retainer and the band into the correct position according to the tooth being restored and transfer it to the dentist (EF). After the matrix is placed, transfer the wedge in cotton pliers (locking is best) or in a hemostat. The dentist places the wedge.
7. When the dentist is ready, prepare the amalgam capsule by twisting the cap, squeezing the capsule together, or placing it in an activator, then placing the capsule in the amalgamator. The amalgamator is set for the specific type of amalgam material and the size of the mix. When the amalgam material has been mixed, remove the capsule from the amalgamator and place it in the amalgam well or a dappen dish. The amalgam is loaded into the amalgam carrier. If the carrier is double ended, both ends are filled and the loaded carrier is passed to the dentist. The carrier and the condenser are used alternately until the restorative material fills the cavity. In some offices, the dental assistant loads the carrier and, at the dentist's direction, places the amalgam into the cavity preparation, eliminating the exchanging of instruments and allowing the dentist to focus on the condensing of the amalgam. After the last exchange, transfer the dentist an explorer to loosen amalgam from the matrix band. While the dentist is using the explorer, clean up any amalgam scraps from the carrier and the well and place them in a sealed container.
8. Receive the explorer and transfer carving and finishing instruments at the dentist's signals. Operate the HVE tip near the site to evacuate amalgam particles. After the dentist completes the preliminary carving, pass the cotton pliers to remove the wedge and then receive the wedge, pliers, and matrix retainer. The cotton pliers may be used again to remove the matrix band. Receive the cotton pliers and band and then transfer the carver of the dentist's choice for finishing the carving of the anatomy in the restoration.
9. The dental dam is carefully removed at this time (EF). Transfer the clamp forceps, receive the forceps with the clamp, and transfer scissors to cut the interseptal dam. Receive the scissors, frame, napkin, and dam material. Rinse and evacuate the patient's mouth.
10. Dry the area and transfer the articulating paper, positioned on the forceps, to the dentist. The assistant may be instructed by the dentist to place the articulating paper over the restoration. The patient is instructed to gently tap the teeth together. Additional carving and checking the occlusion are continued until the dentist is satisfied and the patient is comfortable.
11. The restoration is wiped off with a wet cotton roll to remove any blue marks left by the articulating paper. Rinse and evacuate the patient's mouth thoroughly and clean any debris from the patient's face. The patient is cautioned not to chew on the side of the restoration for a few hours and is then dismissed.

Composite Restorative Materials

Composite restorative materials dominate the field of esthetic restorations. These materials have natural appearances and were used primarily for anterior restorations but are being developed as esthetic restorations for posterior teeth.

Technology is expanding the types of materials available as alternatives to dental amalgam. With concerns over the mercury in amalgam and the desire for a natural appearance of teeth, there is ongoing research and development with composite restorative materials. Composites, glass ionomers, and porcelain materials are used for esthetic restorations.

These direct restorative materials are inserted into the cavity preparation and then self-cured, light-cured, or dual-cured. They are supplied in syringes or single-application cartridges (**compules**) and have a variety of shades or shade modifiers. The location and the size of the cavity determines which material the dentist chooses.

Manipulation Considerations

Shrinkage of composites can be minimized by placing the composite in small layers in the cavity preparation. After each layer is placed, it is light cured to the hardened form. The layering of the composite is also a method to modify the shade of the restoration. The layers can be composed of different types of composites with varying properties to enhance the qualities of the material (Procedure 13–13).

Composites are packaged as one-paste systems that are light cured. The paste may be supplied in a syringe for multiple applications or in single-dose cartridges that are used with a syringe. The pastes also come in a variety of shades. A specific shade guide comes with the composite systems to assist in the selection of a shade that matches the patient's natural dentition.

The pulp is protected with a cavity liner before the acid etching, bonding, and composite placement steps.

Glass Ionomer Restorations

Type II glass ionomer materials are used as an esthetic restoration most often in nonstress-bearing restorations. Examples include restoring the gingival one-third and root surface cavities. These materials are not suitable for areas that require strength or where esthetics are critical.

Resin Ionomers

The combination of the composite resins and glass ionomers have improved the qualities of the glass ionomer restorations. They are used for Class III and V restorations. They are supplied in various shades and are light-cured materials.

The technique for placement is similar to that for composites, with the following exceptions. The tooth is conservatively prepared with no need for

PROCEDURE

13-13 Composite Restoration: Class III

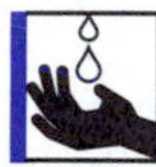
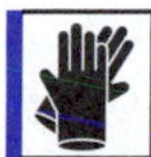
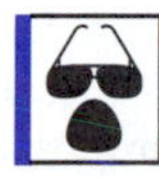
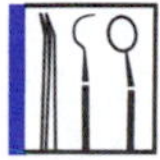

This procedure is completed by the dentist and the dental assistant. The tooth is prepared with the dental handpiece and assorted burs. After the tooth is prepared, it is restored with composite.

EQUIPMENT AND SUPPLIES *(Figure 13–7)*

- Basic setup: mouth mirror, explorer, cotton pliers
- Air-water syringe tip, HVE tip, and saliva ejector
- Cotton rolls, gauze sponges, cotton pellets, cotton tip applicators, and dental floss
- Topical and local anesthetic setup
- Dental dam setup
- High- and low-speed handpieces
- Assortment of dental burs (including diamond and cutting burs)
- Spoon excavator
- Hand cutting instruments (dentist's choice may include binangle chisel and Wedelstaedt chisel)
- Base and liner with mixing materials and placement instruments
- Etchant and applicator, if necessary (usually supplied with composite system)
- Primer (usually supplied with composite system)
- Composite materials, including a shade guide
- Composite placement instrument (plastic filling instrument)
- Curing light with protective shield
- Celluloid matrix strip and wedges
- Locking pliers or hemostat
- Finishing burs or diamonds
- #12 scalpel
- Abrasive strips
- Polishing discs
- Lubricant
- Articulating paper and forceps

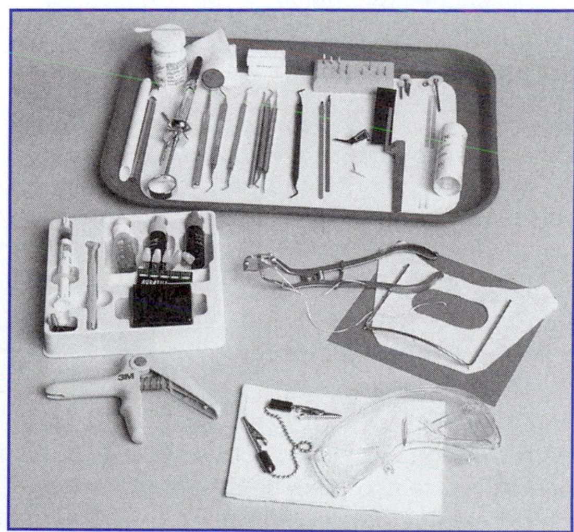

FIGURE 13–7 Composite procedure tray setup.

PROCEDURE STEPS *(Follow aseptic procedures)*

1. The patient is seated and prepared for the procedure. Confirm the procedure and review the medical history.
2. Rinse the patient's mouth, dry the injection site, and place the topical anesthetic (EF). Prepare the syringe. When the dentist enters, remove the topical anesthetic applicator and transfer the mouth mirror and explorer to the dentist. After receiving the mirror and explorer, the anesthetic syringe is transferred to the operator. Following the administration of the local anesthetic, rinse the patient's mouth.

(continued)

3. The shade is determined for the composite material before the placement of the dental dam. Under natural light, the dentist compares a shade guide to the patient's teeth. A shade or combination of shades is selected to match the patient's teeth as closely as possible. The shade is recorded on the patient's chart for further reference.
4. The dental dam is placed by the dental assistant or with the dental assistant helping the dentist.
5. Transfer a mirror, high-speed handpiece, and bur to the dentist. Maintain visibility throughout the procedure by cleaning the mirror, retracting the tissues, and evacuating the area. During the cavity preparation, transfer instruments and change burs as indicated by the dentist.
6. When the cavity preparation is complete, rinse and dry the preparation. How close to the pulp the cavity preparation is determines the type of base or liner needed for protection. Mix the appropriate materials, usually a calcium hydroxide or glass ionomer liner, and hold the mixing pad, applicator, and 2 × 2 gauze near the patient's chin. After each application, wipe the instrument. If the materials need the light for the curing process, the curing light is prepared and positioned.
7. Transfer a brush or applicator tip containing the acid etching materials to the dentist, who applies it to the cavity preparation. The etchant is rinsed thoroughly after the recommended time.
8. The celluloid matrix strip is placed by the dentist. If required, a plastic wedge is also placed (the plastic wedges permit light curing of the bonding agent and the composite).
9. The bonding material is placed according to manufacturer's instructions. With some bonding resins, a **primer** or conditioner is placed before the bonding material.
10. Most composites are applied in a single-application syringe, which can be used to place the material directly into the cavity preparation. Sometimes, a composite placement instrument is used for placement. The matrix is held around the tooth to restore contour. If the material is light cured, it is placed in incremental layers and light cured after each layer is placed. The self-curing composites are mixed and placed in the cavity preparation. Within a few minutes, the material begins to chemically set.
11. Transfer cotton pliers to remove the wedge and the matrix strip. After receiving these items, an explorer is transferred to examine the restoration.
12. Transfer the low-speed handpiece with finishing bur to the dentist. When the dentist is using the handpiece, use the air syringe. Finishing burs, diamonds, and abrasive discs may be used to finish the composite restoration. Abrasive strips may be used to smooth the interproximal areas. Composite polishing points, discs, and cups are then used to smooth the restoration.
13. The dental dam is removed carefully and the oral cavity is rinsed.
14. Transfer the mirror and explorer to the dentist for examination, dry the tooth, receive the mirror and explorer, and pass the articulating paper. The occlusion is checked and any high marks are removed. The patient's mouth is rinsed and the patient is given postoperative instructions.

mechanical retention or bevels. A retraction cord may be placed with the Class V preparations to expose the entire margin of the cavity preparation. The preparation is cleaned with a chlorhexidine soap solution. Follow the manufacturer's directions on the finishing and polishing of the restoration. Some need to be kept moist or have lubricants placed when polishing. A layer of light-cured enamel bonding agent is applied over the finished restoration.

CHAPTER 14

Laboratory Materials and Techniques

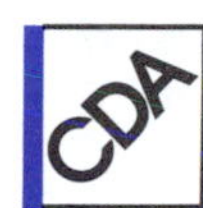

OBJECTIVES

The student should strive to meet the following objectives and demonstrate an understanding of the facts and principles presented in this chapter:

1. Identify the materials used in the dental laboratory and perform the associated procedures.
2. Demonstrate the knowledge and skills needed to prepare, take, and remove alginate impressions and wax bites.
3. Demonstrate the knowledge and skills necessary to prepare elastomeric impression materials such as polysulfide, silicone (polysiloxane and polyvinyl siloxanes), and polyether for the dentist.
4. Demonstrate the knowledge and skills necessary to use gypsum products such as Type I: Impression plaster; Type II: Laboratory or model plaster; Type III: Laboratory stone; Type IV: Die stone; and Type V: High-strength die stone.
5. Demonstrate the knowledge and skills necessary to pour and trim an alginate impression (diagnostic cast).
6. Identify the classifications and uses of waxes used in dentistry.
7. Demonstrate the knowledge and skills necessary to fabricate acrylic tray resin self-curing and vacuum-formed trays.

KEY TERMS

articulator (p. 246)
distortion (p. 230)
exothermic reaction (p. 236)
gypsum (p. 236)
homogenous (p. 250)
imbibition (p. 223)
irreversible hydrocolloid (p. 222)
polysulfide (p. 231)
silicones (p. 232)
syneresis (p. 223)
undercuts (p. 223)

Introduction

Numerous materials are used by dental assistants in the dental laboratory that are not used in the dental treatment room. Some other materials are used initially in the treatment room and then taken by the dental assistant to the laboratory, where a second procedure is completed. Many of the models are taken to an in-office dental laboratory, where the laboratory technician completes the procedures or the models are sent out to a commercial dental laboratory for additional procedures to be completed.

Any dental assistant who has skills in performing laboratory duties is an asset to his or her employer. The better cross-trained the dental team members are, the better the dental office functions. A number of basic functions in the dental laboratory are routinely performed by the dental assistant, such as pouring and trimming study models, fabricating custom trays, and fabricating provisional temporaries. To accomplish these procedures, the dental assistant must understand the materials that are used, the properties of each material, and the steps in each procedure.

Hydrocolloid Impression Materials

Impressions are taken to reproduce an accurate three-dimensional duplicate of a patient's teeth and surrounding tissues. The impression makes a negative reproduction where gypsum material can be poured to create a completed positive model. Varying degrees of accuracy can be obtained depending on the type of impression material and gypsum used. The operator gives directions to the dental assistant on the type of model that is desired. Models can be used for many purposes. One of the most common models the dental assistant makes is the study cast or primary model. Most often, the impression material used is irreversible hydrocolloid, which is commonly called alginate.

Alginate (Irreversible Hydrocolloid) Impression Material

Alginate is a generic name used for a group of **irreversible hydrocolloid** impression materials. Alginate is used when less accuracy is needed. One of the most common areas in which alginate is used is in making diagnostic casts or study models. Alginate impression material is used routinely in making opposing models for fixed and removable prosthetics, orthodontic appliances, mouth guards, bleach trays, provisional restorations, and custom trays.

Advantages and Disadvantages of Alginate. Alginate has a number of advantages that allows it to be widely used in the dental office. They include:

- Ease of manipulation
- Minimal equipment required
- Economical
- Meets the requirements for accuracy for a number of applications
- Rapid setting
- Comfort for the patient
- Can be used for both teeth and tissue impressions
- Withdraws over **undercuts** (recessed areas that are wider on the bottom than on the top) due to its elastic properties

The disadvantages of alginates primarily come from the loss of accuracy due to atmospheric conditions. If the impression is stored prior to pouring, it is susceptible to dimensional change due to loss or gain of water. If the impression loses water content due to heat, dryness, or exposure to air, it causes shrinkage. This condition is known as **syneresis** (sin-er-**EE**-sis). If the reverse happens and the impression takes on additional water and causes swelling, the impression will have a dimensional enlargement, known as **imbibition** (im-bah-**BIH**-shun). The material also can cause some tissue distortion due to its thickened consistency.

Setting Time for Alginate. The time from which the alginate powder material is mixed with water until it is completely set is called the **gelatin time.** The gelatin time differs depending on the type of material used. Most of the materials are supplied in two types: Type I is a fast-set alginate and Type II is a regular-set alginate. The gelatin time for both is broken into two different increments. First is the working time, where the dental assistant mixes the material to the desired consistency, loads it into the tray, and inserts and positions the tray into the patient's mouth. The working time for the regular set is approximately one minute and less than that for fast set. The second phase is the setting time, where the material remains in the patient's mouth and sets until the chemical reaction is completed, the gel is formed completely, and the tray is removed from the patient's mouth. Type I for both the working and setting times ranges from one to two minutes. Type II normally ranges from two to four and one-half minutes for both working and setting times. The setting times can be altered. The most convenient way to control the setting time is to adjust the temperature of the water. The suggested temperature of water to be used is room temperature (70°F or 21°C). If the temperature of the water is higher, there are shorter working and setting times. If the water is cooled, the working and setting times are longer. Warm weather causes the alginate to set more rapidly as well. Some offices refrigerate the water during hot humid weather.

Alginate Powder/Water Ratio. All the alginate materials are supplied with their own specific measuring devices for both the powder and the water. First, read the manufacturer's directions for dispensing the material. The dispensing of each material may be slightly different. For example, some materials direct that the powder be fluffed with the lid on prior to putting it into the powder scoop, while others may indicate that the powder should be packed into the scoop. This makes a significant difference in the amount of powder used. The water measure is usually a plastic cylinder with lines on it to indicate the amount of water for each scoop of powder. Usually it takes two scoops of powder to two increments of water for each mandibular impression. Three of each is normally needed for the maxillary impression. (These may alter depending on the size of the patient's arches.)

It is important that the correct amounts of both powder and water are used. If a lower water-to-powder ratio transpires, a stiffer, thicker mix is produced. Along with being more difficult to use, the material has decreased detail, decreased ability to pull from undercuts, decreased flexibility, increased tissue displacement, rapid setting time, increased strength, and a mix that is not as uniform in consistency. If a higher water-to-powder ratio is used, the impression has a decreased resistance to deformation, decreased strength, and increased setting time. Both increases and decreases in spatulation affect the setting time and decrease the strength of the material.

Trays Used for Alginate Impressions. Several types of trays are available for taking alginate impressions. Those most commonly used are perforated trays made of metal or plastic. The perforations allow the material to ooze through and lock the impression material in the tray.

The operator must make sure that the tray fits correctly in the patient's mouth. Selecting the correct tray is essential to obtain an accurate impression. The trays are made in several sizes. The operator first examines the patient's mouth and identifies a sterilized or disposable tray he or she thinks will fit (Procedure 14–1). The trays should be tried in the patient's mouth to ensure a correct fit and the proper comfort for the patient. The tray should extend 2 or 3 mm beyond the last molar area and below both the lingual and facial tooth surfaces. Keep in mind that there should be enough room for 2 mm of the alginate material between the tray and all surfaces of the teeth and tissue.

Taking Alginate Impressions for Diagnostic Casts (Study Models). In some states, dental assistants are allowed to take the alginate impressions (Procedure 14–2, 14–3, and 14–4). In other states, the dental assistant can select the tray, mix the material, load the material into the tray, and pass the tray for the dentist to place in the patient's mouth.

P R O C E D U R E

14-1 Preparing for an Alginate Impression

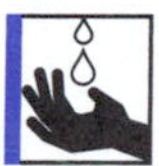 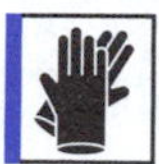 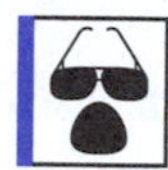

This procedure is performed by the dental assistant in the states where it is allowed. The materials are prepared and the alginate impression is taken on the maxillary and mandibular arches.

EQUIPMENT AND SUPPLIES

- Flexible spatula/broad blade or disposable spatula
- Flexible rubber bowl(s) or disposable bowl
- Alginate material with water and powder measuring devices
- Water
- Impression tray(s) and wax

PROCEDURE STEPS *(Follow aseptic procedures)*

Patient Preparation

1. Health history is reviewed.
2. The patient is seated in an upright position with a patient napkin in place.
3. The patient's mouth is rinsed with water or mouth rinse to remove any food debris and reduce thick saliva.
4. The procedure is explained to the patient.
5. The impression trays are tried in the oral cavity to determine the correct size.

Material Preparation

1. Wax is placed around the borders of the impression trays, if necessary, to extend the borders of the trays or to provide additional patient comfort.
2. The impression water (room temperature) is measured for the mandibular model, normally two calibrations of the water measurement device supplied by the manufacturer. The water is placed in the flexible mixing bowl. NOTE: Place the water in the bowl first to ensure that all the powder is incorporated into the mixture.
3. Fluff the powder prior to opening the powder canister, if the manufacturer's directions indicate.

Taking the mandibular model first allows the patient to build confidence and feel more secure prior to the maxillary impression, which often causes more gagging.

4. Fill the measure of powder by overfilling and then leveling off with the spatula (use the flat blade, not the edge blade of the spatula) to get an accurate measure. Dispense two corresponding scoops into a second flexible rubber bowl.
5. When ready, place the powder in the water.
6. Mix the water and powder first with a stirring motion. Then, mix by holding the bowl in one hand, rotating the bowl occasionally, and using the flat side of the spatula to incorporate the material through pressure against the side of the bowl (Figure 14–1). The mixing for Type I fast set is thirty to forty-five seconds; Type II regular set is one minute.
7. Upon completion, the mixture should be homogeneous and creamy. When the material is mixed thoroughly, load it into the impression tray. On the mandibular tray, the material should be loaded from both lingual sides. Use the flat side of the blade to condense the material firmly into the tray. If necessary to further smooth the surface, take a gloved hand, moisten, and smooth the top.

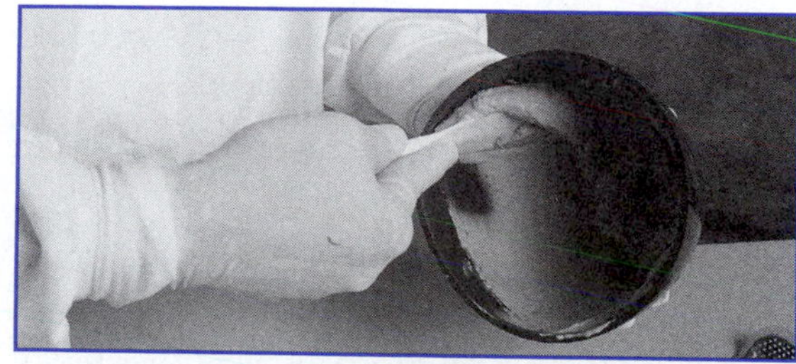

FIGURE 14–1 Mixing the alginate material in a flexible rubber bowl, pushing on the sides of the bowl to eliminate the incorporation of air bubbles.

PROCEDURE

14-2 Taking an Alginate Impression

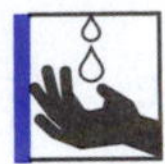 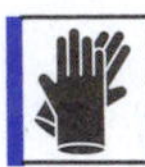 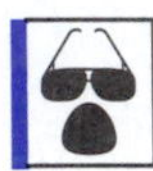

Refer to Procedure 14–1, Preparing for an Alginate Impression, to identify the needed PPE, equipment, and supplies.

PROCEDURE STEPS *(Follow aseptic procedures)*

1. Facing the patient, retract the right cheek slightly.
2. Use the excess alginate material to rub onto the occlusal surfaces of the teeth to obtain more accurate anatomy.
3. Invert the impression tray so that the material is toward the teeth.
4. Turn the tray so that it passes through the lips with one side of the tray entering first, using the other hand to retract the opposite corner of the mouth.
5. When the tray is completely in the patient's mouth, center it above the teeth.
6. Lower the tray onto the teeth, placing the posterior area down first, leaving the impression tray slightly anterior.
7. Have the patient raise the tongue and move it side to side to ensure that the lingual aspect of the alveolar process is defined in the impression.
8. Retract the lip using the other hand.
9. Complete seating the impression tray, pushing it slightly toward the posterior of the mouth with the tray. This guides the impression material down into the patient's anterior vestibule to produce an esthetic model that captures the necessary anatomy. One area that often lacks full detail in an alginate impression is the anterior segment. Leaving the tray slightly anterior and pushing it gently toward the posterior, while keeping the lips out of the way, helps correct this problem.
10. Allow the lip to cover the tray, close to the handle.
11. Hold the tray in the patient's mouth using two fingers on the back of the tray, one on the right side and one on the left, until the alginate has set. Periodically check the excess material around the edges of the impression tray or in the bowl to determine when the material has set. The alginate should feel firm and not change shape when pushed. When torn, it should break free without resistance. When set, remove impression (Procedure 14-3).
12. Load the maxillary alginate impression tray from the posterior, making sure the material completely fills the tray, free of voids (Figure 14–2A). Smooth the material using an index finger (Figure 14–2B). Remove a small amount of alginate from the palatal area to prevent the alginate from oozing down the patient's throat upon insertion (Figure 14–2C). Smear a small amount of excess alginate on the occlusal surfaces of the maxillary teeth with an index finger.
13. Insert the maxillary tray into the patient's mouth by turning the tray so it passes through the lips with one side of the tray entering first, using the other hand to retract the opposite corner of the mouth (Figure 14–2D). Raise the tray to the maxillary arch and retract the lip prior to seating the tray. Hold the tray in position until the material in the bowl has set (Figure 14–2E). When set, remove impression from the mouth (Procedure 14-3).

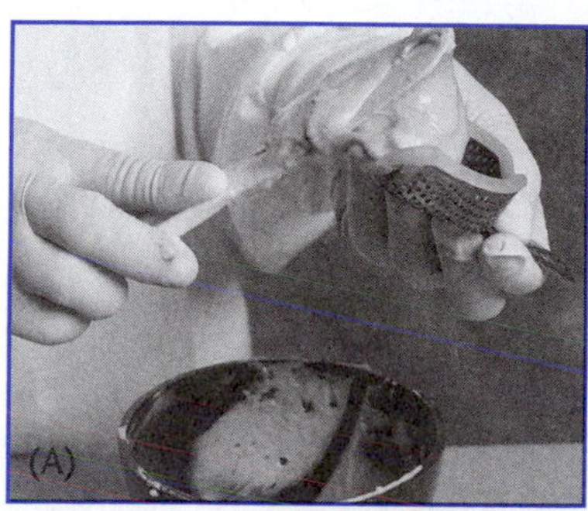
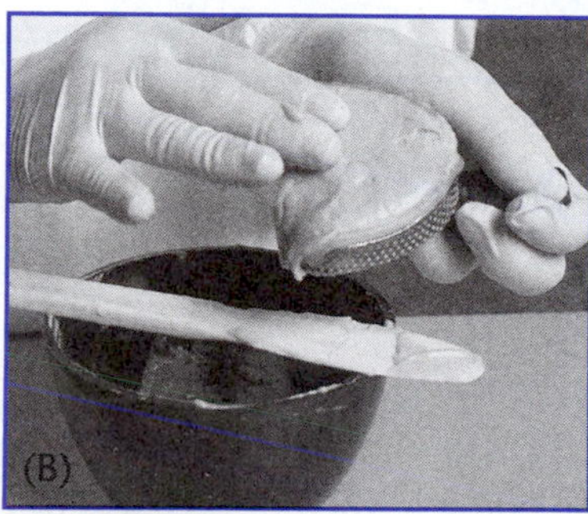
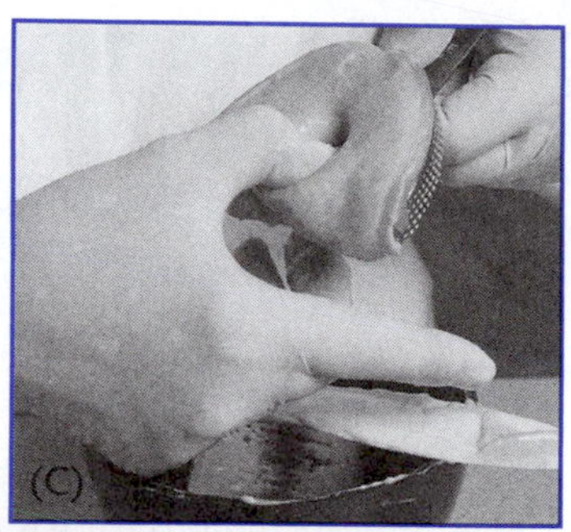
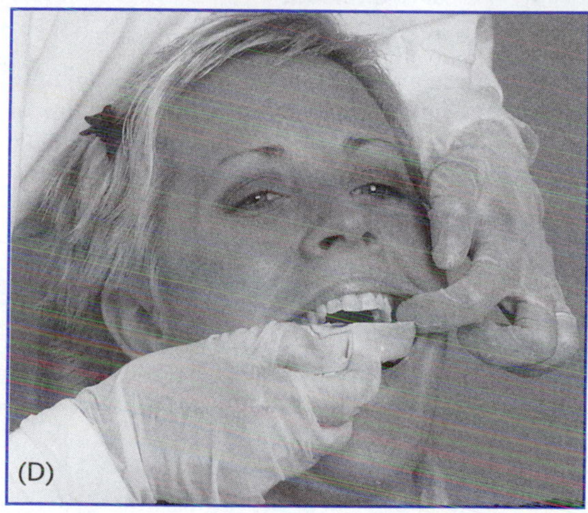
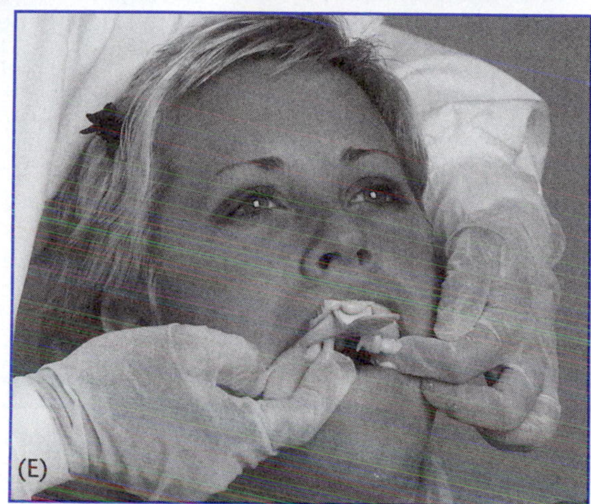

FIGURE 14–2 (A) Load the maxillary alginate tray from the posterior area. (B) Smooth the impression material using the fingers. (C) Remove a small amount of the alginate from the palatal area prior to seating the tray in the patient's mouth. This prevents the alginate material from oozing down into the back of the patient's throat. (D) Insert the impression tray into the patient's mouth. (E) Hold the tray in position until the impression material has set.

Accuracy of an Alginate Impression

- The tray covers all the necessary areas.
- The tray is centered on the central incisors.
- The tray is not pushed down or up too far, allowing the teeth to penetrate through the material to the tray.
- The impression is not torn.
- The impression is free of bubbles and voids.
- The impression shows sharp anatomic detail of all the teeth and tissues.
- The impression has a sufficient peripheral roll and includes all the vestibular areas.
- The mandibular impression shows sharp detail in the retromolar areas and shows the lingual frenum and the mylohyoid ridges.
- The maxillary impression shows sharp detail in the tuberosities and palate.

PROCEDURE

14-3 Removing the Alginate Impression

Refer to Procedure 14–1, Preparing for an Alginate Impression, to identify the needed PPE, equipment, and supplies.

PROCEDURE STEPS *(Follow aseptic procedures)*

1. When the material has completely set, remove it from the mouth by first loosening the tissue of the lips and cheek around the periphery with fingers to break the suctionlike seal.
2. Place fingers of the opposing hand on the opposite arch to protect the adjacent arch as the tray is removed.
3. Remove the tray in an upward or downward motion (depending on the arch) with a quick snap. Turn it to the side to allow it to be removed from the oral cavity.
4. Remove excess alginate material from the patient's mouth with the evacuator and have the patient rinse. Check the patient's face for excess alginate material. If present, give the patient a tissue and mirror to remove the material.
5. Check the impression for accuracy.
6. Rinse the impression gently with water to remove saliva or blood.
7. Spray with approved surface disinfectant.
8. If there is a time lapse (maximum of twenty minutes) prior to pouring, wrap the alginate impression in an airtight container or a moist towel and place it in a plastic bag labeled with the patient's name. If the impression is placed in a wet towel for an extended time, imbibition (taking up of additional moisture) may occur.

PROCEDURE

14-4 Disinfecting Alginate Impressions

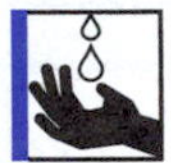
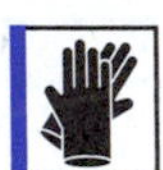
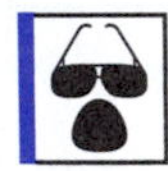

This procedure is performed by the dental assistant immediately after removing alginate impressions from the patient's mouth and caring for the patient.

EQUIPMENT AND SUPPLIES

- Approved disinfectant
- Covered container or resealable plastic sandwich bag

PROCEDURE STEPS *(Follow aseptic procedures)*

1. Rinse the impressions gently under tap water to remove any debris, blood, or saliva.
2. Spray the impressions with an approved disinfectant (See Chapter 6, Infection Control).
3. If not pouring immediately, place the impressions in a covered container or resealable plastic sandwich bag.
4. Label the container or resealable plastic sandwich bag with the patient's name.

Wax Bite Registration

A wax bite registration is taken to establish the occlusal relationship between the maxillary and mandibular teeth (Procedure 14–5). It is used to verify the occlusal relationship when trimming diagnostic casts (study models). The wax is usually folded and formed in the shape of a horseshoe; however, flat sheets of utility wax may also be used to take a bite registration.

Other materials may be used to register a patient's bite. Polysiloxane impression material, specifically designed for occlusal registration, is extruded directly onto the patient's occlusal surfaces using a dispensing gun and cartridge tip. The patient is asked to close the teeth together in the normal biting position and to remain closed until the material sets; this usually takes two minutes. The set material is then removed, disinfected, stored with the patient's other laboratory case materials, and used to establish the patient's occlusal relationship.

PROCEDURE

14-5 Taking a Bite Registration

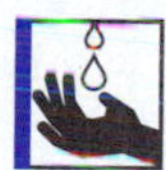
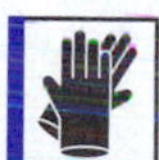
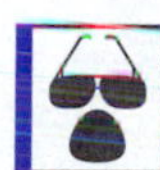

This procedure is performed by the dental assistant under the direction of the dentist or by the dentist with the dental assistant assisting.

EQUIPMENT AND SUPPLIES

- Bite registration wax or wax horseshoe or polysiloxane and extruder gun and disposable tips
- Laboratory knife
- Warm water or torch

PROCEDURE STEPS *(Follow aseptic procedures)*

1. The patient remains seated in an upright position with a patient napkin in place after the impressions are taken.
2. The procedure is explained to the patient.
3. The bite registration wax is tried in to determine correct length. If correction is needed, the laboratory knife is used to trim the excess.
4. The patient is instructed to practice biting to establish occlusion.
5. The bite registration wax is heated in warm water or with a torch to soften.
6. The wax is placed on the mandibular occlusal surface of the patient. If using polysiloxane, the bite registration material is extruded from the disposable tip directly onto the occlusal surface of the mandibular teeth (Figure 14–3A).

(continued)

PROCEDURE 14-5 *continued*

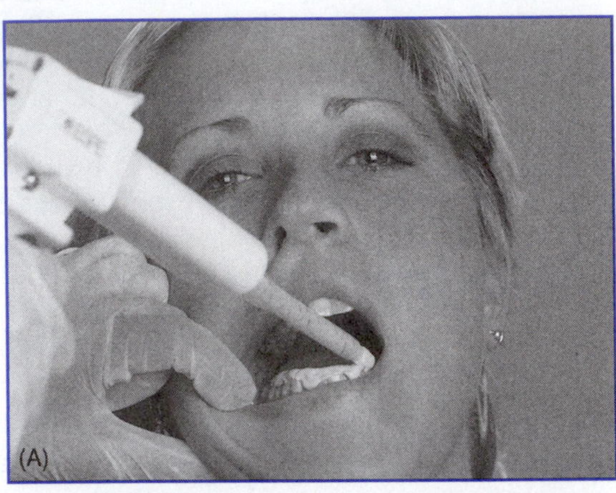

7. The patient is instructed to bite together gently in correct occlusion.
8. The wax will cool in one to two minutes while the patient keeps the teeth together in occlusion. If using polysiloxane, the patient gently occludes until the material sets (Figure 14–3B).
9. The wax or polysiloxane bite is removed gently without distortion.
10. The wax or polysiloxane bite registration is disinfected, labeled and stored for use during trimming of the diagnostic casts (Figure 14–3C).

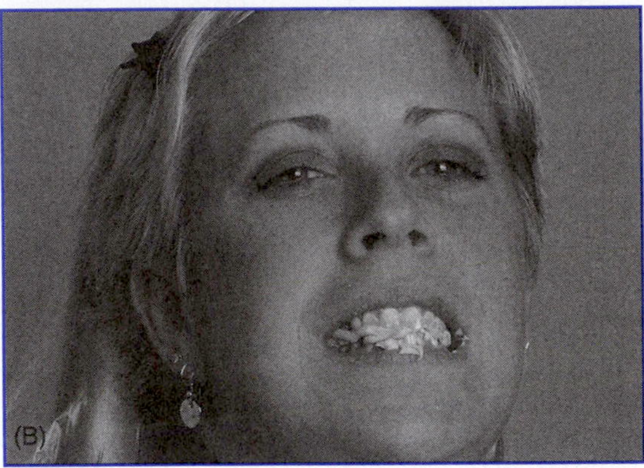

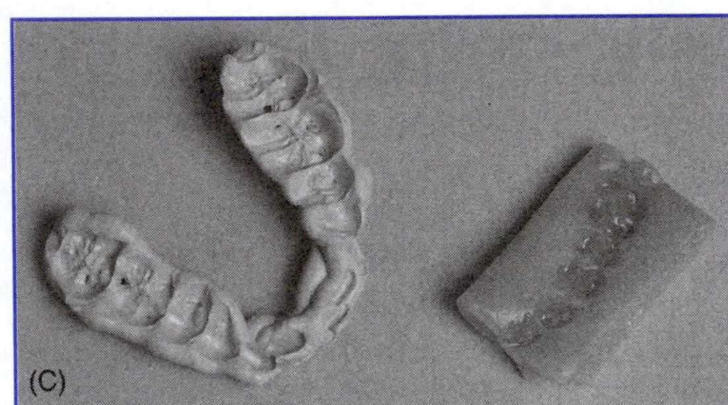

FIGURE 14–3 (A) Bite registration material is extruded from the tip directly onto the occlusal surface of the mandibular teeth. (B) Patient gently occludes until material sets. (C) Polysiloxane bite and wax bite taken on a patient for use in establishing the patient's occlusion.

Elastomeric Impression Materials

Elastomeric impression materials have rubberlike qualities and are used for oral areas that require precise duplication. The materials in this classification are not as affected by the atmospheric changes as the hydrocolloids. They are more elastic and rubberlike when set, therefore allowing the removal from the mouth to take place without tearing and distortion. **Distortion** is a dimensional change in shape. There are three primary groups of materials in this classification: polysulfide, silicone (polysiloxane and polyvinyl siloxanes), and polyether.

Polysulfide

Polysulfide impression materials may be called mercaptan or rubber-base materials (Procedure 14–6). They are supplied in two pastes: a base and a catalyst. The base is the larger tube and the white color of the two pastes.

PROCEDURE

14-6 Taking a Polysulfide Impression

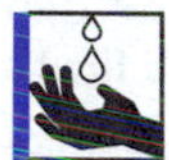
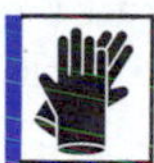
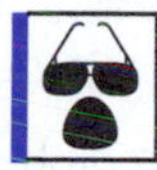

This procedure is performed by the dentist with the dental assistant assisting. This procedure can be a four- or six-handed procedure. Polysulfide is a material used in taking final impressions for which extreme accuracy is required.

EQUIPMENT AND SUPPLIES

- Two rigid, tapered, laboratory spatulas
- Paper pad, provided by the manufacturer
- Two pastes each (two syringes, two trays) from the same manufacturer (a base and an accelerator of the syringe material and a base and an accelerator of the tray material)
- Impression syringe with tip in place and plunger out of the cylinder
- Custom tray that has been painted with corresponding adhesive and permitted to dry

PROCEDURE STEPS *(Follow aseptic procedures)*

1. Health history is reviewed.
2. The patient is seated in an upright position with a patient napkin in place and a large drape over the clothes.
3. The patient's mouth is rinsed with water or a mouth rinse to remove any food debris and aid with removing thick saliva.
4. The procedure is explained to the patient.
5. The material is mixed concurrently by two individuals. The syringe material is mixed slightly ahead of the tray material.
6. Dispense the accelerator onto the pad in a long, even line about four inches long. If more material is needed, additional lines can be placed together on the paper pad. NOTE: Be sure to wipe the end of the tube before placing the lid back on to prevent mess and sticking of the top.
7. Dispense the base onto the pad in a long, even line the same length as the accelerator. Additional lines can be dispensed, however they should not touch the accelerator until the operator wants the process of polymerization to begin.
8. When ready, the individual with the syringe material begins the mixing by first gathering up the accelerator with the spatula and placing it in the base material. Spatulate the pastes together using broad sweeps. After one minute has lapsed, the individual mixing the tray material begins the same process.
9. When the mix is homogeneous and lacks brown or white streaks, it is completely mixed. This process takes forty-five seconds to one minute.
10. The syringe material is then loaded into an impression syringe using the back portion or the working end nozzle of the barrel and

(continued)

PROCEDURE 14-6 *continued*

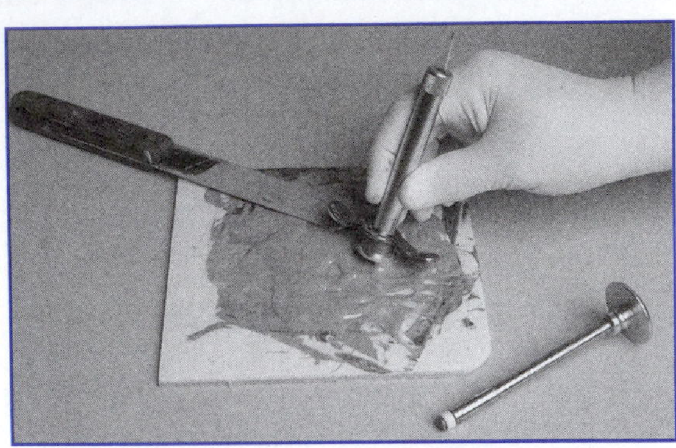

FIGURE 14–4 Loading the mixed polysulfide syringe material into the syringe for placement directly around the prepared tooth.

pushing the syringe over the material repeatedly to force the material into the chamber (Figure 14–4). When the material is in the syringe chamber, wipe the edges quickly and place the plunger in the syringe. Extrude the material slightly to make sure it is working and pass it to the dentist.

11. The tray material is mixed to the same consistency and within the same time frame. The bulk of the tray material is picked up by the spatula and loaded into the impression tray and spread evenly. The tray is then transferred to the dentist after the syringe has been used. The mixing and loading (working time) must be completed within four minutes.
12. The impression must remain in the patient's mouth, held by the operator or the dental assistant, for six minutes to achieve a final set.
13. Cleanup is accomplished after the material has reached the rubber stage. The material peels off the spatula. The paper pad has a corner for the spatula to fit under to aid in removing the soiled top sheet. The disposable impression syringe and paper sheet can be disposed of and the spatula sterilized.
14. Remove the impression after releasing the seal, taking care to protect the opposing teeth from the quick snap.

The advantages of the polysulfide material include relative stability after the final set has been achieved, good accuracy, sharpness of detail, and a relatively long shelf life (two years). The disadvantages of polysulfide are the odor, taste, staining, and the relatively long setting time.

Silicone (Polysiloxane and Polyvinal Siloxanes)

Silicones have the advantages of polysulfide without the disadvantages. They are more expensive than polysulfide, however. Advantages of the material include high accuracy, no shrinkage, dimensional stability, high tear resistance, no taste, and no odor.

The material is supplied in a number of forms. It is available in putty form for making a custom tray, in tubes of base and accelerator (catalyst) for injection, and regular and heavy type for impressions. It also is available in the cartridge form to be used with the mixing tip and extruding gun (automix cartridge system).

The putty material is in two different colors. Each container of putty has a colored scoop used for either the base or the catalyst (Figure 14–5). Do not mix

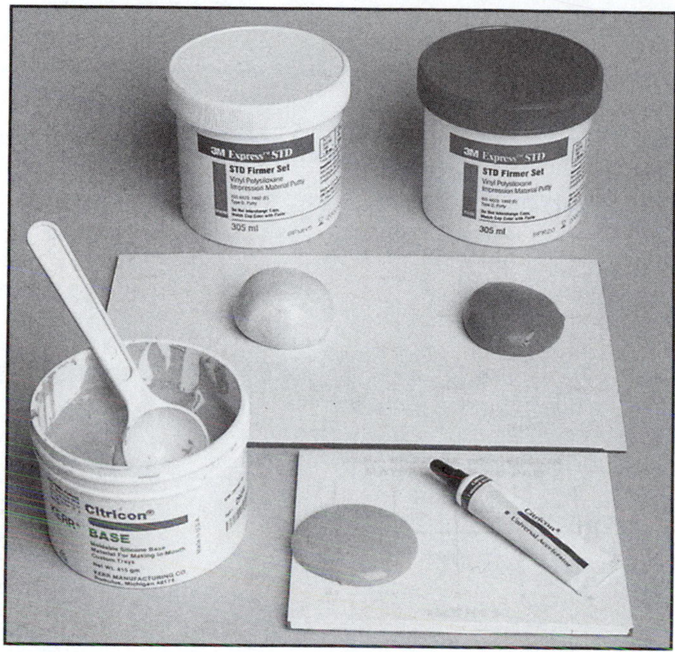

FIGURE 14–5 Two scoops of the putty or putty and tube of accelerator are dispensed for easy incorporation.

up the scoops because doing so will contaminate the material and cause the polymerization process to start, making the material hard and useless. The material is dispensed in an equal volume of base and catalyst putties. The putty is kneaded and mixed quickly until a homogeneous color is achieved; mixing takes about thirty seconds. Mixing putty with latex gloves adversely affects the set of some materials. The silicone is placed in the tray, covered with a thin plastic sheet, and inserted into the patient's mouth or over the model. It takes about three minutes for the material to harden. Remove the plastic, and a custom tray is ready for the impression material. The putty material is not suitable for detailed impressions (Procedure 14–7).

Polyether

Polyether is another impression material used for crowns and bridges. It has excellent accuracy and dimensional stability. It is supplied in tubes as pastes, a larger one for the base and the smaller one for the catalyst. The material comes only in regular body and is stiffer than many of the other materials. It can be used for both the custom tray and the syringe. If used for a custom tray, a tray is chosen that is the correct size, painted with adhesive, and allowed to dry for one minute. The material is dispensed on a paper pad, supplied by the manufacturer, one inch per tooth required for the impression. Equal lengths of material are placed on the pad, not equal amounts. This material is then mixed

PROCEDURE

14-7 Taking a Silicone (Polysiloxane) Two-Step Impression

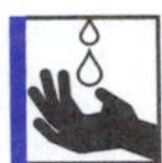 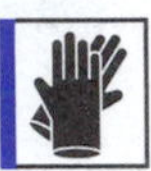 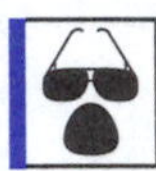

This procedure is performed by the dentist with the dental assistant assisting. Silicone (polysiloxane) is a material used in taking final impressions for which extreme accuracy is required.

EQUIPMENT AND SUPPLIES

- Spatula
- Paper mixing pad
- Vinyl overgloves
- Two containers of putty (one base and one catalyst) with color-coordinated scoops or one putty base and liquid dropper of catalyst (Figure 14–6)
- Stock tray with adhesive painted on the interior
- Plastic sheet for use as a spacer
- Extruder gun, mixing tip with intraoral delivery tip or injection syringe (Figure 14–6)
- Cartridges of impression material (light-body or wash material)

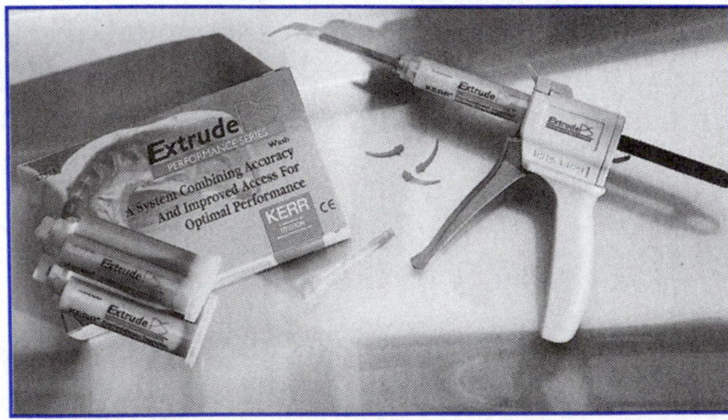

FIGURE 14–6 Extruder gun, mixing tips, and cartridges of impression material. *(Courtesy of Kerr Corporation)*

PROCEDURE STEPS *(Follow aseptic procedures)*

Patient Preparation

1. Health history is reviewed.
2. The patient is seated in an upright position with a bib in place.
3. The retraction cord is placed around the prepared tooth.
4. The procedure is explained to the patient.

Preliminary Putty Impression

1. Don vinyl gloves.
2. Either equal scoops of the putty are mixed together or putty base and drops of catalyst are mixed together. The putty must be kneaded together until a homogenous mixture is obtained within the manufacturer's recommended time; this time is thirty seconds. The mixture must be even with no streaks.
3. After the material is mixed, mold it into a patty and load it into the prepared tray. With the index finger, make a slight indentation where the teeth are located.
4. Place the plastic spacer sheet over the material and insert it into the patient's mouth. The objective is to create 2 mm of space for the final syringeable viscous impression material.
5. The setting of the putty takes about three minutes. The tray is then removed from the patient's mouth, the spacer is removed, and the putty is checked for accuracy and left to set further.

Final Impression

1. After the tooth has been prepared, the area cleaned and dried, the retraction cord placed, and the dentist indicates he or she is ready for the final impression, prepare the material.
2. The tray with the preliminary impression is ready with the spacer removed. The extruder gun is prepared and loaded with the light-body or wash material.
3. The syringe (light-body) material is extruded through the mixing tip and placed in the preliminary impression (Figure 14–7).
4. The tip is wiped off and an intraoral delivery tip placed on for direct injection around the prepared tooth after the retraction cord has been removed. The extruder gun is transferred to the dentist. Instead of using the intraoral delivery tip, some dentists prefer to use an injection syringe, which can be loaded with the mixing tip.
5. The tray is seated by the dentist immediately into place and held steady for three to five minutes, depending on the material used.
6. After the material has set, the impression tray is removed after releasing the seal and taking care to protect the opposing teeth from the quick snap.
7. Immediately rinse the impression under running water and lightly air blow dry. Disinfect according to manufacturer's directions.
8. Impressions should be poured immediately but can be poured up to weeks later and still remain dimensionally stable.

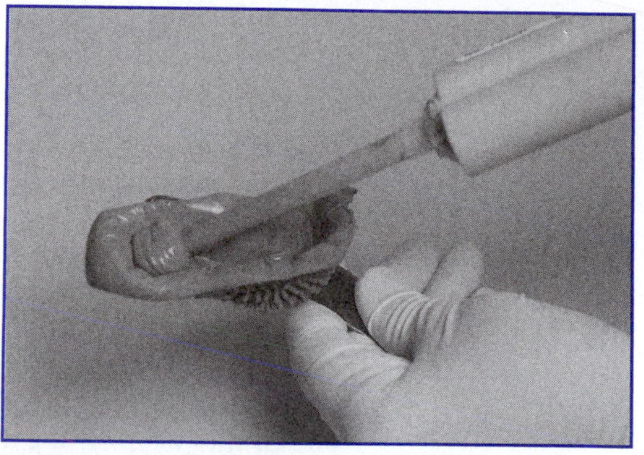

FIGURE 14–7 The syringe material is extruded from the extruding gun into the prepared tray.

by placing the catalyst in the base in a figure-eight motion and obtaining a homogenous mixture free of streaks. Mixing should not take longer than thirty seconds. When mixing is complete, the material is loaded onto the spatula and into the tray. The tray is seated by the dentist in the patient's mouth. After about two minutes of holding the impression in the patient's mouth, agitate the tray in all directions to make room for the final polyether impression material after the teeth are prepared. Remove the tray after three minutes.

To take the final impression after the teeth are prepared with polyether, dispense the material in a similar manner. Less material is needed because of the volume already in the preliminary tray. If a less viscous impression material is desired, a thinner (or body modifier) can be added to the mixture. The catalyst and the modifier are mixed into the base material. The material is loaded into an injection syringe and the excess material is placed in the preliminary impression. The impression tray is then reinserted into the patient's mouth and held for four minutes to obtain an accurate impression. This technique can be accomplished in a one-step technique as well, eliminating the preliminary tray.

After the tray is loosened from the mouth and removed with a quick snapping motion, protecting the opposing arch, it is rinsed with cold water and then completely air dried. The impression is disinfected with a 2 percent solution of glutaraldehyde for ten minutes.

Gypsum Materials

Several different **gypsum** materials are used when pouring an impression to make a model. It is important to identify the application for the material prior to determining the type of gypsum product to use. Gypsum materials vary in strength, dimensional accuracy, resistance, reproduction detail, water/powder ratio, and setting times.

The primary types of gypsum that are used in dentistry are:

- Type I: Impression plaster
- Type II: Model or laboratory plaster
- Orthodontic stone/combination of Type II: Model or laboratory plaster and Type III: Laboratory stone
- Type III: Laboratory stone
- Type IV: Die stone
- Type V: High-strength, high-expansion die stone

The strengths of the gypsum products are determined by the calcination process and the water/powder ratio needed to incorporate the mixture. Plaster (beta hemihydrate) is gypsum particles that are larger and more irregular than the particles of stone (alpha hemihydrate) that have undergone further processing and transformed into more dense particles. It is important to follow the manufacturer's directions when mixing gypsum products. One of the chief obstacles to overcome when mixing gypsum products is the incorporation of air and wetting each particle. Plaster particles are more irregular and require more water to wet each surface of each particle. The ratio of water to powder for plaster is 50 mL of water to 100 grams of powder; stone requires only 30 mL of water to 100 grams of powder. Die stones require even less water because the particles are smaller, less irregular, and more dense.

Avoid whipping the powder and the water together, because doing so increases the air in the mixture. It should be mixed to a creamy, puttylike consistency. The incorporating and spatulating procedure should take about one minute.

Gypsum becomes set when the plaster or stone transforms back to the dihydrate through a chemical reaction. This process gives off heat, called an **exothermic reaction**. The temperature of the water increases or decreases the setting time. The hotter the water, the more rapidly the material sets.

It is important to have the correct water-to-powder ratio. If less water is incorporated, the model can have greater setting expansion. It will have increased strength and hardness but may result in a thick mixture that becomes a dry, crumbly mass that cannot flow into the impression. At this stage, more water cannot be added to the mixture. It will need to be disposed of and a new mixture made. If too much water is incorporated into the mixture, the model will be weak, slow setting, and filled with air spaces. A plaster model sets in ten to twenty minutes and can be determined by feel. If the heat has dissipated, the model is set. It goes through a cycle and heats up and seems to perspire; then, the heat diminishes and the model is cool and dry. The final set occurs after twenty-four hours when the model reaches the optimum hardness. The gypsum powder is measured by weight; the water is calibrated by volume.

All gypsum products are packaged in a plastic bag or container to ensure that they do not become contaminated with moisture. If contaminated, the properties and the setting reaction may be altered. These plastic bags are normally further packaged in a cardboard box for easier handling.

Plaster

Plaster (plaster of paris) is a white gypsum referred to as beta-hemihydrate. It was one of the first gypsum products available to dentistry. It is the weakest and least expensive of the gypsum products. Plaster requires more water to incorporate the powder. After the model dries and the water evaporates, the areas where the water was become air bubbles. This is the primary reason plaster is weaker than stone. Stone is more compact and requires less water, therefore making a stronger model. Plaster is used in areas where detail and strength are not as important. Plaster is used to pour study models, for opposing models, in mounting study models and casts, and for repairing casts (Procedure 14–8, 14–9, 14–10, and 14–11).

Type I: Impression Plaster

Impression plaster (modified Type II: laboratory or model plaster) was used to take impressions prior to the newer, easy-to-manipulate impression materials now on the market. Plaster (Type I), mixed with a water-to-powder ratio of 60 mL of water to 100 grams of powder, is inserted into the mouth carefully on the area to be duplicated, and the operator waits for the plaster to set. After the set (usually four to five minutes), the material is broken apart and reassembled in the laboratory. Because the material is so rigid, it fractures and breaks easily. Today, the material is rarely used for impressions. It is used primarily to mount casts on an articulator because of its quick setting time.

Type II: Laboratory or Model Plaster

Model plaster is used routinely in the dental office by the dental assistant to pour diagnostic casts or study models. It is slightly stronger than the Type I: impression plaster, because it requires a water-to-powder ratio of 50 mL of water to 100 grams of powder, making the material less porous.

PROCEDURE

14-8 Mixing the Plaster to Alginate Impression

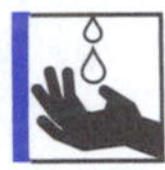
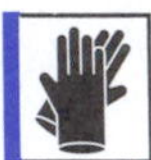

This procedure is performed by the dental assistant in the dental laboratory.

EQUIPMENT AND SUPPLIES *(Figure 14–8)*

- Spatula, metal with rounded end and stiff, straight sides
- Two flexible rubber mixing bowls
- Scale
- Plaster (100 grams)
- Gram measuring device
- Water measuring device (calibrated syringe or vial)

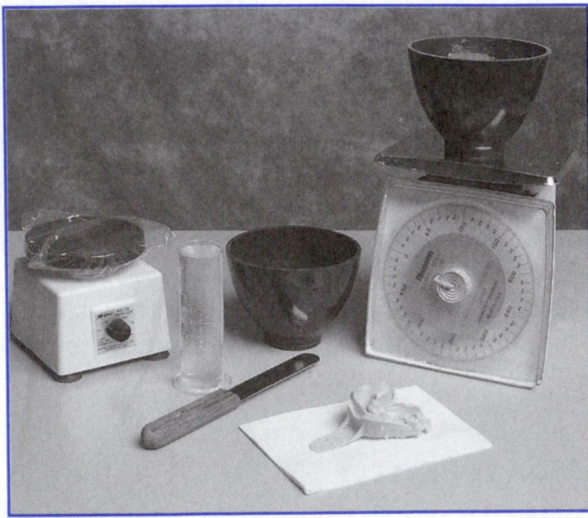

FIGURE 14–8 Equipment needed to pour plaster.

- Vibrator with paper or plastic cover on the platform
- Room-temperature water
- Alginate impression (disinfected)

PROCEDURE STEPS *(Follow aseptic procedures)*

Mixing the Plaster

1. Measure 50 mL of room-temperature water into one of the flexible mixing bowls.
2. Place the second flexible mixing bowl on the scale and set the dial to zero. This allows the plaster powder to be weighed.
3. Weigh out 100 grams of plaster in the second rubber bowl.
4. Add the powder from the second bowl to the water in the first bowl. Pouring the water in first allows all the powder to become incorporated into the mixture. Allow several seconds for the powder to dissolve into the water.
5. Use the spatula to slowly mix the particles together. The initial mixing should be completed in twenty seconds. The total mixing procedure should take about one minute.
6. Turn on the vibrator to medium or low speed.
7. Place the rubber bowl on the vibrator platform, pressing lightly.
8. Rotate the bowl on the vibrator to allow the air bubbles to rise to the top surface (Figure 14–9). Mixing and vibrating should be completed within two minutes. The mixture is ready if the spatula can cut through it and it

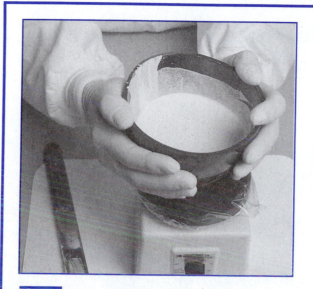

FIGURE 14–9 The vibrator brings the air bubbles to the surface of the plaster.

stays to the sides without changing positions. It will appear like whipped cream with a smooth, creamy texture. Another way to check whether the powder/water is in correct ratio is to place a spoonful on the spatula and turn it upside down. If the material remains in place, the mixture is ready.

Note: If the spatula is held sideways, any mixture will fall from it.

Type III: Laboratory Stone

Type III: laboratory stone is stronger than plaster and is used where more strength is needed. It requires 30 mL of water to 100 grams of powder, making it denser, harder, and stronger. It is normally yellow due to the manufacturer's added pigments, more expensive than plaster, and referred to as alpha-hemihydrate. It is used for study models (diagnostic casts) that require more strength, working casts, and models for partial and full dentures.

Orthodontic Stone

Orthodontic stone is a mixture of laboratory or model plaster and laboratory stone. This white stone allows for a stronger model to be used for the diagnosis and treatment of orthodontic cases.

Type IV: Die Stone

Type IV: die stone requires much less water (less than 24 mL to 100 grams of powder) to incorporate its small, uniform particles. More stone with less water and air makes the model strong and resistant to abrasion. It is used most often for dies or where a very strong model or cast is needed.

PROCEDURE

14-9 Pouring an Alginate Impression for a Study Model

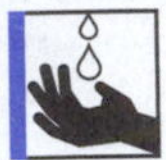 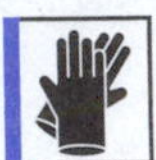 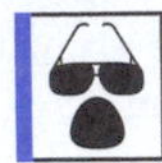

This procedure is performed by the dental assistant in the dental laboratory immediately after mixing the plaster. The impression is ready to pour, the excess moisture is removed, and a laboratory knife has been used to eliminate any excess impression material that will hamper the pouring of the model.

EQUIPMENT AND SUPPLIES

- Metal spatula (stiff blade with rounded end) or disposable spatula
- Mixed plaster from Procedure 14–8, Pouring an Alginate Impression with Plaster
- Vibrator with paper towel or plastic cover on platform

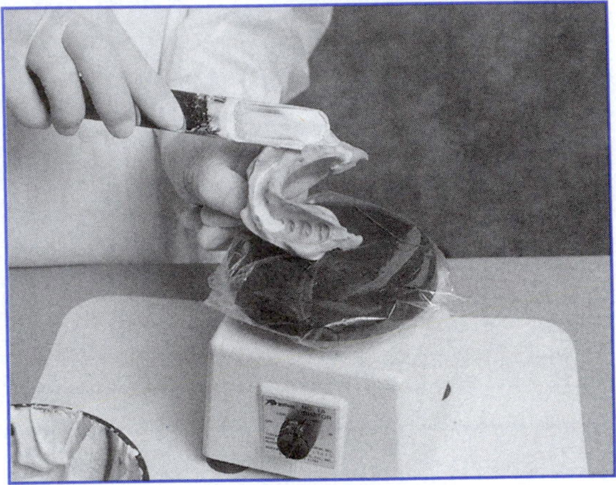

FIGURE 14–10 The mixed plaster is vibrated into the alginate impression, starting at the posterior area of an arch and continuing to fill from that area while the material rotates around to the opposite side of the arch.

PROCEDURE STEPS *(Follow aseptic procedures)*

1. Use the vibrator at low or medium speed.
2. Hold the impression by the handle with the tray portion on the platform of the vibrator. Allow a small amount of plaster to touch the most distal surface of one side of the arch in the impression (Figure 14–10).
3. When the plaster touches the impression that is on the vibrating platform, it flows down the back of the impression and into the anatomy of the teeth. Continue to add small increments of the plaster in the same area as the plaster flows around toward the anterior teeth and to the other side of the arch. (Using this technique allows the air to push ahead of the plaster material and eliminates bubbles. This produces a model that has detailed anatomy qualities.)
4. Add the plaster in this manner until it flows out the other side of the impression and fills the anatomic portion of the model. Rotating the impression around on the platform of the vibrator allows the material to travel around the arch.
5. After the anatomy portion is filled with plaster, use larger increments to fill the entire impression, off the vibrator. When filled, place lightly on the vibrator to coalesce (combine). Overvibration can cause bubbles to form.
6. If a two-pour method is to be used, small blobs should be left on the top of the plaster so that it can attach to the art portion of the model. (A flat surface may break apart at a later date.)

PROCEDURE

14-10 Pouring the Art Portion of a Plaster Study Model Using the Two-Pour Method

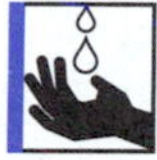 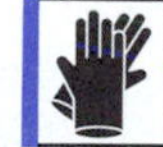

This procedure is performed by the dental assistant in the dental laboratory after the anatomical portion of the study model has set.

EQUIPMENT AND SUPPLIES

- Metal spatula (stiff blade with rounded end) or disposable spatula
- Flexible rubber bowl or disposable bowl
- Vibrator with a paper towel or plastic cover on the platform
- Paper towels
- Plaster
- Calibration measurement device
- Room-temperature water
- Water measuring device

PROCEDURE STEPS *(Follow aseptic procedures)*

1. After pouring the anatomical portion of the impression, allow it to set for five to ten minutes.
2. Wipe the rubber bowl and spatula with paper towel and dispose of the material. Wash, clean, and ready the rubber bowl and spatula for a second pour of plaster.
3. The ratio of powder to water can be altered to create a thicker mix, which is desirable for bases. If pouring the bases or art portion of both the maxillary and the mandibular casts, use 100 grams of powder to 40 mL of water. If pouring only one model, mix half the amount of powder and water.
4. Mix the plaster in the same manner as before. It will appear much thicker. This part of the model is not as crucial as the anatomical portion. Areas that have bubbles can be repaired easily.
5. Gather the plaster on the spatula and place it on a glass slab or a paper towel (Figure 14–11). It is important to allow the material to mass upward and not to spread out.

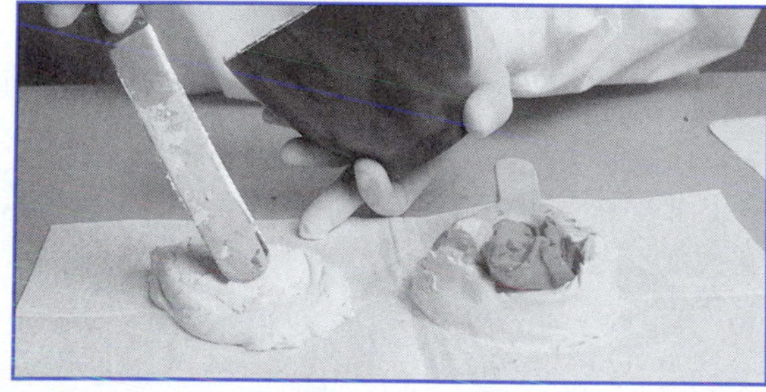

FIGURE 14–11 Plaster is gathered to make a base. It must have enough body so that it does not flatten out.

6. After all the material is on the paper towel, invert the poured anatomy portion onto the base material.
7. Hold the tray steady and situate the handle so that it is parallel to the paper surface or glass slab. It is important to get a base that is even and uniform in thickness. This makes it easier to trim the model later.
8. Carefully drag the excess plaster up over the edges of the cast, filling in any voided areas. Try not to cover any margins of the impression tray while doing this. This locks the plaster onto the tray and may cause the cast to fracture when removing the impression material and the tray.

Note: If using a one- or single-pour method, the base is poured immediately after the anatomical portion is poured. The two-pour method allows the material to initially set in the anatomical portion prior to inverting it and allows even the slightest plaster to flow from any crucial areas.

PROCEDURE

14-11 Separating the Plaster Model from the Alginate Impression

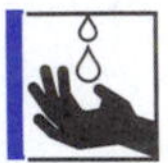 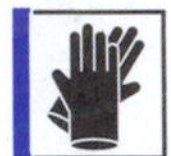

This procedure is performed by the dental assistant in the dental laboratory after the study model has set.

EQUIPMENT AND SUPPLIES

- Laboratory knife
- Maxillary and mandibular plaster models, set in the alginate impressions

PROCEDURE STEPS *(Follow aseptic procedures)*

1. Allow the plaster to set for forty to sixty minutes before removing the impression material and the tray. The exothermic heat should be gone from the plaster material to indicate it has set.
2. Using a laboratory knife, gently remove any plaster that is up on the margin of the tray.
3. Holding the handle of the impression tray, lift the tray straight upward.
4. If the tray does not come off, identify the area holding it back. Remove the necessary plaster in that area to release the tray and impression material. Be sure to lift in an upward motion to remove the tray. Wiggling side to side or lifting sideways may fracture the teeth and anatomical portion of the cast.

Type V: High-Strength, High-Expansion Die Stone

Type V: die stone requires from 18 to 22 mL of water to 100 grams of powder, making it the strongest accepted gypsum product available for use in the dental office.

Water-to-Powder Ratio Recommendations

Type I: Impression plaster	100 grams powder	to	60 mL water
Type II: Laboratory or model plaster	100 grams powder	to	50 mL water
Type III: Laboratory stone	100 grams powder	to	30 mL water
Type IV: Die stone	100 grams powder	to	24 mL water
Type V: Die stone	100 grams powder	to	18–22 mL water

Trimming and Finishing Diagnostic Casts

Diagnostic casts (study models) are used to present the case to the patient. It is important that they have an attractive appearance. They can be trimmed in a geometric form that is pleasing in appearance. Standard guidelines are used in trimming the casts.

PROCEDURE

14-12 Trimming Diagnostic Casts/ Study Models

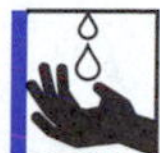 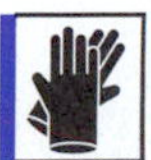 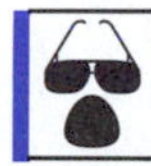

This procedure is performed by the dental assistant in the dental laboratory after the study model has set, been separated from the alginate impression, and prepared for trimming.

EQUIPMENT AND SUPPLIES

- Safety glasses
- Maxillary and mandibular models
- Two flexible rubber mixing bowls
- Laboratory knife
- Pencil
- Measuring straight edge

PROCEDURE STEPS *(Follow aseptic procedures)*

1. If the maxillary and mandibular plaster models are dry, soak them in water-filled rubber mixing bowls for five minutes prior to trimming. The trimming wheel on the model trimmer is more effective if the models are wet prior to trimming.
2. Place on safety glasses and adjust the model trimmer so the water runs freely over the grinding wheel when the trimmer is on.
3. Invert the models so the teeth are resting on the counter. Evaluate whether the base is parallel to the counter. Keep in mind that the art portion is one-half inch when completed.
4. Turn on the model trimmer and trim the base so it is parallel to the occlusal plane. The model trimmer works most effectively when light, even pressure is applied to the grinding wheel. Hold the model as level as possible during this procedure (Figure 14–12).

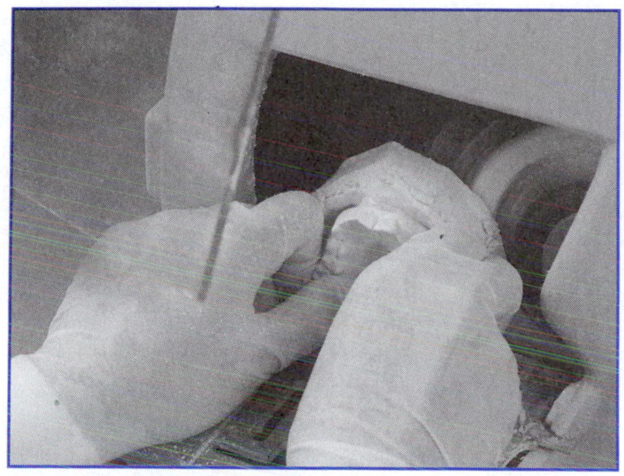

FIGURE 14–12 The base of the study model is trimmed as the operator maintains even pressure on the trimming wheel.

5. Rest hands on the table of the model trimmer and keep fingers away from the grinding wheel.
6. The model may have to be returned to the counter for re-evaluation and then again to the model trimmer to achieve a parallel surface. Trim both models to this stage.

Note: Move the models back and forth once across the grinding surface as the model comes off the grinding wheel. This eliminates the circular grinding marks made as the wheel rotates.

7. Place the models together in occlusion (a wax bite may be necessary) and again evaluate whether the objective of obtaining parallel models has been achieved. If not, grind to get the models to this stage.

(continued)

8. When the cut maxillary and mandibular models as a pair are parallel, keep them in occlusion and evaluate which posterior teeth are the most distal: the maxillary or the mandibular. When that has been determined, take that model and draw with pencil a line behind the retromolar area indicating where to trim.

9. Place the base surface of that model on the model trimmer table guide and cut the posterior area at a right angle with the base up to the indicated lines.

10. Put the two models back into occlusion and place the cut model on the top, whether it is the maxillary or the mandibular. Place the opposite base on the model trimmer table guide holding the models together and trim the posterior at a right angle to the base (Figure 14–13). The trimmed model acts as a guide to follow while trimming. When small particles of plaster are trimmed off the first base, it indicates that they are trimmed to the same plane. To evaluate this, the models are taken off the grinding wheel and placed on their backs (Figure 14–14). The occlusal plane is at a right angle to the counter. If the models stay in occlusion, the objective has been met. If they fall apart and out of occlusion, place them back onto the grinding wheel until they stay in the correct position.

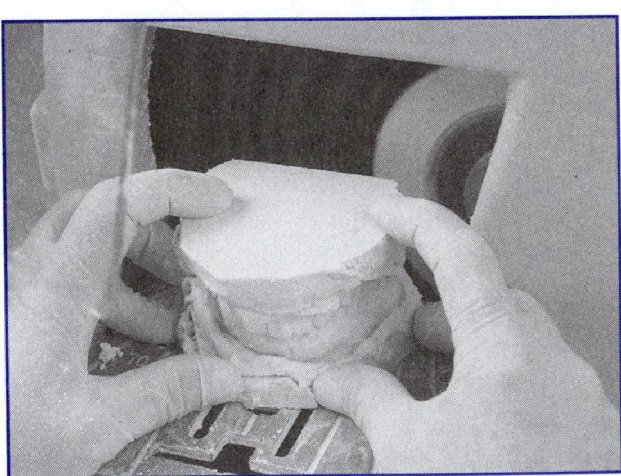

FIGURE 14–13 The models are placed together to trim the back cut.

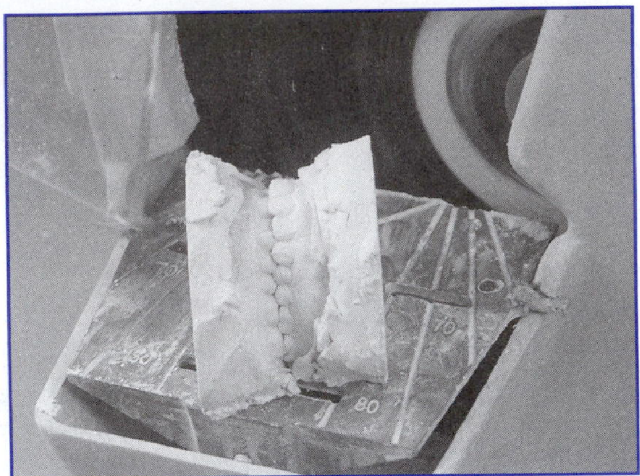

FIGURE 14–14 The models are placed on their backs on a hard, flat surface in occlusion to verify whether the back cuts are correct.

11. The top, bottom, and back now are trimmed. Left to trim are the heel, side, and anterior cuts. The first to be cut are the side angles. Take the pencil and mark the following areas: outward from the middle of the mandibular premolars to the edge of the model and the maxillary cuspids in the same manner. Draw a line running parallel to the teeth at the greatest depth of the buccal vestibule, from the molars to the premolars. This line will be about 5 mm from the buccal surface of the teeth. Mark both sides of the maxillary and the mandibular models in this manner.

12. Place the model base back on the model trimmer table guide and trim the model to the pencil lines on both sides. Repeat this procedure with both models.

13. Mark with pencil a dot at the midline of the maxillary model in the vestibule area. Using the straight edge of the measuring device, draw a line from the dot to the canine/cuspid line on each quadrant. Cut both of the anterior cuts, forming a pointed area at the midline and the center of both cuspids. If the

teeth are highly irregular, adjustments may have to be done. After the lines are drawn, make sure that the cuts will not trim away the protruding teeth. If it appears that this may happen, move the lines out on each side to accommodate this. The model should appear symmetrical.

14. The mandibular model is marked in a rounded manner from the middle of the canine/cuspid on one side to the middle of the canine/cuspid on the other side. A pencil line can be drawn at the depth of the anterior vestibule as a guide for trimming.

15. The heel cuts on both the maxillary and mandibular models are three-eighths to five-eighths inches wide and should appear symmetric in length. They can be drawn on the model by turning the base upward and placing an imaginary diagonal line from the cuspid (maxillary) premolar (mandibular) to where the side and back cuts meet. Draw a 90° angle across the base, opposite the anterior area. The heel cuts are small cuts on both the maxillary and the mandibular models that finish the trimming of the models.

16. After the models are trimmed symmetrically, a laboratory knife is used to trim the tongue area flat and smooth other areas on the art portion. Take care not to destroy the anatomy of the diagnostic casts. Any air bubbles can be filled with plaster. Use dry plaster on the finger, and push it into the wet model to fill small air bubbles. To complete the smoothing of the flat surfaces, a fine wet/dry sandpaper can be used under water. Any small beads of plaster can be removed carefully from the surfaces of the teeth.

17. Place the models in a model gloss for 10 minutes or spray with gloss to provide a professional appearance and add strength. The models need to be polished with a dry cloth to buff the surface in order to achieve the desired high gloss.

18. Label both the models with the patient's name and the date the models were taken. In an orthodontic office, the patient's age may also be identified on the models.

Two-thirds of the trimmed model is made from the anatomic portion of the cast. The anatomic portion includes the teeth, the mucosa, and frenum attachments and is about one inch wide. This area was duplicated from the oral cavity. The remaining one-third is the base or the art portion of the cast. This portion is trimmed in a geometric form with specific angles and is about one-half inch wide. When maxillary and mandibular models are trimmed and in occlusion, they should have an overall height of three inches.

Trimmed Diagnostic Casts (Study Models) Evaluation (Figure 14–15)

- Both maxillary and mandibular models are trimmed symmetrically following specific cut angles indicated.
- All the anatomic portions of the models are accurate.
- The trimmed models sit on end and maintain occlusion.
- Models exhibit a one-half inch base each and a one inch anatomic portion each.
- Final finishing is accomplished and the models present a professional appearance.

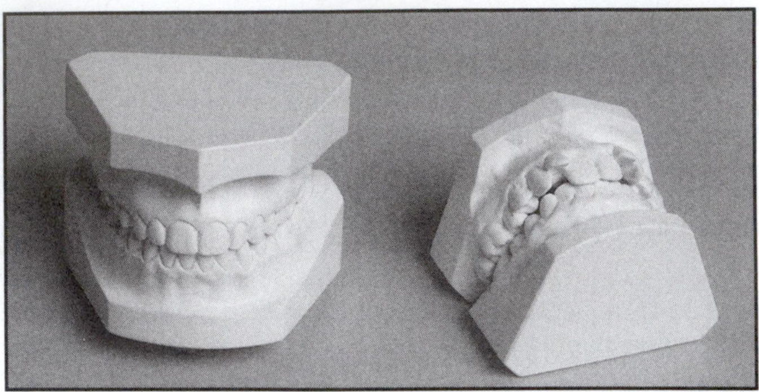

FIGURE 14–15 Trimmed study models.

Articulating Casts or Study Models

An articulator is used to duplicate the patient's occlusion on models. An **articulator** is a frame that holds models of the patient's teeth in to maintain the patient's occlusion and represent his or her jaws.

Articulators can be used to study malocclusion, to wax and carve teeth for crowns and bridges, and to demonstrate to the patient the action that is of concern. The dental assistant may perform the task of mounting models or assist the dentist in this task.

Dental Waxes

Waxes are among the oldest materials used in dentistry. Dental waxes are derived from a number of sources, including bees, plants, and minerals.

Groups of Waxes

Waxes are classified into three broad groups: pattern, processing, and impression. Pattern waxes are hard waxes used in crown and bridge casting (inlay wax) and the construction of the baseplate tray (baseplate wax). Processing and impression waxes have many uses in dentistry.

Pattern Wax

Pattern, or inlay, wax is supplied in dark-colored sticks (Figure 14–16A). It is used on a die, a positive replica of the prepared tooth made from stone. The wax is melted and applied to the die, making a wax pattern used to create the metal and/or porcelain restoration.

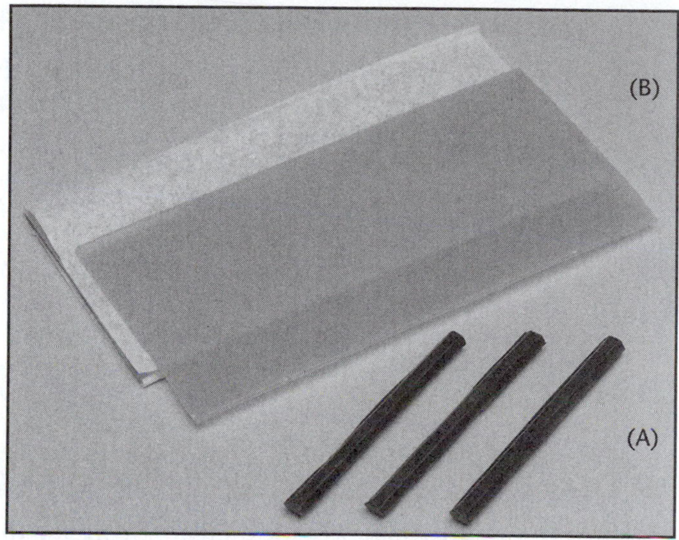

FIGURE 14–16 Pattern waxes. (A) Inlay wax. (B) Baseplate wax.

Baseplate wax is a hard wax that can be heated to make the initial base on which to form a denture (Figure 14–16B). It comes in Types I, II, and III; Type III is the hardest. Type II is most often used in the fabrication of baseplates.

Processing Wax

Several waxes used in dentistry fall into the processing wax category. Boxing wax is a soft, pliable wax used to form a box around an impression prior to pouring it with gypsum. It is supplied in strips one and one-half inches wide and can be reused to extend the periphery around the impression to hold the gypsum in place until it has set.

Sticky wax is another type of processing wax. It is very brittle at room temperature but when melted with a flame source becomes soft and sticky. It adheres to a number of surfaces, such as metal, gypsum, and porcelain. It is used to hold two fractured pieces together until they can be repaired.

Utility wax, also called periphery or bending wax, is a soft wax that is adhesive and pliable. It does not require additional heat and can be molded to most surfaces. This is used to bead around trays to extend them and assist in patient comfort. This wax is also used for orthodontic patients to cover the brackets and uncomfortable areas until the cheeks and lips can adjust. It is supplied in long ropes or strips and in a number of colors.

Impression or Bite Registration Waxes

Normally containing copper or aluminum particles, impression waxes are used to take bite registrations. They are supplied in horsehoe shapes for obtaining the maxillary and mandibular biting surfaces.

Additional Waxes

Other waxes used in dentistry that are not in the three primary classifications are study wax and undercut wax. Study wax is hard wax supplied in blocks used for carving teeth and anatomy. Undercut wax is a putty-type wax used to fill in the undercuts prior to the impression being taken.

Custom Trays

The dentist may ask for a custom tray for the patient to obtain an accurate impression. This may be because a stock tray does not fit. The stock tray will not allow a minimum amount of space for the material to flow around the prepared area, or it may require that an overabundance of impression material be used to obtain the impression, therefore risking an inferior impression. In any case, a custom tray can be fabricated to meet the need. Several materials are available to make a custom tray. It can be constructed from self- or light-curing acrylic resin, a vacuum resin, or a thermoplastic material. All materials must be rigid enough to provide subsistence for the material as it is inserted into and removed from the mouth. It is important that the material adapts well during the construction so that the final tray meets the required criteria.

Required Criteria for a Custom Tray

- Stable enough to hold the material rigid during placement and removal
- Can be smoothed and contoured to the arch
- Can be adapted to an edentulous, a partially edentulous, and a full dentition
- Can be adapted to allow uniform thickness of impression material in all areas of the arch
- Can be altered and contoured to any irregular area
- Can be designed so stops are in the spacer, holding the material in a stable, specifically determined area, providing a more accurate impression

Constructing a Custom Tray

Regardless of the material type used, the custom tray model is prepared in the same manner.

Outlining the Margins of the Tray

If a full custom tray is desired on an edentulous arch, draw a blue line at the bottom of the vestibule area around the facial surface, across the palate area on the maxillary model, around the posterior retromolar area, along the bottom of the vestibule area, and across the opposite posterior retramolar area on the mandibular model. From that first marking, make a red line 2 mm upward (toward the ridge). This gives a definite line to follow when adapting the spacer. A **spacer** is placed on the model to allow room in the tray for the impression material. This spacer is made of pink baseplate wax, however a commercial nonstick molding material may be used (especially when using the vacuum-formed custom tray because of the heating element) or a moist paper towel can be used. When the spacer is placed, the **undercuts** are filled in. Undercuts are recessed areas in the model that make it impossible to seat or remove the custom tray properly. Undercuts are caused by bubbles in the plaster, cavities, or the shape of the arch or dentition. If using baseplate wax for the spacer, it can be heated with warm water and conformed to the model. Cut it back to the red line in an angle-forming manner (see Procedure 14–13). This provides a smoother tissue side to the custom tray and is more comfortable to patients than a blunt-edge cut. After the spacer is in place, take a warm plastic instrument to lute (secure) the edges of the wax to the cast. Cut into the crest of the wax with a laboratory knife, making small rectangular or round holes. These **stops** (holes on the spacer that allow bumps to be formed on the tissue side of the tray) allow the tray to be seated 2 to 3 mm from the teeth or tissue and to not seat too deeply. This allows an adequate amount of impression material to flow around the prepared teeth or the tissue. There should be a minimum of four stops on an edentulous model, two on each first molar and cuspid area. When making a custom tray for crowns and bridges, the stops should be placed one tooth distal and mesial from the prepared tooth.

After the cast is prepared, the custom tray material is mixed according to the manufacturer's directions and formed to the cast. In the doughy stage, the maxillary material can be shaped into a patty and the mandibular can be rolled into a log shape prior to placing the materials on the cast. A handle can be made from the remaining material. It is placed on the anterior of the tray near the midline of the arch. It is secured by wiping the anterior area and the handle area that is to be attached with the resin liquid and then placing it on the custom tray. Because the handle is still soft when it is applied to the cast, it must be held in place until initially set up. Make sure the handle is large and strong enough to allow for leverage in placing and removing the custom tray from the mouth. When working on edentulous custom trays, the handles should extend upward and outward from the model. If this is not done, the handle is placed so that it protrudes directly through the lip of the patient.

PROCEDURE

14-13 Constructing a Self-Cured Acrylic Resin Custom Tray

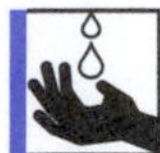 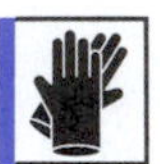 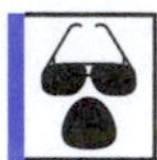

This procedure is performed by the dental assistant in the dental laboratory on a working cast.

EQUIPMENT AND SUPPLIES

- Maxillary and/or mandibular casts
- Laboratory knife
- Pencil (plain or red and blue)
- Wax spatula
- Baseplate wax and heating source (warm water or laboratory torch)
- Tray resin with measuring devices
- Separating medium with brush
- Wooden tongue blade and wax-lined paper cup
- Petroleum jelly
- Tray adhesive

PROCEDURE STEPS *(Follow aseptic procedures)*

Preparing the Cast

1. Outline the area of the cast for the spacer to be placed. This is 2 to 3 mm below the margin of the prepared tooth or 2 to 3 mm above the lowest point in the vestibule if the arch is edentulous.
2. Fill any undercuts in the cast or cover with the spacer material. Heat the spacer material and contour to the pencil line.
3. Using a laboratory knife, trim the wax or spacer to the line using an angled cut instead of a blunt cut.
4. Cut the appropriate stops in the spacer (Figure 14–17).
5. Cover the spacer with aluminum foil or paint it with separating medium.

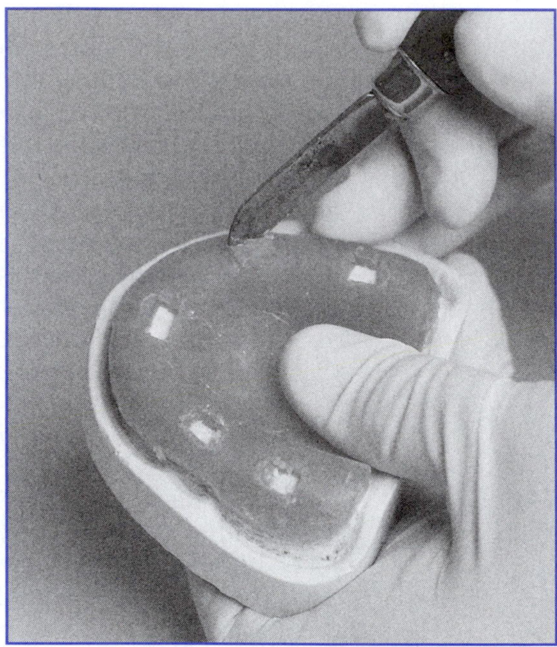

FIGURE 14–17 Stops are cut into the wax spacer. These allow room for the impression material.

Mixing the Custom Tray Acrylic Self-Curing Resin

1. Measure the powder and the liquid to the correct calibrations on the measuring devices according to the manufacturer's directions.
2. Mix the powder and liquid together in the wax-lined paper cup with the wooden tongue blade until **homogenous** (uniformly mixed).
3. Allow the mixture to go through initial polymerization for two to three minutes. Some manufacturers indicate that a cover be placed over the material during the polymerization.

4. During this time, place petroleum jelly over the cast and on the palms of your hands.

Contouring the Custom Tray Acrylic Self-Curing Resin

1. The material is ready to conform to the tray after the initial set when the material is no longer sticky and can be gathered into a ball. Knead the material to further mix the material and set a small amount aside for the handle. This doughy stage allows the material to be formed into a patty for the maxillary arch or a roll for the mandibular arch.
2. Place the dough-like patty for the maxillary cast, covering the wax spacer. Contour and adapt it to extend 1 to 2 mm over the wax spacer (Figure 14–18A). Try to complete the adaptation with a rolled edge at the designated area. If unable to accomplish this, a laboratory knife can be used to trim the material back. (Doing this causes rough edges that need to be smoothed back later.)
3. The material set aside for the handle is shaped and a drop of the monomer liquid placed on the tray where the handle is to be adapted and then on the handle where it will be placed on the custom tray. This allows the materials to join together for a better outcome.
4. Place the handle in the midline area of the arch (Figure 14–18B). If making an edentulous custom tray, the handle should come up from the ridge and then outward. A custom tray handle that is made for an area that has teeth can come directly outward.
5. Place the handle and hold it in the proper position until the material becomes firm.

Finishing the Custom Tray Acrylic Self-Curing Resin

1. The setting takes eight to ten minutes. Remove the custom tray from the cast and take out the spacer material.
2. If foil has been used, the cleaning will not take a great deal of time. If only wax was used, melt it. A wax spatula is used to remove it, along with hot water and an old toothbrush.
3. After the final set (thirty minutes minimum), use an acrylic bur or an arbor band to trim the edges of the custom tray. Do not trim the inside of the tray.
4. Clean and disinfect the custom tray according to the manufacturer's directions. Write the patient's name on the tray.
5. Apply the adhesive provided by the manufacturer of the impression material to the inside of the custom tray and along the margins.

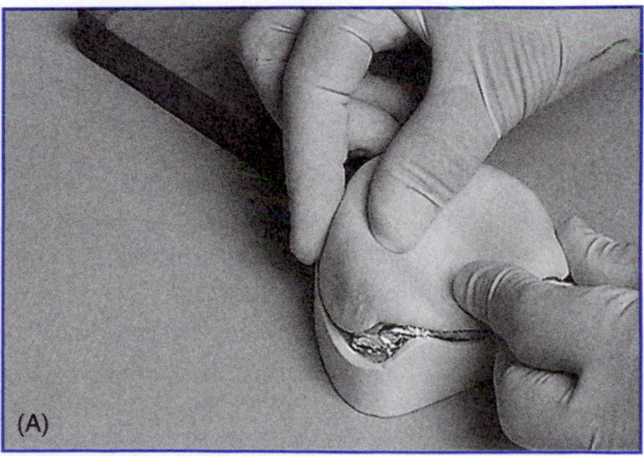

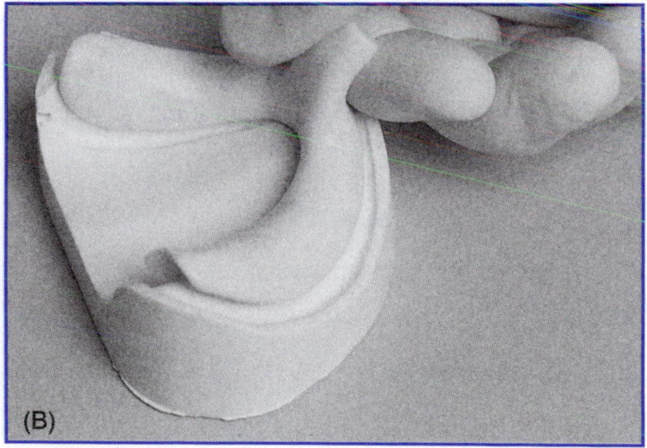

FIGURE 14–18 (A) The custom tray material is adapted to the model over the wax spacer. (B) The handle is attached to the adapted custom tray.

When the exothermic reaction has completed and the model has cooled (about ten minutes), remove the spacer and evaluate the tray. The inside of the tray does not need to be smooth because the impression material covers this area. Any rough areas on the margins and on the outside of the tray can be smoothed for patient comfort. This can be accomplished by using an acrylic bur in a straight handpiece or with an arbor band on the laboratory lathe. Wear protective glasses when performing either of these trimming procedures. When completed, clean and disinfect the custom tray according to manufacturer's directions and place it in a barrier ready for patient use.

Vacuum-Formed Tray

Trays that are vacuum formed (Procedure 14–14) can be used for a number of applications in dentistry. Most often they are used for custom trays, bleaching trays, night guards, mouth guards, and matrices for provisional restorations. The material comes in several gauges and thicknesses for specific applications. Custom tray material is much more thick and rigid than the other applications. All use a vacuum former with a heating element, a cast, and material that can be heated and adapted using vacuum pressure.

PROCEDURE

14-14 Constructing a Vacuum-Formed Acrylic Resin Custom Tray

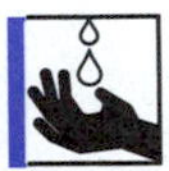
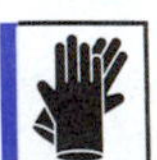

This procedure is performed by the dental assistant in the dental laboratory on a working cast.

EQUIPMENT AND SUPPLIES

- Maxillary and/or mandibular casts
- Laboratory knife
- Laboratory scissors
- Spacer material (optional)
- Vacuum former with heating element
- Acrylic sheets

PROCEDURE STEPS *(Follow aseptic procedures)*

Preparing the Cast

1. The cast is soaked in warm water for up to thirty minutes prior to forming a custom tray on it. This eliminates small air bubbles. (These air bubbles coming to the surface [**percolating**] cause small spaces between the cast and the acrylic sheet. Then, the custom tray does not have the accuracy desired.)
2. Place the spacer, if indicated. (A wax spacer will melt under the heating element, if used.)
3. Mark the desired outer margin of the custom tray.

4. Place the cast on the platform of the vacuum-forming unit.

Contouring the Acrylic Resin Sheets During the Vacuum-Forming Process

1. Select the appropriate acrylic resin sheets to be used for the procedure.
2. Place the acrylic resin sheets between the heater frame and the gasket frame and tighten the anterior knob to secure the material in place. Place the cast on the platform (Figure 14–19).

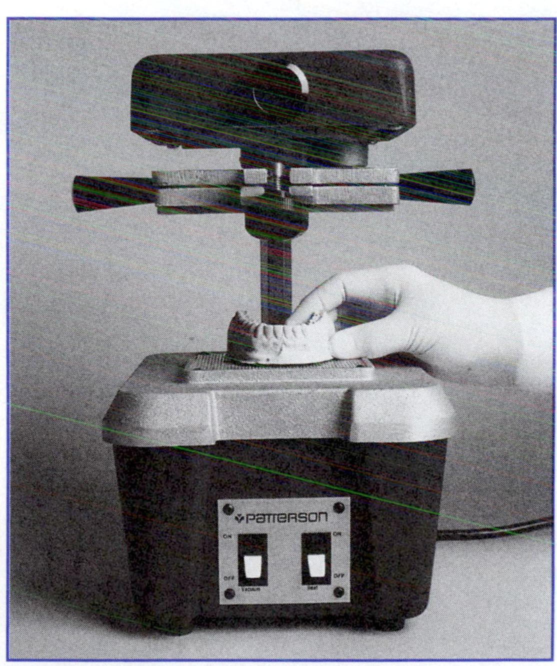

FIGURE 14–19 The resin sheets are secured in place and the cast is placed on the platform of the vacuum-forming unit.

3. Make sure the heating element is in the correct place above the acrylic resin sheet and turn it on.
4. Watch the resin as it heats. It will begin to sag. Allow this to continue until the resin droops downward about one inch. (Overheating causes air bubbles to form on the surface of the acrylic resin.)
5. After the material is heated properly, grasp both handles on the frame and pull the frame down-ward, over the cast. Only touch the handles because the entire area is extremely hot.
6. Turn on the vacuum immediately after the resin sheet is entirely over the cast.
7. Turn off the heating unit.
8. Allow the vacuum to continue for one to two minutes to cool the resin so it becomes firm again.

Finishing the Vacuum-Formed Acrylic Resin Custom Tray

1. After the resin material is cooled, remove it from the vacuum form frame.
2. Separate the resin-formed custom tray from the cast. Using laboratory scissors, trim to the desired form.
3. Use a torch to heat and apply a cutout handle section to the custom tray.
4. Clean and disinfect the custom tray according to the manufacturer's directions and write the patient's name on it.

CHAPTER 15

Endodontics

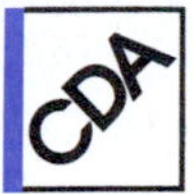

OBJECTIVES

The student should strive to meet the following objectives and demonstrate an understanding of the facts and principles presented in this chapter:

1. Define endodontics and the role of the endodontist.
2. Identify instruments used in endodontic procedures and describe their functions.
3. Identify materials used in endodontics and describe their functions.
4. Describe endodontic procedures and the responsibilities of the dental assistant.
5. Explain surgical endodontic procedures and the instruments used.

KEY TERMS

apical periodontitis (p. 257)
apicoectomy (p. 266)
barbed broaches (p. 259)
endodontics (p. 256)
exudate (p. 256)
files (p. 259)
Glick #1 (p. 262)
gutta percha (p. 258)
intracanal instruments (p. 259)
irreversible pulpitis (p. 256)
master cone (p. 265)
nonvital pulp (p. 256)
obturating (p. 261)
percussion (p. 257)
periapical abscess (p. 257)
pulpal necrosis (p. 256)
radiographs (p. 257)
reamers (p. 260)
retrograde filling (p. 267)
reversible pulpitis (p. 256)
root canal sealer (p. 260)
rubber stops (p. 260)
spreaders (p. 261)
vital pulp (p. 256)

Introduction

Endodontics is the branch of dentistry concerned with the diagnosis and treatment of diseases of the pulp and the periapical tissues. Endodontic procedures include diagnosis, root canal treatment, and periapical surgery.

The Endodontic Team

The staff in the endodontist's office shares similar responsibilities as the general dental office staff, except there is an increase in communication with other dental offices because most of the patients are referrals.

The endodontist is assisted by dental assistants who perform traditional assisting responsibilities in addition to expanded duties specific to endodontics as allowed by the state Dental Practice Act.

Progress of Pulpal and Periapical Diseases

The healthy pulp is said to be **vital pulp**. When the pulp or periapical tissues are irritated or injured, the result is inflammation. Advanced dental decay is one of the primary sources of pulpal irritation. Other irritations or injuries include impact trauma, fractures, invasive restorative procedures, and adverse reactions to dental materials. The degree of pulpal inflammation depends on the severity and duration of the irritation or injury and the ability of the tissues to respond. The patient may or may not have symptoms that indicate the degree of the inflammation of the **nonvital pulp**.

Pulpal Diseases

Pulpal diseases include reversible pulpitis, irreversible pulpitis, and pulpal necrosis.

- **Reversible pulpitis**—The pulp is inflamed but able to heal when the irritant is removed. Causes include incipient caries, enamel fractures, and occlusal attrition. Symptoms include sensitivity to hot and cold. Treatment involves removing the irritant and placing sedative materials to soothe and heal the pulp.
- **Irreversible pulpitis**—The inflammation continues until the pulpal tissue cannot recover. Symptoms include pain to the patient that may be short and sharp or dull and continual. The treatment for irreversible pulpitis is root canal therapy or extraction.
- **Pulpal necrosis**—The death of the pulpal cells, which often results from irreversible pulpitis. As the pulp inflammation progresses, **exudate** (**ECKS**-you-dayt), or pus, and gas form in the pulp chamber. If the tooth is sealed and the exudate cannot escape, pulpal necrosis is rapid. If the exudate drains through caries or exposure to the oral cavity, the process is slowed. A fistula is a tubelike passage that forms occasionally to drain an abscess from the apex of a tooth into the oral cavity.

Periapical Diseases

When the infection in the pulp reaches the apex of the tooth, it continues into the periapical area. The intensities of the inflammation and the host response determine the extent of the infection. Periapical disease includes apical periodontitis and periapical abscess.

- **Apical periodontitis**—Pulpal inflammation extends into the periapical tissues. This acute condition subsides if the irritation is removed. If the process continues and the irritant is not removed, the apical periodontitis becomes a chronic inflammation.
- **Periapical abscess**—A localized destruction of tissue and accumulation of exudate in the periapical region. The patient's reaction can range from moderate to severe discomfort and/or swelling. The treatment includes releasing the pressure by creating an opening into the pulp chamber, removal of the necrotic pulp, and root canal therapy.

Endodontic Diagnosis

Endodontic diagnosis includes patient medical and dental history; clinical examination, including pulp testing; and review of communication from the referring dentist about the case.

The Clinical Examination

The clinical examination, or the *objective examination,* includes evaluation of the extraoral tissues. Facial asymmetry, swelling, redness, and external fistulas are some of the indications to the problem the patient may be experiencing.

A visual examination of the teeth may reveal caries, discoloration, or fractures; however, clinical tests are commonly performed for a complete diagnosis. Clinical tests are performed by the dentist to diagnose the patient's situation correctly. Following are some of the testing procedures.

Radiographs. **Radiographs** are the most useful of the diagnostic tools. Radiographs are taken and processed immediately so the dentist can refer to them.

Palpation. Pressure is applied to the mucosal tissue near the apex of the root of the suspicious tooth. The area around the affected tooth may be soft and raised because it is filled with pus.

Percussion. **Percussion** is performed by tapping on the occlusal surface or incisal edge of the tooth. The dentist or endodontist often uses the handle of a mouth mirror to perform percussion testing. Tapping is performed first on a control (healthy) tooth and then on the symptomatic tooth.

Mobility. Tooth mobility is tested by placing the handle of an instrument or a finger on the lingual surface and the handle of another instrument on the facial surface of the tooth and applying pressure.

Cold Test. Cold testing is performed by using either dry ice, ethyl chloride, or a piece of ice. The tooth is isolated and dried; then the ice is applied to the facial surface of the tooth.

Heat Test. Heat testing uses several heat sources. Examples include a small ball of **gutta percha** heated by a flame, the heated end of a ball burnisher, or frictional heat from running a rubber cup on the tooth surface. Heat is applied to the tooth and, if the pain increases and lasts, there is a distinct possibility of irreversible pulpitis.

> Gutta percha is a thermoplastic material used to fill the canal and it is used as a heat source when testing the sensitivity of a tooth.

Electronic Pulp Testing/Digital Pulp Testing. Electronic pulp testing determines if the tooth is vital. Pulp testing units are battery operated and calibrated to deliver variable, high-frequency currents. The current creates an electrical stimulus to the tooth (Procedure 15–1).

Selective Anesthesia. Sometimes the patient is unable to identify which tooth or which arch is causing the problem. In these cases, after talking with the patient and completing the clinical examination, **selective anesthesia** is used. One area of the patient's mouth is selected and an injection is given. If anesthetic in this area alleviates the discomfort, the problematic quadrant has been determined.

PROCEDURE

15-1 Electronic Pulp Testing

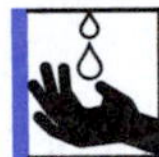
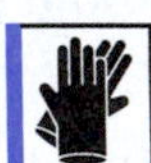
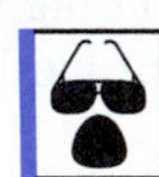
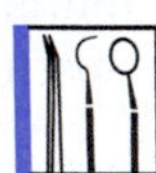

EQUIPMENT AND SUPPLIES

- Basic setup: mouth mirror, explorer, and cotton pliers
- Electronic pulp tester
- Conducting medium, such as toothpaste

PROCEDURE STEPS

Follow these steps to electronically test the pulp (test control tooth first):

1. Place a small amount of toothpaste on the tip of the electrode (the toothpaste acts a conducting medium). Dry the tooth before using the electrode.
2. Ask the patient to signal when he or she notices a sensation, which is usually a tingling or hot feeling.
3. Place the tip on the facial surface of the tooth and gradually increase the power. **CAUTION:** Do not place the electrode on a metal restoration.
4. If the patient feels any sensation, some degree of tooth vitality is indicated. If no sensation is felt, the pulp may be necrotic.

Endodontic Instruments

Characteristics of Intracanal Instruments

Endodontic **intracanal instruments** are made of stainless steel and nickel titanium alloy wire. They are flexible, fracture resistant, smooth, able to maintain sharp cutting edges, and corrosion resistant. The wire is twisted and tapered into instruments called files and reamers. To ensure consistency in the sizes and lengths of the intracanal instruments, the ADA and manufacturers have standardized numbers and a color-code system.

Barbed Broaches

Barbed broaches are made of fine metal wire with tiny, sharp projections or barbs along the instrument shaft. The barbs are angled to allow a smooth entry but catch tissue when retracted. Broaches are used for removal of soft tissue from the pulp canal.

Files

Endodontic **files** are used to enlarge and smooth the canal. They are long, tapered, twisted instruments that are moved in an up-and-down motion inside the canal.

Standard files are known as **K-type files** (Figure 15–1A). These tightly twisted files are used to scrape the walls of the canal, widen them, and remove necrotic tissue.

Hedström files are manufactured by a different process than K-type files (Figure 15–1B). The edges of the Hedström files are very sharp and cut more aggressively. These files are only used in a push-and-pull motion.

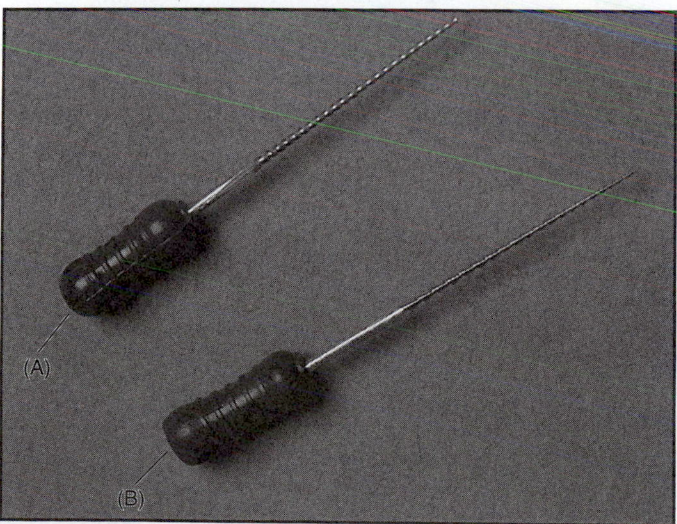

FIGURE 15–1 (A) K-type file. (B) Hedström file.

Reamers

Reamers are used with a "reaming" or twisting motion. They have long twisted shanks similar to the files, but the blades are spaced much farther apart. The cutting action is completed as the reamer is revolved out of the canal. They are color-coded and numbered according to size, similar to files.

Different methods are available to store and organize reamers and files. Some of the storage containers can be sterilized and are designed to hold a range of the intracanal instruments.

Rubber Stops

Rubber stops (also called file stops, endo stops, or markers) are placed on reamers and files to mark the length of the root canal (Figure 15–2). These small, circular, silicone disks have prepunched holes in the center for easy application. The length is determined by holding a file with a rubber stop against a radiograph and adjusting the stop to match the incisal or cusp edge.

Gates-Glidden Drills

Gates-Glidden drills are used with latch attachments on slow-speed handpieces. The drills are long-shanked and elliptically shaped with blunt, football-shaped ends. They run in a clockwise direction. Gates-Glidden drills are used in the upper portion of the canal to prepare the opening access by removing the obstructing dentin.

Peeso Reamers

The Peeso reamers have parallel cutting sides rather than the elliptical shape of the Gates-Glidden drills. They are used with latch attachments on slow-speed handpieces. Peeso reamers are used to prepare the canal for a post and to reduce the curvature of the canal orifice for straight-line access.

Lentulo Spirals

The Lentulo spiral is a long, twisted, wire instrument used to spin **root canal sealer**, or cement, into the canal. Spirals are used with slow-speed handpieces and latch attachments.

Endodontic Spoon Excavator

The spoon excavator has a very long shank that allows the instruments to reach into the coronal portion of the tooth. The spoon-ended excavator removes deep caries, pulp tissue, and temporary cement.

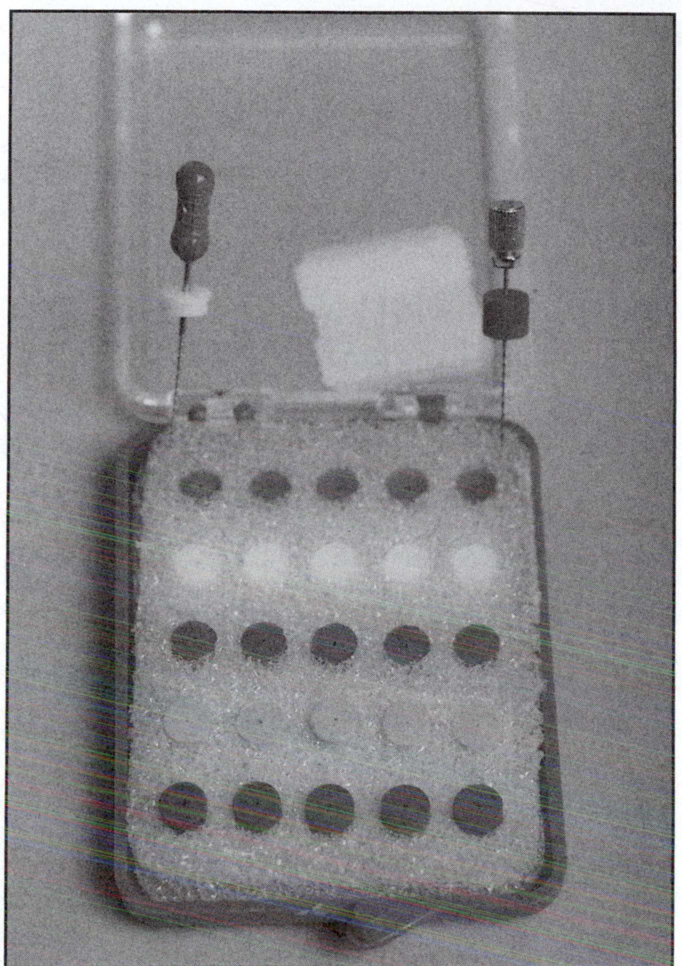

FIGURE 15–2 Examples of rubber stops and how they are positioned on a file.

Endodontic Explorer

The endodontic explorer is designed to aid in locating the orifices (opening) of the canals. This long, pointed explorer is designed specifically for endodontic procedures.

Endodontic Spreaders, Pluggers, and the Glick #1

Spreaders and pluggers (condensors) are instruments used to laterally condense materials when **obturating** (sealing/filling) the canal. Both of these instruments have long, tapered working ends. The spreaders are pointed on the ends, while the pluggers are flat. Spreaders are used to adapt the gutta percha into the canal (lateral condensation), and pluggers are used to condense the filling material to provide space for additional gutta percha cones.

The **Glick #1** instrument is used to remove the excess gutta percha from the coronal portion of the canal and to condense the remaining gutta percha in the canal opening.

Endodontic Materials

Absorbent Paper Points

Paper points are used to dry canals, place medications, and take cultures of the canal. Paper points are absorbent and are supplied in various sizes, from x-fine to coarse.

Gutta Percha

Gutta percha is used to obturate the canal. It is a thermoplastic material that is flexible at room temperature yet stiff enough to be placed into the root canal. Gutta percha cones are supplied in graduated sizes.

Irrigation Solutions

During the root canal treatment, the root canal is frequently irrigated to remove debris. Sterile water can be used for irrigating; however, the most common biomechanical cleaner is **sodium hypochlorite,** which is household bleach. This solution is mixed with water (50/50) and loaded into a Luer-Lock syringe. The canal is irrigated with the sodium hypochlorite/water solution, which disinfects and dissolves necrotic tissue. During the irrigation process, the dental assistant places the evacuator close to the tooth to remove the debris and solution.

Root Canal Sealers and Cements

Root canal sealers used with obturating materials prevent microleakage in the canal. A variety of materials are used as sealers, including zinc oxide-eugenol, calcium hydroxide, and glass ionomer. Sealers are mixed to a thick consistency and then inserted into the canal using paper points, the Lentulo spiral, or files or by placing the sealer directly onto the gutta percha.

Sterilization Procedures

Endodontic instruments must be sterilized before they are used and/or during the course of cleaning and shaping the canal. Sometimes instruments are sterilized at chairside, using a small glass bead or salt sterilizing unit.

Endodontic Procedures

Root Canal Treatment

Root canal treatment is usually completed in two appointments. However, this varies depending upon the degree of infection and the dentist's judgment.

The procedure begins with the dentist opening the coronal portion of the tooth with a dental high-speed handpiece and burs. This is followed by cleaning and enlarging the canal. Restoring of the canal is also known as obturation. During this phase of treatment, the pulp canal is permanently sterilized, filled, and sealed (Procedure 15–2).

PROCEDURE

15-2 Root Canal Treatment

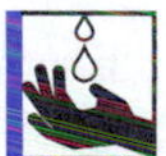
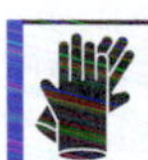
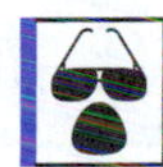
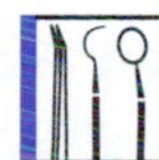
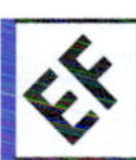

This procedure is performed by the dentist or endodontist, who is assisted by the dental assistant. The following sequence indicates steps involved in a root canal treatment that requires two appointments.

EQUIPMENT AND SUPPLIES

- Basic setup: mouth mirror, explorer, and cotton pliers
- Endodontic explorer and spoon excavator
- Locking cotton pliers
- Saliva ejector, evacuator tip (HVE), air-water syringe tip
- Cotton rolls, cotton pellets, and gauze sponges
- Anesthetic setup
- Dental dam setup
- High-speed handpiece and assortment of burs
- Low-speed handpiece
- Irrigating syringe and solution (sodium hypochlorite or hydrogen peroxide)
- Barbed broach, assorted reamers and files, and rubber stops
- Paper points (assortment)
- Temporization materials
- Permanent obturating materials (gutta percha or silver points and root canal sealer)
- Heat source
- Endodontic spreaders, pluggers, and Glick #1
- Articulating forceps and paper

PROCEDURE STEPS *(Follow aseptic procedures)*

Administer Anesthetic

1. Administer topical and local anesthetic for endodontic treatment as with restorative procedures in general dentistry.
2. Usually the dentist or endodontist anesthetizes the patient at every appointment, but it is up to the dentist's discretion. After the first appointment, when the pulp chamber has been opened and the canals have been cleaned, the dentist may determine that anesthetic is unnecessary.

(continued)

PROCEDURE 15-2 *continued*

3. If anesthetic is used, prepare the syringe and assist during the administration of the anesthetic.

Isolate the Area

1. Place the dental dam, isolating the tooth being endodonically treated. In addition to isolating the tooth, the dam improves visibility and protects the tooth from saliva and solutions used in endodontic treatment.
2. Once the dental dam is placed, the dental assistant wipes the area with a disinfectant to remove bacterial contaminants.

Gain Access to the Pulp

1. The dentist or endodontist uses the high-speed handpiece and a round or fissure bur to gain access to the pulp. The opening is made through the crown of the tooth and should be sufficient to expose the pulp chamber and permit access for intracanal instruments.
2. Evacuate and maintain good visibility for the dentist.
3. Once access to the pulp has been gained, the endodontic explorer is used to locate the main and accessory canals.

Remove the Pulpal Tissues

1. The dentist inserts a barbed broach into the canal and removes the pulpal tissues.
2. Receive the barber broach in a gauze sponge and discard in a SHARPS or biohazard container.

Enlarge and Smooth the Root Canal

1. Using the periapical radiograph, the dentist or endodontist estimates the length of the root of the tooth (Figure 15–3). An apex finder may also be used. Rubber stops are used to mark the length of the tooth on files and reamers. A series of small files are used to remove debris and enlarge the canals. Canals must be at least a #25 file before Gates-Glidden burs can be used. As the files enlarge, the diameter of the canal, the size of the files, and/or the Gates-Glidden burs increase, respectively.

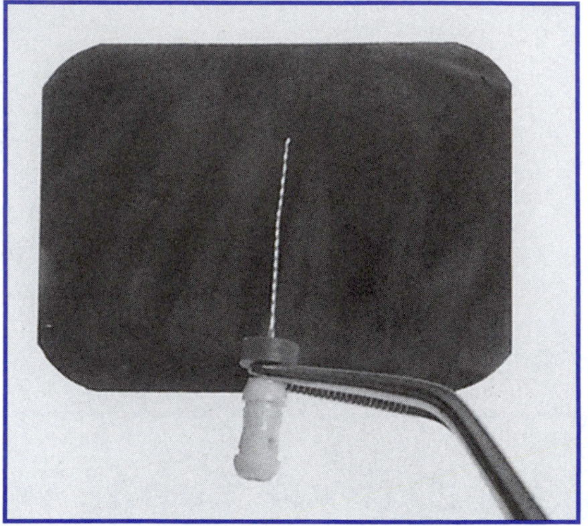

FIGURE 15–3 Measuring the length of the root using a radiograph and reamer.

2. Prepare the stops on the files and reamers according to the dentist's or endodontist's instructions. This measurement must be precise for each hand instrument. (The duties of the assistant may vary greatly depending on the preferences of the dentist or endodontist. For example, some may want the assistant to sterilize the reamers and files at chairside, or they may want radiographs taken periodically.)
3. Keep the files and reamers in order and free from debris.

Irrigate the Root Canal

1. Periodically, the canal is irrigated to remove debris (Figure 15–4). After the canal is flushed, it is dried with paper points.
2. Prepare the solution in the disposable syringe and transfer it to the operator. As the operator flushes the solution into the canal, evacuate the area. Then, transfer paper points in locking pliers to the operator and receive the used saturated points in a gauze sponge.

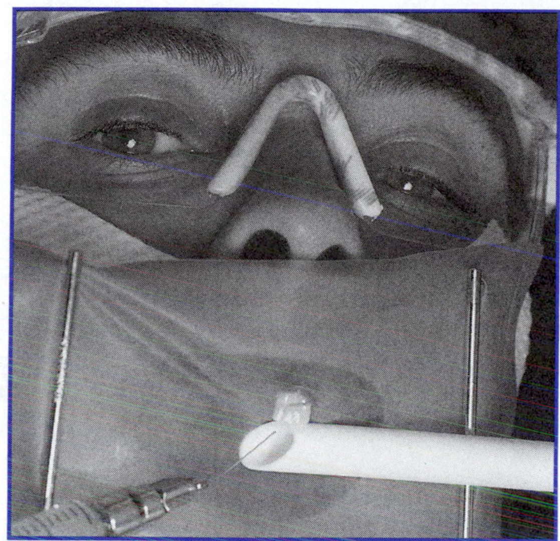

FIGURE 15–4 Irrigating the root canal.

Note: At this time, the dentist or endodontist may decide to place a temporary restoration and reappoint the patient in several days to two weeks.

3. Prepare the temporary restorative materials and either place the temporary or assist the dentist in placement.
4. Remove the dental dam and dismiss the patient.

Obturate the Root Canal

1. Obturation of the root canal is routinely performed at the second appointment. After the patient is seated, the temporary filling is removed and the canal is flushed to remove debris.
2. Radiographs are taken periodically throughout the procedure for the dentist or endodontist to evaluate the progress. Once the canal is adequately enlarged and free of disease, it is permanently filled to prevent debris, fluids, and bacteria from entering the canal. There are many materials and techniques available to fill the canal; however, gutta percha materials are most common.
3. The dentist or endodontist selects a gutta percha point as the **master cone**. The cone should be no more than 1 mm short of the prepared length. The operator inserts the cone into the canal to check the fit. If the master cone is the correct length and fits snugly near the apex, the cone is removed, the canal is dried, and the root canal sealer is prepared.
4. The root canal sealer is mixed and then placed in the canal with a Lentulo spiral and/or a master cone dipped in the sealer and placed in the canal.
5. A spreader is used to create space for additional accessory gutta percha cone. Dip each accessory gutta percha cone into the root canal sealer and transfer it to the dentist for placement. Transfer the spreader to create space for the subsequent cones. Repeat this procedure until the canal is filled.
6. Once the canal is filled, the excess gutta percha in the crown of the tooth is removed with a hot Glick #1 or a heated plugger. The warm gutta percha is vertically condensed into the cervical portion.
7. Hold a 2 × 2 gauze to remove any excess gutta percha from the instruments.
8. A final radiograph is taken.
9. The coronal portion of the tooth is sealed with a permanent restoration or a temporary restoration if a fixed prosthesis is the treatment choice.
10. The dental dam is removed and the patient's mouth is rinsed.
11. The patient's occlusion is checked with articulating paper.
12. The patient is given postoperative instructions and is dismissed.

Note: The patient returns to the general dentist for the final restoration of the tooth. Follow-up radiographs may be taken at six months and at one-year intervals.

Surgical Endodontics

Endodontic treatment has a high rate of success; however, situations arise where surgical endodontic treatment is necessary to save the involved tooth from extraction. Surgery is performed in the area surrounding the roots of the teeth. These surgeries involve a facial surface incision through the tissue to expose the underlying bone. An opening through the alveolar bone is made to expose the root area where surgical endodontic treatment is performed.

Apicoectomy

One of the most common endodontic surgical procedures is an **apicoectomy** (a-pee-koh-**ECK**-toh-me). In this procedure, the apex of the root and infection surrounding the area are surgically removed (Procedure 15–3).

PROCEDURE

15-3 Apicoectomy

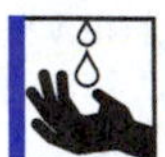
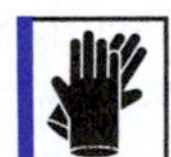
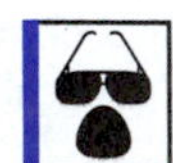
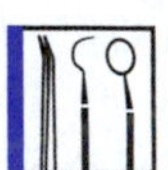

This procedure is performed by the dentist or endodontist, who is assisted by the dental assistant.

EQUIPMENT AND SUPPLIES

- Basic setup: mouth mirror, explorer, and cotton pliers
- Endodontic explorer and spoon excavator
- Locking cotton pliers
- Saliva ejector, surgical evacuator tip, and air-water syringe tip
- Cotton rolls and gauze sponges
- Anesthetic setup
- Scalpel and blades
- Periosteal elevator and tissue retractors
- High-speed handpiece and assortment of burs (handpiece is specifically designed with a very small head)
- Surgical curettes
- Irrigating syringe and a sterile saline solution
- Hemostat and surgical scissors
- Amalgam setup
- Suture setup

PROCEDURE STEPS *(Follow aseptic procedures)*

1. Anesthetic is administered.
2. The operator makes a flap incision with the scalpel and lifts the tissue away from the bone with a periosteal elevator. Retract the tissue for the dentist throughout the procedure.

3. Transfer instruments and keep the site clear and clean using the surgical evacuator and tissue retractors.
4. The high-speed handpiece is used by the operator to gain access to the root apex through the bone.
5. The dentist removes debris and infection around the apex of the root with a surgical curette (apical curettage).
6. Evacuate and remove debris from instruments with a gauze sponge.
7. Prepare the handpiece and the sterile saline irrigation syringe.
8. The high-speed handpiece and burs are used to remove a section of the exposed root tip. The root tip is beveled for better access. The area is rinsed with the sterile saline to prepare the root to receive the **retrograde filling** material.
9. Retrograde filling material is placed in the prepared cavity (Figure 15–5). Amalgam is commonly used, however gutta percha, zinc oxide eugenol, and composites are also used.
10. Flap replacement and suturing are the final steps of this procedure. The flap is returned to position and held in place for a few minutes. The operator then sutures the flap into place.

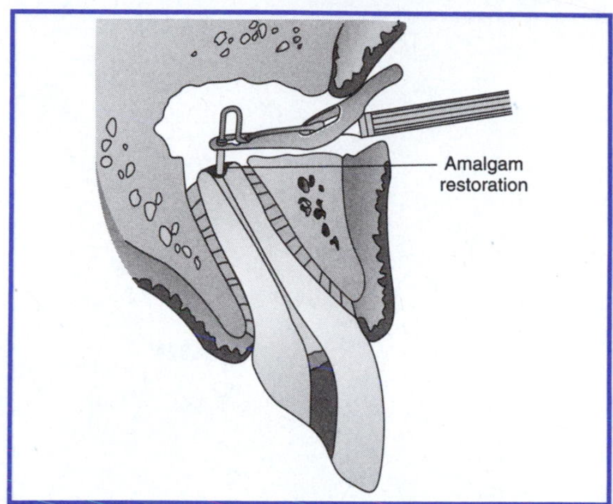

FIGURE 15–5 Retrofill being placed in root canal at the apex of the tooth.

11. Prepare the sutures and assist during placement. Once the suturing procedure is completed, give the patient postoperative instructions, a prescription for pain medication, and dismiss him or her.

CHAPTER 16

Oral and Maxillofacial Surgery

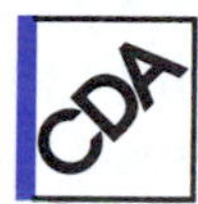

OBJECTIVES

The student should strive to meet the following objectives and demonstrate an understanding of the facts and principles presented in this chapter:

1. Describe the scope of oral and maxillofacial surgery.
2. Identify the various surgical instruments used in oral and maxillofacial surgery and describe their functions.
3. Describe how to prepare the patient for oral/maxillofacial surgical treatment.
4. Explain surgical procedures, including tray setups and assisting responsibilities.
5. List postoperative instructions given to patients.
6. List and describe the types of dental implants and explain the procedures they are used with.
7. Explain the function of sutures and when they are placed.
8. List the equipment and supplies needed for suture removal.
9. List the basic criteria for suture removal.
10. Explain the steps of suture removal.
11. Explain postoperative patient care.

KEY TERMS

alveolitis (p. 286)
alveoplasty (p. 279)
biopsy (p. 281)
debride (p. 290)
dental implants (p. 287)
elevators (p. 273)
extraction forceps (p. 273)
hemostats (p. 272)
luxates (p. 279)
maxillofacial (p. 270)
mouth props (p. 271)
mucoperiosteum (p. 273)
needle holders (p. 272)
osseointegration (p. 287)
periosteal elevator (p. 273)
retractors (p. 271)
rongeurs (p. 273)
root tip picks (p. 273)
surgical aspirating tips (p. 272)
surgical bone files (p. 272)
surgical chisels (p. 272)
surgical curettes (p. 272)
surgical mallet (p. 272)
surgical scalpels (p. 271)
surgical scissors (p. 272)

INTRODUCTION

Oral and **maxillofacial** surgery is the branch of dentistry that focuses on the diagnosis and treatment of diseases, injuries, and malformations. It involves surgery for both functional and esthetic aspects of the face, jaws, mouth, neck, and head. This specialty is sometimes referred to as oral surgery.

The oral and maxillofacial surgeon performs the following: patient examination; diagnosis; teeth extraction; cyst and tumor removal; temporomandibular joint treatment; biopsies; and emergency, reconstructive, and implant surgeries. The oral surgeon works primarily in the office setting but also goes to the hospital to perform complicated surgeries and to treatment emergencies.

The surgical dental assistant's responsibilities often vary depending on the size of the practice.

Typical responsibilities of a surgical dental assistant include:

- Perform traditional duties, such as instrument transfer and maintaining the operating field during the procedure
- Assist with the administration of intravenous sedation and analgesics
- Take and record vital signs
- Prepare treatment rooms
- Sterilize instruments
- Ensure that all presurgery steps are completed and all materials or prosthetics required are ready
- Prepare the patient for treatment
- Maintain asepsis throughout the procedure
- Stabilize the patient's head and mandible during surgery, if necessary

- Provide postoperative instructions to the patient
- Clean the treatment room
- 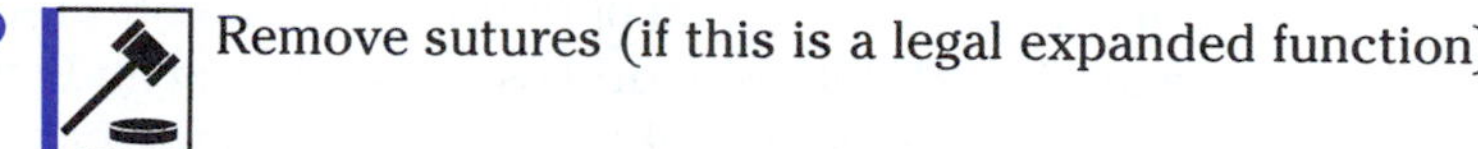 Remove sutures (if this is a legal expanded function)

ORAL SURGERY INSTRUMENTS

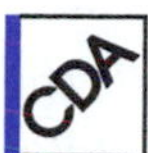

Surgical instruments are designed to apply adequate pressure in specific areas of the oral cavity to remove bone tissue or teeth. Surgical instruments are made of stainless steel (so they can be sterilized after each use).

Scalpel

Surgical scalpels are surgical knives used to *incise* or *excise* the soft tissue in a precise manner with the least amount of trauma.

Scalpels are designed in two sections: the handle and the blade. The metal handle is slim and straight and is designed to accommodate detachable, disposable blades. A common handle is the Bard Parker style. This handle is flat and has a metric ruler. The blades are very sharp and are supplied in a variety of lengths and designs. The blades are used once and then disposed of in the sharps container.

> When removing or replacing blades on the scalpel handle, use cotton pliers, a hemostat, or a blade protector to avoid injury. Disposable surgical blade removers are available. The scalpel blade is placed in a plastic cap of the removers and removed from the handle. The blade is left in the cap and discarded.

Retractors

Retractors are used to deflect tissue from the surgical site so that the operator's view is unobstructed. There are several types of retractors: tissue retractors, cheek and lip retractors, and tongue retractors.

Mouth Props

Mouth props are used to prevent the patient from closing during the procedure. Sometimes, a long appointment, the type of anesthesia administered, or the physical condition of the patient requires the use of props. Mouth props are made of hard rubber, silicone, plastic, or stainless steel. They are supplied in child and adult sizes. The prop is inserted into the patient's mouth with the tapered end toward the posterior teeth. This allows the muscles to relax while keeping the mouth open.

Hemostats

Hemostats have multiple uses during surgical procedures. They are used to retract tissue, remove small root tips, clamp off blood vessels, and grasp loose objects. A hemostat is a forceps with working ends that are not sharp but long, serrated, or grooved beaks. They have locking handles that can be manipulated with one hand.

Needle Holders

Needle holders are similar to hemostats and function in much the same manner. They are forceps with straight beaks; however, needle-holder beaks are shorter than hemostat beaks. The needle holder has fine serrations with a groove down the center of each beak to hold the suture needle.

Surgical Scissors

Surgical scissors are used to cut sutures and to trim soft tissue. They are made of stainless steel and should be used only for surgical procedures to maintain their sharp edges. Surgical scissors have pointed beaks with either straight or angled blades.

Surgical Aspirating Tips

Surgical aspirating tips are made of metal or plastic. The surgical aspirating tips are long tubes that are either very slender or taper to small openings. The tips are used to aspirate blood and debris from the surgical site.

Surgical Curettes

Surgical curettes are used for curettage and debridement of the tooth socket or the diseased tissue. They are double-ended and have either straight or curved shanks; the working end of the instrument is spoon shaped.

Surgical Chisels and Mallets

Surgical chisels are used to remove or shape the bone. They can be used alone if the bone is soft, but if the bone is dense; a **surgical mallet** is used with the chisel. The chisel is positioned on the bone, and mallets are used to gently tap the end of the chisel. Chisels and mallets also are used to split teeth into smaller portions for easier removal.

Surgical Bone Files

Surgical bone files are used in a back-and-forth motion to smooth the edges of alveolar bone. They trim and smooth the bone after the teeth have been extracted and the rongeurs have contoured the bone.

Rongeurs

Rongeurs (**RON**-jeers) are hinged forceps that have springs in the handle. They are used to trim and shape the alveolar bone after extractions. The beaks are sharp and have cutting edges, similar to fingernail trimmers. When multiple teeth are removed and a denture is to be seated, rongeurs are necessary to contour the ridges of the alveolar bone and eliminate sharp edges.

Periosteal Elevator

The **periosteal elevator** is an instrument of many uses. It is often used to detach the **periosteum** (bone covering) and gingival tissues from around the tooth prior to the use of extraction forceps. The periosteal elevator is also used to reflect and lift the **mucoperiosteum** (mucosa and periosteum) from the bone.

Elevators

Elevators are used by the surgeon to loosen and remove teeth, retained roots, and root fragments. Elevators are designed in different shapes and sizes to accommodate a variety of tasks, operating techniques, and tooth morphology.

Apical elevators are similar to the elevators with the large handle but have smaller working ends. They are either straight or angular and have longer, narrower blades to loosen and remove roots or root or bone fragments.

Root tip picks or elevators are thinner and longer than the apical elevators. They are paired left and right and are also either straight or angled. Root tip picks are designed to tease the root tips or fragments out of the bone socket.

Forceps

Extraction forceps are used to remove teeth from the alveolar bone. They are hinged instruments with a variety of handles and beak styles. Specific forceps are used on certain teeth or in certain areas of the mouth (Figures 16–1 and 16–2). Each instrument has a number imprinted on the handle and is labeled with an "L" or "R" for left or right. For example, a #88R is used on the maxillary right first and second molars.

Some forceps are **universal forceps** and can be used on any of the four quadrants.

Asepsis in Oral Surgery

Like all dental offices, the oral and maxillofacial surgery office follows a plan for infection control. It is critical to prevent cross-contamination. The oral surgery office is at a higher risk because of the increased possibility of contact with blood.

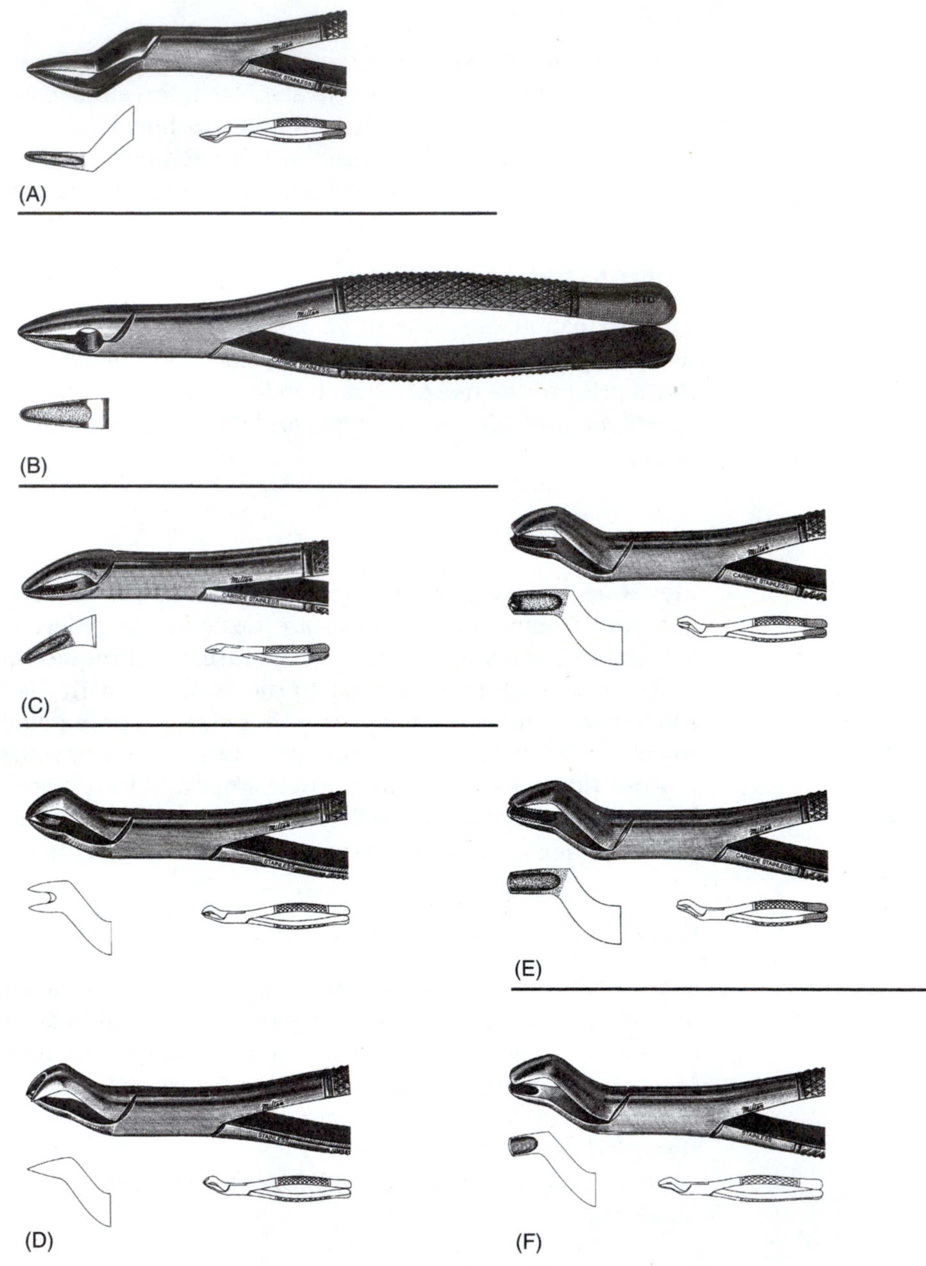

FIGURE 16–1 Maxillary extraction forceps. (A) Incisors and root tips. (B) Incisors and cuspids. (C) #150 incisors, cuspids, bicuspids and roots—universal. (D) #88R and #88L first and second molars. (E) #53R and #53L first and second molars. (F) #210 third molars—universal. *(Courtesy Miltex Instrument Co., Inc., Lake Success, NY)*

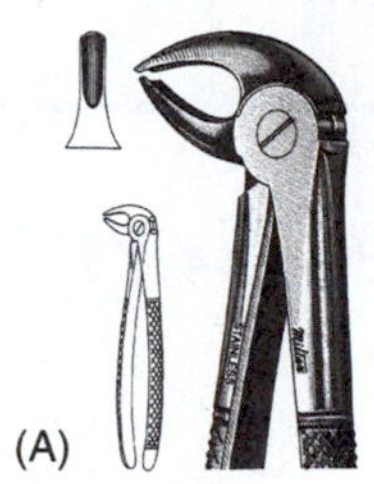

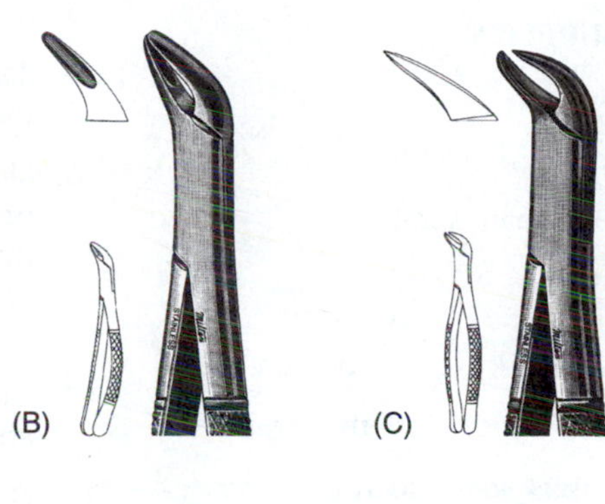

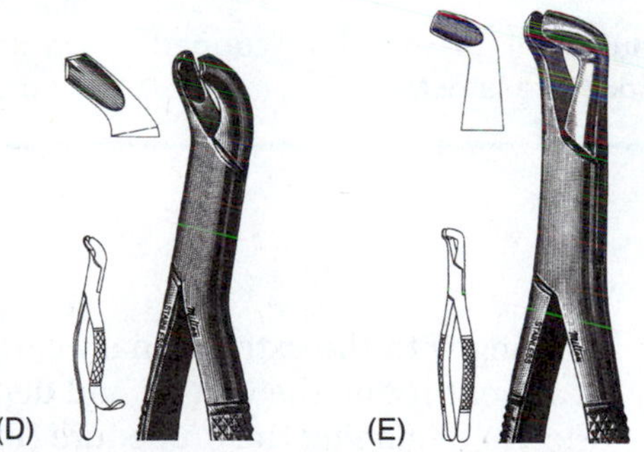

FIGURE 16–2 Mandibular extraction forceps. (A) Incisors, bicuspid, cuspids, and roots. (B) #151 incisors, cuspids, and roots—universal. (C) #23 first and second molars—universal "cow horns". (D) #15 first and second molars—universal with finger ring. (E) #222 third molars—universal. *(Courtesy Miltex Instrument Co., Inc., Lake Success, NY)*

PROCEDURE

16-1 Surgical Scrub

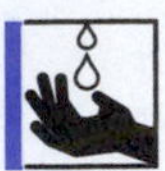

This procedure is performed by the oral surgeon and the dental assistant prior to donning sterile gloves for a surgical procedure.

EQUIPMENT AND SUPPLIES

- Handwashing sink
- Antimicrobial soap
- Sterile scrub brush or foam sponge
- Disposable sterile towels

PROCEDURE STEPS *(Follow aseptic procedure)*

1. Remove watch and rings before the scrub.
2. Use an antimicrobial soap, such as *chlorhexidine gluconate.*
3. Wet hands and forearms up to the elbows with warm water.
4. Dispense about 5 mL of soap into cupped hands and work into a lather.
5. Beginning with the fingernails, scrub the fingers, hands, and forearms with a surgical scrub brush.
6. Rinse thoroughly with warm water.
7. Repeat the procedure with soap but without the scrub brush.
8. Rinse with warm water, beginning at the fingertips and moving hands and forearms through the water and up so that the water drains off the forearms last. This prevents the hands from being recontaminated.
9. Dry hands and arms thoroughly with disposable sterile towels.
10. Don sterile surgical gloves.

Note: The surgical scrub was commonly referred to as the "five-minute scrub." Follow scrub product manufacturer's instructions and OSHA guidelines. Do not use a brush so stiff that it creates microscopic abrasions on the skin.

Along with the extraordinary care of the surgical instruments, supplies, and treatment room, the dentist and dental assistant also perform a surgical scrub prior to beginning the procedure (Procedure 16–1).

The Dentist and the Dental Assistant

The dentist and the dental assistant must follow the routine requirements of personal protective equipment (PPE) for all surgical procedures. The surgical hand scrub is completed before donning sterile gloves.

PATIENT PREPARATION

Whether a general anesthetic is administered will determine the preoperative instructions given to the patient. It is important for the patient to follow the instructions carefully, prior to his or her appointment.

Typical Preoperative Instructions for the Patient

1. Wear loose-fitting clothing and low-heeled shoes. Your shirt should be short sleeved or easy to roll up.
2. Remove contact lenses before surgery.
3. Notify the dentist if a cold, a sore throat, a fever, or another illness develops prior to surgery.
4. Do not consume alcoholic beverages twenty-four hours before surgery.
5. Arrange transportation to and from the office on the day of the surgery.
6. When a physical examination is requested by the oral surgeon, have the physician send written approval prior to surgery.
7. Some medical conditions, such as rheumatic heart disease or artificial heart valves, require prophylactic antibiotics to be taken prior to surgery.
8. If the surgery is in the morning, do not eat anything after midnight. This includes medicines, food, and all fluids.*
9. If the surgery is in the afternoon, drink only water, juice, tea, or coffee prior to six a.m. After six a.m., take absolutely nothing by mouth.*

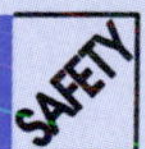

*Food, liquids, or medications in the stomach when general anesthesia is administered may cause vomiting. The vomit may then be aspirated into the lungs.

Patient Preparation

1. The patient should be asked to empty his/her bladder.
2. The patient is escorted to the treatment room. The dental assistant checks the following: any changes in the medical history, whether the patient followed the preoperative instructions, and whether prescribed medication was taken as directed.
3. The patient is given an antimicrobial rinse.
4. The patient is seated and a full-length drape is placed on him or her. The patient is then reclined to a routine position for the dentist.
5. A sterile towel is placed over the patient's chest.
6. Vital signs are taken and recorded. The patient is prepared for administration of the intravenous sedation.

Oral Surgery Procedures

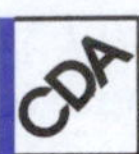

Procedures frequently performed in the oral surgeon's office are routine extractions, multiple extractions and alveoplasty, surgical removal of impacted third molars, biopsy procedures, and dental implant surgery.

Routine or Uncomplicated Extractions

Routine or uncomplicated extractions include the removal of permanent or primary teeth that are erupted into the oral cavity. The dental assistant prepares the tray setup and selects forceps and elevators for the specific tooth to be extracted (Procedure 16–2).

Multiple Extractions and Alveoplasty

Multiple extractions are needed when the patient is to have a full or partial denture. The extraction process is similar for one tooth or for several teeth, how-

PROCEDURE

16-2 Routine or Uncomplicated Extraction

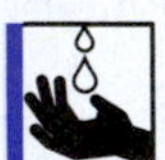
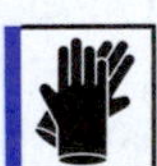
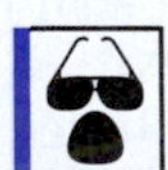
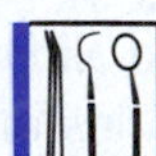

The dental assistant assists the oral surgeon throughout this procedure. The dental assistant must be prepared to anticipate the surgeon's needs.

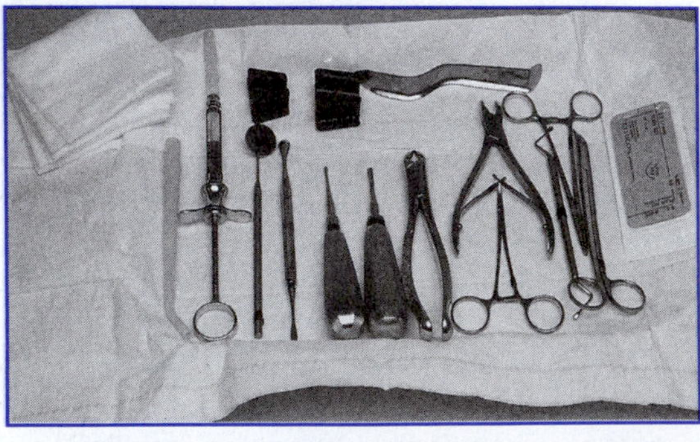

FIGURE 16–3 Tray setup for uncomplicated extraction.

EQUIPMENT AND SUPPLIES *(Figure 16–3)*

- Mouth mirror, explorer
- Gauze sponges
- Surgical HVE tip
- Retractor for the tongue and the cheek
- Local anesthetic setup
- Nitrous oxide setup (optional)
- Periosteal elevator
- Straight elevator
- Extraction forceps
- Hemostat/needle holder
- Surgical curette
- Suture setup

PROCEDURE STEPS *(Follow aseptic procedures)*

1. The surgeon examines the site of extraction. The dental assistant transfers the mouth mirror and explorer to the surgeon. The patient's x-rays are mounted on the viewbox for the dentist to review.

2. Topical anesthetic is placed on the mucosa and local anesthetic is administered. The dental assistant prepares the topical anesthetic and transfers it to the surgeon. The syringe is prepared and transferred to the surgeon. The dental assistant then observes the patient.

3. Either the periosteal or a straight elevator is used by the oral surgeon to determine whether the patient is adequately numb, to separate epithelial attachment from around the tooth, and to initiate alveolar bone expansion around the neck of the tooth (to accommodate forceps placement). The dental assistant transfers and receives elevators and has gauze ready to remove blood or debris from the instruments. The dental assistant maintains the operating field, adjusts the light, and retracts tissues as needed.

4. Once the tooth is loosened in the alveolus, forceps are placed securely on the tooth and, with a firm grasp, the surgeon **luxates** (moves or dislocates) the tooth and then removes it from the socket. This may be easy, or the tooth may have to be subluxated (rocked back and forth), rotated, and lifted several times before the bone around the tooth is spread enough to lift the tooth out of the socket. During this time, the dental assistant transfers forceps and elevators as needed by the surgeon, keeps the instruments clean of debris, and retracts the cheek or tongue. The dental assistant should observe the patient for signs of anxiety or syncope. Once the tooth is extracted, the forceps beaks and tooth are received in the palm of the dental assistant's hand while transferring gauze to the surgeon. Once the forceps and tooth are placed on the tray, the tooth is examined for fractured roots.

5. The alveolus (socket) is examined for fractured root tips and debris. A surgical curette is used to remove bone chips, granulation tissue, and abscesses/cysts. The dental assistant evacuates the alveolus using the surgical HVE tip, then transfers the surgical curette. A gauze is held close to the patient's chin to remove debris from the curette.

6. Once the tooth and any fragments are removed, the area is debrided and the would is covered with a folded, moistened gauze as a pressure pack. The patient is instructed to bite down on the gauze to apply pressure. This aids in controlling the bleeding and the formation of the blood clot.

7. The dentist may place sutures. The dental assistant prepares the sutures and assists during placement. The dental assistant debrides the site with the HVE and has the moistened gauze folded and ready to place.

8. The dental assistant checks and cleans the patient's face, returns the patient to a sitting position, and allows a few minutes before giving postoperative instructions. The patient is then dismissed.

9. The dental assistant gives postoperative instructions.

ever after several teeth have been removed, the bone and soft tissue must be contoured and smoothed. The contouring process is called an **alveoplasty**. The alveolar ridge must be free of any sharp edges or points to achieve the best comfort and function for the patient. If both the maxillary and the mandibular teeth are to be extracted at one appointment, the maxillary teeth are extracted first. This prevents hemorrhage and debris from contaminating the mandibular extraction site during surgery. Routinely, the dentist starts at the most posterior tooth and moves anteriorly (Procedure 16–3).

PROCEDURE

16-3 Multiple Extractions and Alveoplasty

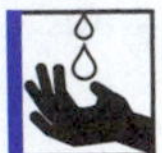 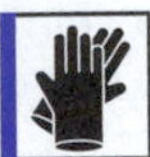 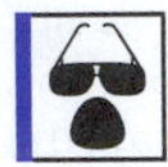 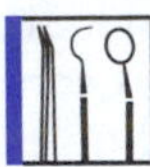

The procedure is performed by the oral surgeon, who is assisted by the dental assistant. This sterile procedure involves the removal of several teeth and contouring the bone. Responsibilities of the dental assistant include evacuation and instrument transfer.

EQUIPMENT AND SUPPLIES *(Figure 16–4)*

- Mouth mirror
- Gauze sponges
- Surgical HVE tip
- Luer lok syringe and sterile saline solution
- Retractor for the tongue and cheeks
- Local anesthetic setup
- Nitrous oxide setup (optional)
- Scalpel and blades
- Hemostat and tissue retractors

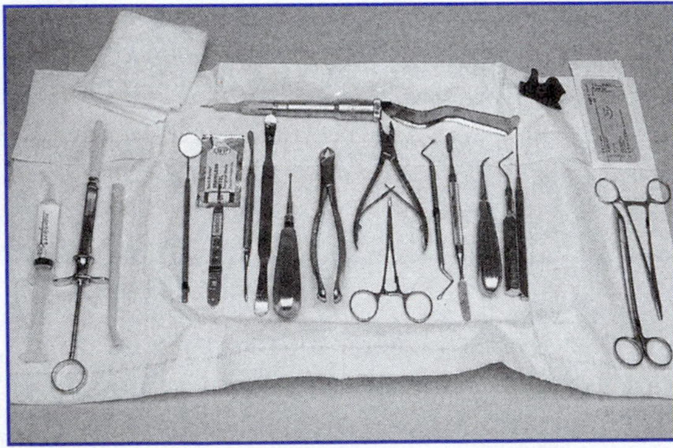

FIGURE 16–4 Tray setup for multiple extractions and alveoplasty.

- Periosteal elevator
- Straight elevator
- Extraction forceps (selected for the teeth being extracted)
- Surgical curette
- Root tip picks
- Rongeurs
- Bone file
- Low-speed handpiece and surgical burs
- Suture setup

PROCEDURE STEPS *(Follow aseptic procedures)*

1. The surgeon examines the teeth to be extracted.
2. When several teeth are to be extracted, the patient may request general anesthesia. The patient will be prepared for intravenous sedation, which is followed by local anesthetic. The local anesthetic reduces bleeding at the extraction site and postoperative pain. The dental assistant prepares the materials necessary for the local and intravenous anesthetic and then assists in the administration.
3. The teeth are removed using the same techniques described for the routine extraction.
4. After the teeth have been extracted and root tips or debris removed, the alveoplasty procedure begins. The alveoplasty usually is accomplished one quadrant at a time. The surgeon makes an incision on the buccal and lingual surface, to remove the interdental papillae and to expose the crest of the alveolar bone. The flap of tissue is reflected for clear vision.

The dental assistant transfers the scalpel and evacuates the area as necessary, receives the scalpel, and transfers the periosteal elevator to reflect the soft tissue. The dental assistant uses tissue forceps to retract the tissue and maintain the operating area.

5. Rongeurs and/or surgical burs are used for the initial trimming and contouring of the alveolar bone. The dental assistant transfers the rongeurs and/or the low-speed handpiece with surgical burs and keeps them free of debris. The dental assistant intermittently uses the HVE and the irrigation syringe with sterile saline solution to maintain the operating field.
6. Final contouring and smoothing are done with the bone file. The area is rinsed with sterile saline solution. At this point, a **plastic stint** (clear denture base material, molded to the same shape and size as the denture) is placed in the patient's mouth. Areas that impinge on the stint can be seen by the surgeon. The surgeon continues to contour the bone until all interferences are removed. The dental assistant transfers instruments and continues to maintain the surgical site. The stint needs to be kept clean, so the dental assistant removes blood and debris from it between placements.
7. The buccal and lingual flaps are repositioned and sutured into position. The dental assistant prepares the suture materials and, once the tissue is in position, the suture is transferred for placement. The dental assistant assists during the suture procedure and holds the tissue as the surgeon places the sutures
8. A folded, moist gauze pack is placed over the surgical site or the immediate denture is seated. The dental assistant prepares the gauze pack and transfers it to the surgeon. If the patient receives an immediate denture, the dental assistant readies the denture and transfers it to the surgeon for placement.
9. The patient is allowed to recover and then postoperative instructions are given both verbally and in writing.
10. The patient is scheduled for a postoperative examination and suture removal.

Impacted Teeth Extractions

Extracting impacted teeth is one of the most common procedures the oral surgeon performs, especially third molar extractions. There are many factors that determine the difficulty of the impacted tooth extraction, including the depth, position, or angulation of the tooth in the bone. The teeth may be impacted in soft tissue or in the bone. If the teeth are impacted in bone, dental hand pieces and surgical burs are required to gain access. Additional surgical instruments are utilized to facilitate the removal of the tooth from the bone. Often, all third molars are removed at one appointment (Procedure 16–4).

Biopsy Procedures

With every patient, the dentist and staff must be aware of any abnormal tissue. Through the clinical examination, x-rays, or patient complaints, the presence of pathology may be discovered. Once the suspicious lesion or area is recognized, the dentist will order a **biopsy**. The biopsy procedure, performed by an oral surgeon, involves removal of tissue from a suspicious area, either totally or partially, for microscopic examination and diagnosis (Procedure 16–5).

PROCEDURE

16-4 Removal of Impacted Third Molars

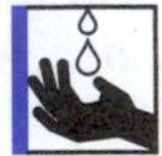
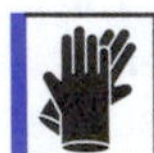
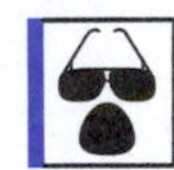
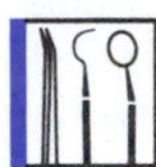

This procedure is performed by the oral surgeon, who is assisted by the dental assistant. Because the teeth are impacted, the surgeon will first have to expose the teeth by incising the tissue and removing the bone. The dental assistant transfers instruments and maintains the operating site.

EQUIPMENT AND SUPPLIES

- Basic setup: mouth mirror, explorer, and cotton pliers
- Gauze sponges
- Surgical HVE tip
- Irrigating syringe and sterile saline solution
- Retractor for the tongue and the cheek
- Local anesthetic setup
- Nitrous oxide setup (optional)
- Scalpel and blades
- Hemostat and tissue retractors
- Periosteal elevator
- Straight elevator
- Extraction forceps (if needed)
- Root tip picks
- Surgical curette
- Rongeurs
- Bone file
- Low-speed handpiece and surgical burs
- Suture setup

PROCEDURE STEPS *(Follow aseptic procedures)*

1. The anesthetic is administered. Oral sedation may be used with local anesthetic, but the most common is intravenous (IV) anesthesia. The dental assistant prepares and transfers the anesthetic and/or assists with the IV.
2. When the patient is adequately anesthetized, an incision is made along the ridge, distal to the second molar. The scalpel incises the mucoperiosteum to the underlying bone. Depending on where the impacted tooth lies, a flap incision may be made to ensure adequate vision for the surgeon. The dental assistant transfers the scalpel and maintains the operating field with the surgical HVE.
3. The periosteal elevator is used to retract the tissue from the alveolar bone. Once the tissue is incised, it must be reflected from the bone. The dental assistant transfers the periosteal elevator and evacuates. When the flap is completed, the dental assistant retracts the tissue.
4. The surgeon uses a surgical bur and handpiece or a chisel and mallet to remove the bone over the tooth. The dental assistant receives the periosteal elevator and transfers the handpiece and bur or the chisel. The dental assistant continues to evacuate as needed.
5. Once the tooth is exposed, it can often be luxated and lifted from the socket with elevators or forceps. If this is not possible, the tooth may be sectioned or divided for removal. This involves sectioning the tooth into two or more parts. Burs and/or the chisel are used to separate the tooth in half to remove part or all of the crown of the tooth from the root portion. The dental assistant passes elevators and forceps. The dental assistant keeps the area clear with the HVE and periodically transfers new gauze to the surgeon.

6. When the tooth is removed, it is placed on a flat surface and examined to ensure that all of the tooth has been removed.
7. Curettes are used to remove the follicle (sac of thickened membrane) and debride the socket. The rongeurs, bone files, or burs may be used to contour the bone margins. The area is then irrigated with sterile water and evacuated. The dental assistant transfers instruments and removes debris from the working ends with gauze. The dental assistant prepares the irrigating syringe with sterile water and evacuates the area thoroughly.
8. The tissue flap is replaced to its normal position over the wound, and the operator sutures the area. The dental assistant prepares the suture and places it in the needle holder and transfers it to the oral surgeon. The cheeks are then retracted so the surgeon can place the sutures. The dental assistant has a folded, moist gauze ready to place when suturing is completed.
9. The patient is allowed to recover and is given postoperative instructions, an ice pack, and a prescription for pain before being dismissed. The patient will need to schedule an appointment for suture removal. The dental assistant stays with the patient during recovery. When the patient is ready to leave, the dental assistant notifies the patient's escort and verifies that the patient has the necessary prescription(s) and postoperative instructions.

PROCEDURE

16-5 Biopsy

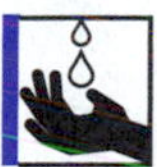
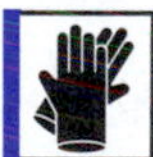
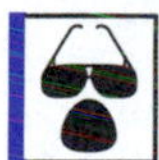
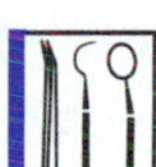

This procedure is performed by the oral surgeon, who is assisted by the dental assistant. The dental assistant readies all materials that are sent to the laboratory as well as the tray setup.

EQUIPMENT AND SUPPLIES

- Mouth mirror
- Local anesthetic setup
- Retractors (tongue, cheek, and tissue)
- Gauze sponges
- Surgical HVE tip
- Scalpel and blades
- Tissue scissors and hemostat
- Small container with a preservative solution, such as formalin
- Suture setup

PROCEDURE STEPS *(Follow aseptic procedures)*

1. The patient is anesthetized with local anesthetic.
2. A scalpel blade is used to incise or excise the lesion and a border of normal tissue. The dental assistant transfers the scalpel with the specific blade the surgeon prefers and has the HVE ready for use, if necessary. The dental assistant uses caution to remove only blood and saliva and not the tissue being removed for biopsy.

(continued)

PROCEDURE 16-5 *continued*

3. Tissue forceps are used to lift the biopsy specimen once freed from the underlying tissue and to place it in a small, covered container. The dental assistant retracts the cheeks and tongue, if needed, and uses gauze to control hemorrhage. The dental assistant has the specimen container ready for the surgeon. Care is taken not to touch the outside of the specimen container in order to prevent contamination. Once the tissue biopsy in placed in the container, the dental assistant replaces the cap tightly.
4. The biopsy site is closed with sutures. The surgeon then prepares the biopsy and the necessary information to be sent to the pathology laboratory. The dental assistant assists during the placement of sutures by transferring the suture needle and thread on needle forceps, retracting tissues, and transferring the suture scissors.
5. The patient is dismissed and scheduled for an appointment in one week for the results of the biopsy and suture removal. The dental assistant gives the patient postoperative instructions. The dental assistant gathers the pertinent information and prepares the biopsy container for pickup by the pathology laboratory.

Postoperative Care of the Patient

Following oral surgery, the patient is given postoperative home-care instructions. The instructions are given routinely by a dental assistant at the direction of the surgeon.

Postoperative Home-Care Instructions

It is important to carefully read and follow these instructions to prevent needless worry. Have someone with you for twenty-four hours following the surgery. Treatment continues until the healing process is completed.

What to expect:

1. **Discomfort** reaches a peak when the anesthetic wears off and sensation returns.
2. **Swelling** is normal following a surgical procedure. The swelling will continue up to twenty-four hours after surgery and can persist for four to five days. Facial discoloration may appear but will disappear.
3. **Bleeding** or oozing may occur for the first twelve to twenty-four hours after surgery. The surgeon will place a sterile gauze in your mouth to bite on immediately following surgery. Remove the gauze when the oozing has stopped.
4. **Difficulty opening mouth, a sore throat,** and **earaches** are not uncommon, especially if third molars were removed.

What to do:

1. Begin taking pain medication before the discomfort begins and the anesthetic wears off. Over-the-counter analgesics are suggested for minor discomfort, and the surgeon will prescribe a stronger medication for pain control, if necessary. Take medications as directed to avoid nausea and vomiting.
2. Use an ice pack to reduce the swelling as soon as possible. Apply the pack to the face over the extraction site for twenty minutes and then remove for twenty minutes (twenty minutes on, twenty minutes off). Continue this cycle intermittently throughout the first twelve to twenty-four hours. After forty-eight hours if the swelling has not subsided, use moist heat.
3. The best way to control bleeding is pressure. To accomplish the pressure needed, place a folded gauze over the surgical site and bite down. Change the sterile gauze pads as needed. If the bleeding persists, insert a wet tea bag over the surgical site and bite down for about twenty minutes. (Tea contains tannic acid, which facilitates in the clotting process.)
4. A soft diet should be followed for twenty-four hours. Eat a well-balanced diet with soups, fruit juices, milk shakes, and other foods, as tolerated. Drink fluids to prevent dehydration and temperature elevation.
5. Take medications to prevent infection as directed.
6. Continue brushing and flossing areas not involved in surgery.
7. Sleep with your head elevated to reduce swelling.
8. Avoid vigorous physical exercise.
9. Rest as much as possible for the first couple of days following surgery to promote healing.

Things to avoid:

1. Avoid strenuous physical activity for forty-eight hours.
2. Do not suck through a straw and avoid spitting.
3. Do not smoke or chew gum.
4. Do not drive, drink alcohol, or operate machinery while taking pain medication.
5. If immediate dentures have been inserted, do not remove them until your next appointment, usually within twenty-four hours of surgery.
6. Do not rinse vigorously for forty-eight hours after surgery. After this time, rinse gently with warm salt-water solution.

IF YOU HAVE ANY QUESTIONS OR PROBLEMS, PLEASE CALL THE OFFICE.

DR. ______________________ TELEPHONE # ________________

Postsurgical Complications

Alveolitis (alveolar osteitis), or **dry socket,** is the most common complication following an extraction. The loss of the blood clot leaves a dry socket, which is very painful. Alveolitis usually develops between the third and the fifth day after surgery (Procedure 16–6).

PROCEDURE

16-6 Treatment for Alveolitis

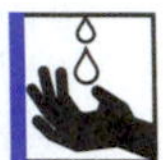 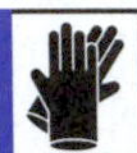 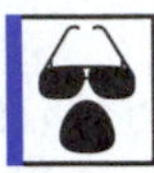 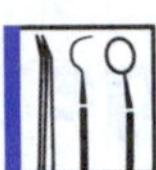

This procedure is performed by the oral surgeon who is assisted by the dental assistant.

EQUIPMENT AND SUPPLIES *(Figure 16–5)*

- Mouth mirror
- Surgical HVE tip
- Local anesthetic setup (may be required)
- Surgical scissors
- Surgical curettes
- Irrigating syringe and warm, sterile, saline solution
- Iodoform gauze or sponge

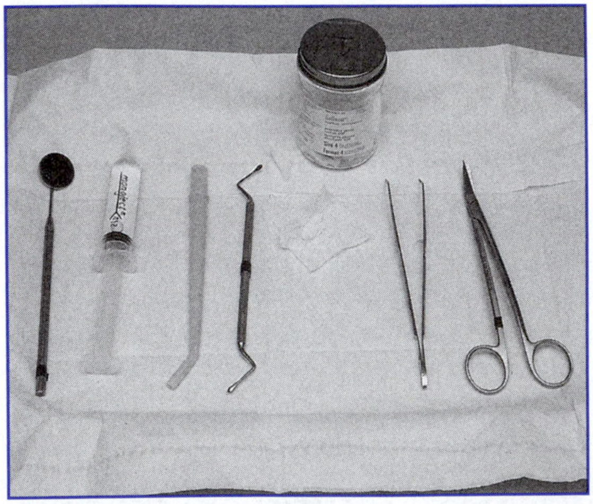

FIGURE 16–5 Tray setup for alveolitis treatment.

PROCEDURE STEPS *(Follow aseptic procedures)*

1. Anesthetic may be administered. The sutures are removed.
2. The surgeon may gently curettage the area inside the socket to stimulate the formation of a new blood clot.
3. The alveolus (socket) is gently irrigated with the warm saline solution. The dental assistant prepares the syringe and maintains the area with retraction and evacuation.
4. The alveolus is gently packed with a medicated dressing. Narrow strips of iodoform gauze or iodoform sponge are used for packing the socket. The dental assistant prepares and transfers the materials to the surgeon for placement.
5. The surgeon prescribes medication for pain control, and the patient is scheduled to return in one to two days.

DENTAL IMPLANTS

Dental implants are becoming an increasingly popular procedure to replace missing teeth. The implant is a metal screw or metal framework surgically embedded in the bone. Titanium is used because it is compatible with human tissue. The implant becomes fused with the bone tissue. This process is called **osseointegration**. Once the implant is integrated and stable in the bone, a fixed or removable prosthesis is fabricated. The prosthesis may be a single crown, bridge, partial, or full denture (Procedure 16–7).

PROCEDURE

16-7 Dental Implant Surgery

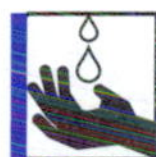
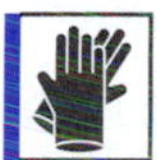
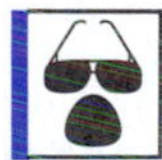
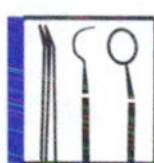

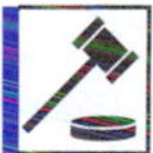

The following procedure is for the surgical placement of an endosteal implant for a single tooth replacement. This is a two-stage procedure in which the appointments are scheduled three to four months apart. During the presurgery appointment, the treatment is explained in detail and the patient signs a written consent for the implant surgery. Radiographs are taken, impressions for diagnostic casts are made, surgical templates (guides) are fabricated, and financial arrangements are completed. The patient is given intravenous sedation for this procedure.

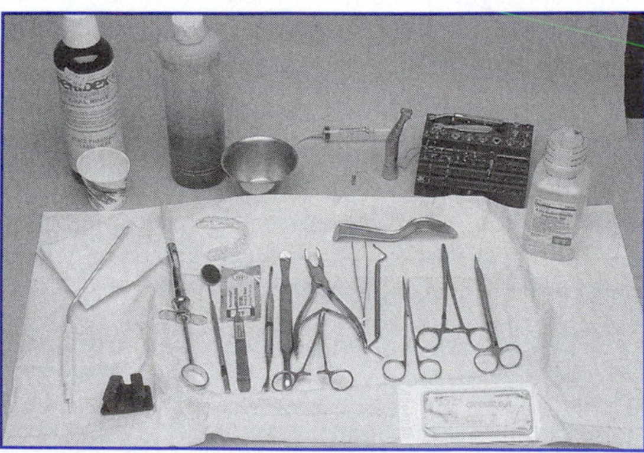

FIGURE 16–6 Tray setup for implant surgery.

EQUIPMENT AND SUPPLIES *(Figure 16–6)*

For first surgical procedure:

- Intravenous sedation and local anesthetic setup
- Mouth mirror
- Surgical HVE tip
- Sterile gauze and cotton pellets
- Irrigation syringe and sterile saline solution
- Low-speed handpiece
- Sterile template
- Sterile surgical drilling unit
- Scalpel and blades
- Periosteal elevator
- Rongeurs
- Surgical currette
- Tissue forceps and scissors
- Cheek and tongue retractors
- Hemostat
- Bite-block

(continued)

PROCEDURE 16-7 *continued*

- Oral rinse
- Betadine
- Implant instrument kit
- Implant kit
- Suture setup

For second surgical procedure:

- First seven items from first procedure
- Electrosurgical (cautery) unit and tips
- Hydrogen peroxide

PROCEDURE STEPS

First Surgery for Endosteal Implants

1. The patient is prepared and IV sedation is administered. Local anesthetic is administered. The dental assistant prepares and assists during the administration of sedation and anesthetic.
2. The surgical template is seated in the patient's mouth. The target is marked through the template into the soft tissues.
3. The template is removed and the oral surgeon incises the tissue to expose the ridge of bone. The dental assistant prepares and transfers the scalpel and blade while maintaining the operating site.
4. A periosteal elevator is used to reflect the overlying tissues. Special spiral burs are used to prepare for the implant. The dental assistant changes burs as size increases and irrigates with the sterile saline solution.
5. The implant is partially placed and then tapped or threaded into position. The dental assistant opens the sterile implant and transfers it to the surgeon. A special inserting mallet or ratchet wrench is transferred, and the dental assistant readies the healing cap and contra-angle screwdriver.
6. A healing cap is screwed into the implant. The dental assistant passes the healing cap and the contra-angle screwdriver.
7. Once the implant and healing cap are positioned, the flap is repositioned and sutured.
8. The patient is allowed to recover and given postoperative instructions.

Second Surgical Procedure

1. Local anesthetic is administered.
2. The template is positioned over the osseointegrated implant and a sharp pointed instrument is used to mark the site.
3. The template is removed and the soft tissue is excised with an electrosurgical loop. Once the healing screw is exposed, it is removed. The dental assistant receives the template and evacuates as the electrosurgical loop is used. Once the tissue is excised, the dental assistant receives the healing screw in a gauze sponge.
4. The inside of the implant is cleaned with hydrogen peroxide on a sterile cotton pellet. The dental assistant prepares the cotton pellet and transfers it to the surgeon.
5. The implant abutment is placed so that it extends slightly beyond the mucosa. The mucosa is then sutured around the abutment. The abutment is transferred to the surgeon and the dental assistant prepares the suture material and assists during the suturing.
6. The patient is given postoperative instructions and is dismissed.

SUTURES

Sutures hold displaced or incised tissue in its original position. Sutures close the wound to promote healing and limit contamination by bacteria and food debris. The dental assistant helps the dentist in the placement of sutures and observes the type and number of sutures, then records this information on the patient's chart for later reference. In five to seven days, the patient returns to the office for the sutures to be removed. In some states, qualified dental assistants are allowed to remove the sutures under the supervision of the dentist. It is the responsibility of the dental assistant to gain the knowledge and the experience necessary to perform this task to the highest standard. The dentist must be aware of the patient's status and be notified immediately if diagnostic decisions are required.

PROCEDURES PRIOR TO REMOVAL OF SUTURES

Prior to the suture removal, several steps and considerations are necessary to ensure patient comfort and safety. Included are reviewing the patient's chart, preparing the equipment and supplies, evaluating the suture site, and consulting with the dentist.

A. Suture Removal Equipment and Supplies

Before the patient's appointment, the tray is set up with the following items: mouth mirror, explorer, cotton pliers, suture scissors, gauze sponges, air-water syringe tip, and evacuator. All aseptic guidelines are followed.

B. Review the Patient's Chart

After the patient has been seated and before the procedure has begun, check the patient's chart for information concerning the sutures. Ask the patient if any problems have occurred with the sutures since the last appointment.

C. Examine the Suture Site

Check the suture site for the following information:

1. Location of the sutures
2. Number of sutures
3. Type or pattern of the sutures
4. Healing of the tissues in the wound area

Healing of the Tissues

The healing of the tissues depends on a number of factors, including the extent of the wound, the healing capabilities of the patient, whether a periodontal dressing was applied, and the amount of healing time. To evaluate the healing process, the dental assistant should **debride** (remove debris from) the suture site. Once the tissues have been cleaned, the suture site is evaluated for progress of healing and signs of infection.

Methods to Debride the Suture Site

1. Use light air and a warm water spray.
2. Use a cotton tip applicator moistened with warm water or diluted hydrogen peroxide.
3. Use a moist cotton gauze and gently dab the suture site.

Suture Removal Criteria

The following are basic criteria to guide the dental assistant when removing sutures:

- Explain the procedure to the patient.
- The healing process should not be disturbed when removing the sutures.
- The suture is removed with the least amount of trauma to the tissues.
- All sutures are removed from the suture site.
- The knot is not cut.
- The suture is cut as closely to the tissue as possible.
- A suture that has been exposed in the mouth is not pulled through the tissue. (This suture is contaminated with saliva, food, and bacteria.)
- The knot is not pulled through the tissue.
- The hemorrhage is controlled following established procedures.
- The sutures are placed on a gauze so they can be counted.

Suture Removal

Each type of suture is placed in a specific pattern. To remove the sutures, identify the pattern and determine where the cuts are to be made. Then, follow the basic criteria and remove the sutures from the suture site (Procedure 16–8 and 16–9).

PROCEDURE

16-8 Removal of the Simple Suture and Continuous Simple Sutures

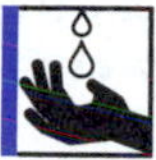 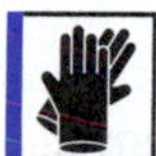 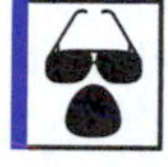 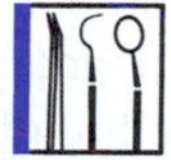 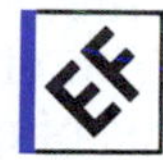

This procedure is performed by the dentist or the expanded-function dental assistant. The patient returns to the office for suture removal. The dental assistant prepares the materials needed and the patient before beginning the procedure.

EQUIPMENT AND SUPPLIES

- Basic setup: mouth mirror, explorer, cotton pliers
- Suture scissors
- Hemostat
- Gauze sponges
- Air-water syringe tip, HVE tip

PROCEDURE STEPS *(Follow aseptic procedures)*

1. Using cotton pliers, gently lift the suture away from the tissues.
2. Take the suture scissors and cut the thread below the knot, close to the tissue.
3. Secure the knot with the cotton pliers and gently pull, lifting the suture out of the tissues.
4. Place the suture on a gauze sponge.
5. For continuous simple sutures, cut each suture and remove individually. Begin with one end and then proceed with each suture stitch.

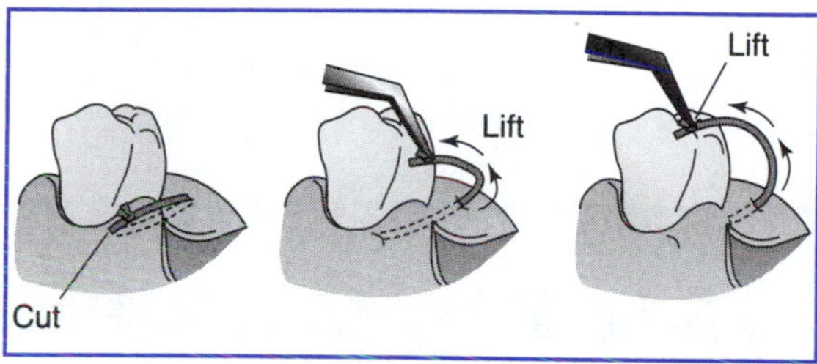

FIGURE 16–7 Removal of simple and continuous simple sutures.

6. Loosen the suture with the cotton pliers and, while still holding the suture thread with the cotton pliers, cut the thread close to the tissue (Figure 16–7).
7. As each suture is removed, place it on a gauze sponge so it can be counted when finished with the procedure.

Always carefully evaluate the sutures before cutting them to be sure sutures exposed in the oral cavity are not pulled through the tissue during removal.

Post Suture Removal

If bleeding resulted when the sutures were removed, apply pressure with gauze sponge for a few minutes until the bleeding stops. Check the patient's mouth for debris and wipe around the outside of the patient's mouth if necessary. After the sutures are removed, the dental assistant should instruct the patient to continue with a soft diet and rinse with warm saltwater for several days. Before the patient is dismissed, the dental assistant should document the procedure on the patient's chart. The chart entry should include any complications encountered and the degree of healing of the suture site.

PROCEDURE

16-9 Removal of Sling Sutures and Continuous Sling Sutures

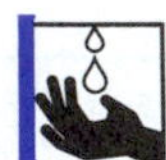
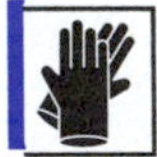
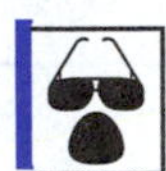
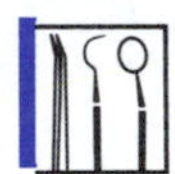
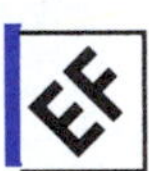

This procedure is performed by the dentist or the expanded-function dental assistant. The patient returns to the office for suture removal. The dental assistant prepares the materials needed and the patient before beginning the procedure.

PROCEDURE STEPS *(Follow aseptic procedures)*

1. The sling suture is cut in two places. With cotton pliers, lift the suture gently on each side of the tooth to loosen the suture from the tissue (Figures 16–8A and B).
2. Lift the knot gently and cut below the knot, near the tissue.
3. Lift the suture thread on the other side of the tooth, near the tissue, and cut it as close to the tissue as possible without cutting the tissue.

Note: When removing a continuous sling suture, this process is repeated, cutting on each side of the tooth until all sutures have been removed.

4. Using cotton pliers, remove each thread carefully, pulling toward the opposite surface, away from the flap. If the suture is taken on the facial and wrapped around the lingual, pull toward the lingual to remove the sutures.
5. Place each thread of the suture on a gauze sponge to be counted.
6. Examine the suture site.

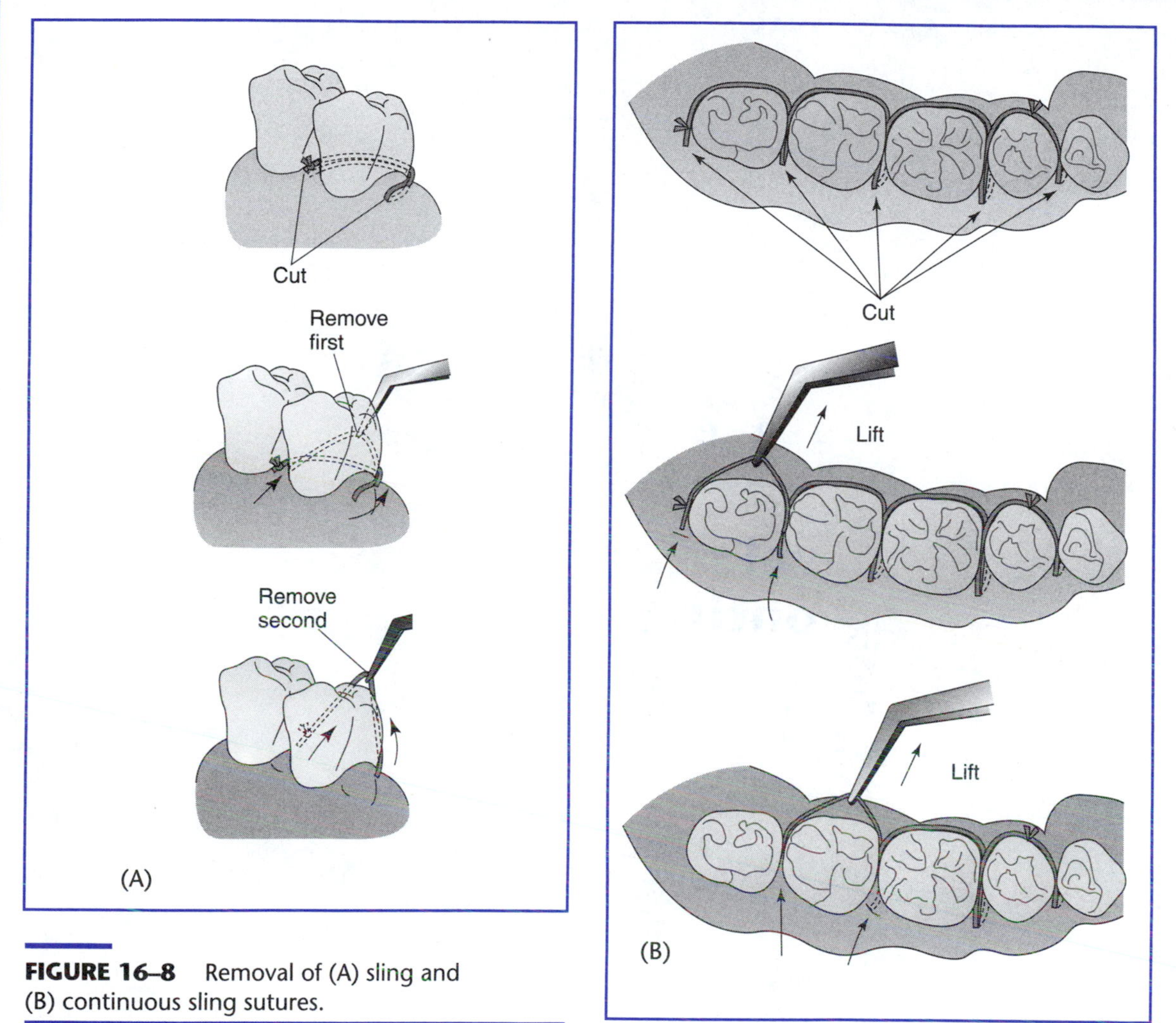

FIGURE 16–8 Removal of (A) sling and (B) continuous sling sutures.

CHAPTER 17

Orthodontics

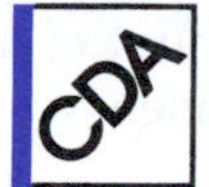

OBJECTIVES

The student should strive to meet the following objectives and demonstrate an understanding of the facts and principles presented in this chapter:

1. Define orthodontics and describe the orthodontic office setting.
2. Describe preventive, interceptive, and corrective orthodontics.
3. Describe the preorthodontic appointment to obtain diagnostic records.
4. Describe the consultation appointment and the role of the patient and the orthodontist.
5. Differentiate between fixed and removable appliances.
6. Identify and describe the function of the basic orthodontic instruments.
7. Describe the stages of orthodontic treatment.
8. Explain the procedure for removing orthodontic appliances and how the teeth are retained in position after removal of appliances.

KEY TERMS

arch wires (p. 299)
brackets (p. 299)
buccal tubes (p. 299)
elastics (p. 299)
ligature wire (p. 299)
orthodontic bands (p. 299)
plastic rings (p. 299)
separators (p. 301)
springs (p. 299)

Introduction

Orthodontics is a specialty of dentistry concerned with the recognition, prevention, and treatment of malalignment and irregularities of the teeth, jaws, and face. Patients seek orthodontic treatment for esthetic and functional reasons.

> *Ortho* means straight; *odont* means tooth.

The Orthodontic Assistant

The orthodontic assistant has a variety of responsibilities depending on the size of the practice and the number of assistants. The functions also vary with each state's Dental Practice Act. Generally, the orthodontic assistant has the following responsibilities:

- Seats and dismisses the patient
- Takes study model impressions
- Takes and processes intraoral radiographs (if not provided by the general dentist)
- Takes and processes extraoral radiographs (panoramic and cephalometric)
- Does the tracing on cephalometric radiographs
- Performs general chairside assisting responsibilities during the treatment appointments
- Maintains and sterilizes instruments
- Maintains inventory and supplies
- Performs routine maintenance of equipment
- Gives oral hygiene instructions
- Gives instructions on appliance wear and care
- Prefits bands before cementation*
- Removes excess cement from bands and brackets*
- Applies sealants to teeth to be bonded*
- Checks for loose and broken appliances at each appointment*
- Places and removes arch wires and ligatures*
- Removes bands and brackets*

*(Where allowed by the state Dental Practice Act)

TYPES OF ORTHODONTIC TREATMENT

Orthodontic treatment involves much more than straightening teeth. The scope of treatments in orthodontics includes:

- Maintaining or establishing a normal, functional occlusion
- Improving the esthetic appearance of the face
- Eliminating problems that may disrupt normal development of the teeth and facial structures
- Correcting facial and oral deformities

Orthodontic treatments are divided into cases where malocclusion may be prevented or intercepted and cases where malocclusion already exists and correction is needed.

PREORTHODONTIC TREATMENT

Often, the patient's first visit to the orthodontist is for a preliminary examination. This enables the orthodontist to make an initial recommendation to determine whether treatment is advisable at that time or should be delayed until further dental development. If treatment is delayed, follow-up appointments may be scheduled periodically to reevaluate the patient's growth patterns. If treatment is advised, an appointment is scheduled for diagnostic records.

Diagnostic Records

Diagnostic records for orthodontic treatment include a medical and dental history, clinical examination, panoramic x-rays, cephalometric (**SEF**-ah-loh-meh-trick) x-rays, intraoral and facial photographs, and study models of the teeth.

Clinical Examination

The orthodontist evaluates the results of an extensive examination of the face, jaws, and teeth, looking for symmetry between them. The teeth are evaluated for size, shape, and position. The jaws are examined for size, shape, and relationship to one another.

The oral cavity is also examined for abnormal functional and neuromuscular patterns, such as tongue sucking, tongue thrusting, mouth breathing, and bruxism.

Radiographs

The orthodontic assistant takes radiographs as part of the diagnostic procedure. The most common type of radiographs for orthodontics are panoramic and cephalometric. Some intraoral films are also taken for more detail of a particular area.

Panoramic x-rays are taken for an overall view of the dentition and surrounding area. Impacted teeth, abscesses, supernumerary teeth, or disorders of the temporomandibular joint can be determined from the panoramic film.

Cephalometric films are taken to evaluate growth patterns and to determine the course of treatment. The cephalometric radiograph is a lateral view of the patient's head that shows the jaw and the teeth. Cephalometric radiograph tracings are done to determine the relationship of certain landmarks.

Photographs

Intraoral and extraoral photographs are taken as part of the patient's records before and after treatment. Facial photographs include a full frontal view and a profile. These are used to evaluate the symmetry and balance of the face.

Study Models

Study models or diagnostic casts are part of the patient's record. They show how the teeth, mouth, and arches relate to each another. Study casts provide information about the sizes and positions of the teeth, along with the widths and lengths of the arches.

The Consultation Appointment

After the diagnostic appointment, the patient (and a parent if the patient is under the age of 18) is scheduled for a consultation appointment. The orthodontist studies the information gathered, makes a diagnosis, and prepares a treatment plan before the patient's appointment. Radiographs, photographs, study models, and other visual aids are used in the presentation. During the consultation, the treatment, duration of treatment, involvement, and fees are explained. The responsibility of the patient is reviewed at this time so it is understood what he or she must do to facilitate treatment progress as planned. If the patient accepts the treatment plan, consent papers are signed and financial arrangements are made.

Orthodontic Appliances

Orthodontic appliances are classified into two categories: fixed and removable.

Fixed Appliances

Fixed appliances are attached to the teeth and cannot be removed by the patient. The appliances are directly bonded onto the tooth or cemented into place. Fixed appliances are commonly known as **braces.**

Orthodontic Bands. **Orthodontic bands** are thin bands of stainless steel carefully fitted around each tooth. Bands are supplied in a variety of sizes and are presized on the patient's model before cementation. Glass ionomer, polycarboxylate, or zinc phosphate cement is commonly used to cement orthodontic bands. Bands are used on the posterior teeth to hold and control tooth movement. Depending on the individual case, various attachments such as brackets or buccal tubes are placed on the bands.

Brackets. **Brackets** are attachments that are either welded to the bands or bonded directly to the teeth. Brackets for the posterior teeth are made of stainless steel and are welded directly to the band. Brackets for the anterior teeth are made of stainless steel, ceramic, or acrylic and are cemented or directly bonded to the teeth.

The functions of brackets are to hold the arch wire in place and to transmit the force of the arch wire to move the tooth.

Arch Wires. **Arch wires** fit into brackets and are secured by ligature ties or elastics. The arch wire is placed in the bracket and through a buccal tube on a posterior molar and then at each bracket; ligature wire or elastics are wrapped around the bracket. Arch wires are supplied in different shapes (square, round, and rectangular), diameters, and compositions, which alter the treatment outcome.

The function of the arch wire is to apply force to either move the teeth or to hold them in the desired positions.

Ligature Wire and Plastic Rings. **Ligature wire** and **plastic rings** are used to hold the arch wire to the brackets. Ligature wire is very thin, flexible wire supplied in precut lengths or on spools. The wire is wrapped around the brackets and then tightened by twisting the wire, which ties or ligates the arch wire to the bracket. Plastic rings, also called elastic ties, are small bands that slip over the bracket to secure the arch wire. Elastic chains are also commonly used. The chain is a continuous chain of *O*s. The elastic chain attaches several adjacent teeth together. This continuous pressure brings the teeth into alignment.

Buccal Tubes. **Buccal tubes** are small cylinders of metal welded to the molar bands, usually on the buccal surface. They provide a method of attachment for the arch wire to connect to the band in the posterior of the mouth.

Springs. **Springs** are specially bent or shaped wires that are attached to the main arch wire. The finger spring provides gentle pressure to individual teeth. The coil springs exert a pressure to expand and compress spaces without losing the working force.

Elastics. **Elastics** are rubber bands or elastic threads available in a variety of sizes. Elastics provide force for movement. They are often used between the upper and lower arches. Elastics are attached to hooks or buttons that are secured on the band or brackets.

TECH

A new advancement in ligature ties is the fluoride-releasing tie that reduces decalcification of the tooth.

Removable Appliances

Removable appliances are designed to be inserted into the mouth and removed by the patient. The more commonly used removable appliances include headgear, functional appliances, retainers, and positioners.

Orthodontic Instruments

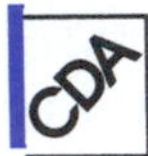

Following are commonly used orthodontic instruments and their functions (Figure 17–1):

- Coons ligature tying pliers—Manipulate ligature wire
- Mathieu needle holder—Tie ligature wire and place elastic ligatures
- Ligature director—Tucks twisted ligature wire ends into the interproximal spaces (a small condenser may also be used)
- Pin and ligature cutter or light wire cutter—Cut thin ligature wire
- Howe pliers—Utility pliers to manipulate ligature wire
- Band seater—Seats posterior metal bands
- Bite stick band seater—Uses force of occlusion to seat the band
- Band driver—Pushes the band into place
- Posterior band removing pliers—Removes posterior bands
- Band contouring pliers—Stretch and shape the posterior bands to adapt to the tooth

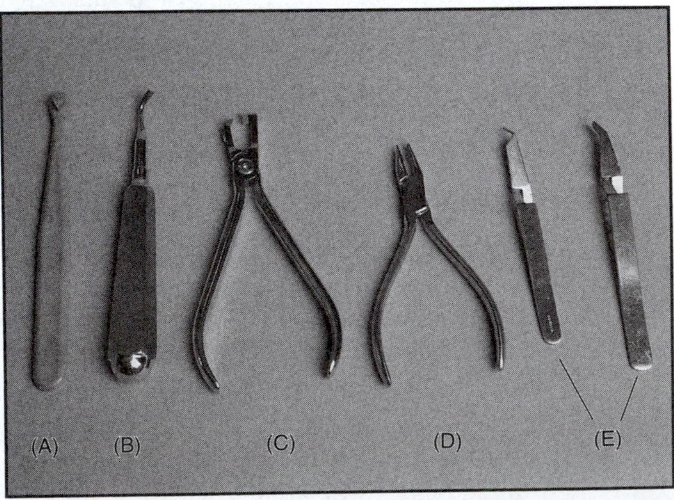

FIGURE 17–1 Orthodontic instruments. (A) Band biter. (B) Band driver (pusher). (C) Posterior band removing pliers. (D) Band contouring pliers. (E) Bracket forceps.

- Bracket forceps—Hold brackets for placement and positioning
- "Bird beak" pliers—Contour wire and form springs
- Three-prong pliers—Adjust and bend wire and clasps
- Weingart utility pliers—Place the arch wire
- Tweed-loop pliers—Form loops and springs in wire
- Distal-end cutting pliers—Cut the distal ends of the arch wire

ORTHODONTIC TREATMENTS

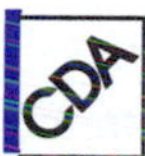

Orthodontic treatment begins after the patient has finished the consultation appointment, the general dentist has restored all areas of decay, and the patient has been given a prophylaxis and fluoride treatment.

Separators

A few days before the bands are placed on the posterior teeth, the patient is scheduled for placement of **separators**. Separators are placed in the contact areas between the teeth, forcing the teeth to spread apart to accommodate the orthodontic bands (Procedure 17–1).

Selection of Orthodontic Bands

The patient returns to the office in a few days to have the separators removed and the orthodontic bands placed. The bands may be selected and sized on the patient's study model before the appointment, or the selection may take place directly on the patient, during the appointment.

Band Cementation

Orthodontic bands are cemented using a variety of cements, including glass ionomer, polycarboxylate, and zinc phosphate. Although zinc phosphate cement has been used for many years, glass ionomer cement is becoming the preferred cement because it releases fluoride, which helps prevent decay under the bands during treatment (Procedure 17–2).

Direct Bonding Brackets

The placement of brackets directly on the anterior teeth is a popular choice of treatment. The bracket kit includes brackets from the left second bicuspid to right second bicuspid on both arches.

The brackets are bonded to the tooth surface with a similar composite resin material and technique that is used to restore anterior teeth (Procedure 17–3).

PROCEDURE

17-1 Placement and Removal of Elastic Separators

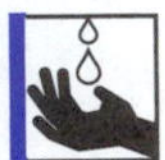
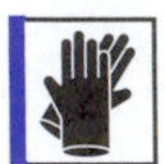
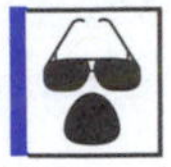
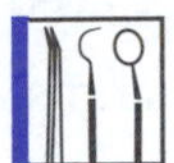
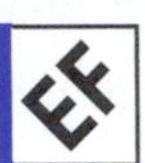

After the diagnosis, the first treatment appointment is to place separators to prepare the teeth for the orthodontic bands. Following the dentist's directions, the dental assistant places the separators. The patient has the separators removed and the bands placed several days following this procedure.

EQUIPMENT AND SUPPLIES *(Figure 17–2)*

- Basic setup: mouth mirror, explorer, and cotton pliers
- Separation pliers
- Separators (wire or elastic)
- Dental floss or tape (optional technique)
- Scaler

PROCEDURE STEPS *(Follow aseptic procedures)*

Placement of Elastic Separators with Separating Pliers

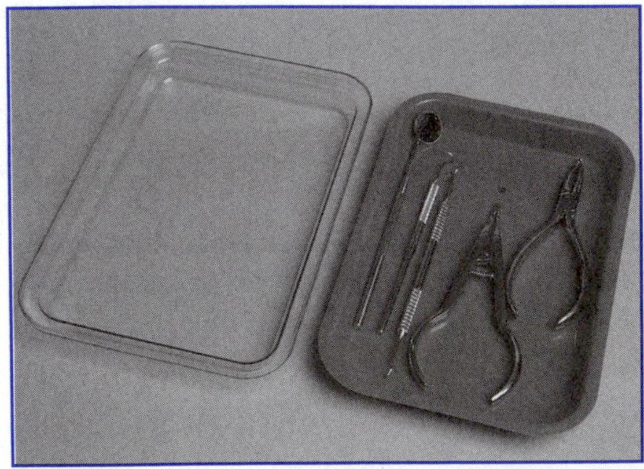

FIGURE 17–2 Separating pliers, Howe pliers, and elastics.

1. First, examine the patient's mouth using the mouth mirror.
2. Place the elastic separator over the beaks of the separating pliers. Squeeze the pliers to secure the elastic on the pliers.
3. Further squeeze the pliers to stretch the elastic separator and place it between two teeth in a back-and-forth motion similar to the motion used when flossing. Insert one side of the elastic band below the contact in the interproximal space.
4. Release the tension on the separating pliers and remove the pliers. Repeat this process on all interproximal spaces around the teeth that are going to receive metal bands.

Placement of Separators with Dental Floss

1. Place two lengths of dental floss through an elastic separator.
2. Fold over each floss length until the ends meet. Pull each piece of floss by the ends to stretch the elastic.
3. Using the back-and-forth motion, insert the separator into place.
4. Once the separator is in place, release the floss and pull free.

Removal of Elastic Separators

1. Using a scaler or an explorer, insert one end into the ring of the elastic separator.
2. Place a finger over the top of the separator to prevent the separator from snapping and injuring the patient.
3. Pull gently on the instrument toward the occlusal until the elastic is free of the contact.

17-2 Cementation of Orthodontic Bands

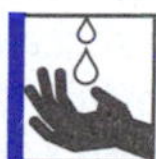  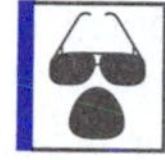 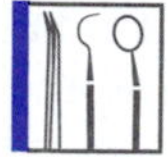 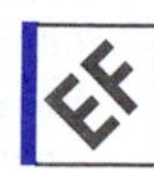

The orthodontic bands are prepared specifically for the patient. The orthodontist places the bands on the teeth to correct the patient's malocclusion. The dental assistant mixes the cement and prepares the band for seating.

EQUIPMENT AND SUPPLIES *(Figure 17-3)*

- Basic setup: mouth mirror, explorer, and cotton pliers
- Cotton rolls and gauze
- Saliva ejector and HVE
- Slow-speed handpiece with rubber cup and prophy paste
- Selected and prepared bands
- Band pusher
- Bite stick
- Scaler
- Cement of choice
- Paper pad or glass slab
- Cement spatula
- Plastic filling instrument (PFI)

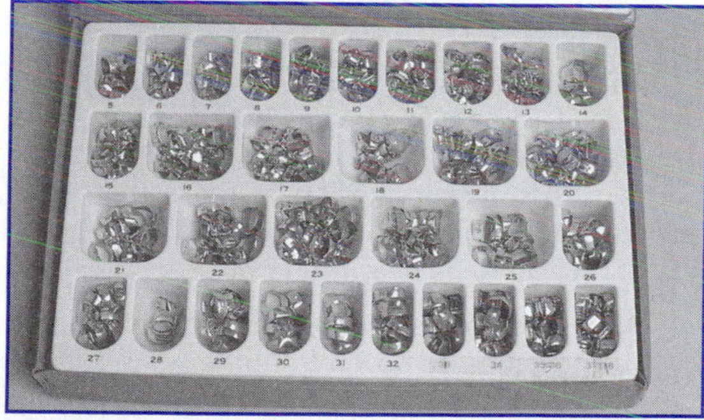

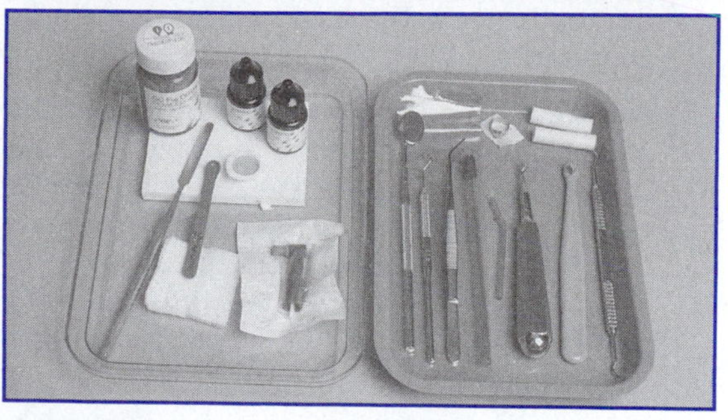

FIGURE 17–3 Selection of bands and armamentarium for cementation.

PROCEDURE STEPS *(Follow aseptic procedures)*

1. Once the separators are removed, the teeth are polished using a rubber cup.
2. The patient's mouth is rinsed thoroughly. The teeth are dried and cotton rolls are placed for isolation in the areas where the bands are to be placed.
3. Mix the cement according to the manufacturer's directions and load the first band. Place cement from the gingival edge, covering the inside of the band. Once the band is ready, transfer it to the orthodontist. Some orthodontists prefer placement on the mixing slab or pad in order. Others like the bands passed on the end of the spatula or on a piece of wax or masking tape. Position the bands so that the orthodontist can pick them up in the order of sequence of placement.
4. The orthodontist seats the band on the tooth. Transfer the band driver and any other instrument the orthodontist might request until the band is properly seated.
5. The banding procedure is repeated. Continue to fill the bands and transfer them to the operator until all bands have been cemented or until the cement becomes too thick and a new mix is required. If a new mix is required, clean

(continued)

PROCEDURE 17-2 *continued*

the instruments with a wet gauze or an alcohol wipe and mix additional cement.

6. Once all bands are in place, the cement is allowed to set. During this time, clean the cement off all used instruments.
7. After the cement is set, remove the excess cement from around the bands with a scaler. When all the cement has been removed, the protective pins or wax is (are) removed from the brackets and the patient's mouth is rinsed.

PROCEDURE

17-3 Direct Bonding of Brackets

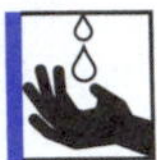
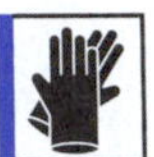
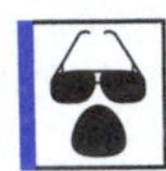
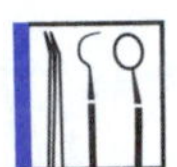
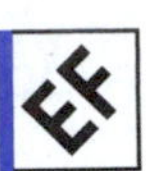

This procedure involves bonding the brackets to the teeth.

EQUIPMENT AND SUPPLIES

- Basic setup: mouth mirror, explorer, and cotton pliers
- Cotton rolls and gauze
- Saliva ejector and HVE
- Slow-speed handpiece with rubber cup and pumice
- Bracket kit
- Retractors for the cheeks and lips
- Bracket forceps
- Acid etchant
- Bonding agent
- Scaler

PROCEDURE STEPS *(Follow aseptic procedures)*

1. Polish the teeth that are to receive brackets with a rubber cup and pumice. (Polishing paste with fluoride is not used because some of the ingredients will interfere with the bonding process.)
2. The patient's mouth is rinsed and dried. Cotton rolls are placed in the area where brackets are to be bonded and retractors are positioned.
3. The acid etchant is placed on the enamel surface. The etchant remains on the tooth for a specific amount of time, following the manufacturer's directions. Prepare the etchant and transfer it to the operator. Maintain the operating field to be sure it stays dry.
4. Rinse the patient's mouth to ensure that all the etchant is removed from the tooth surface (approximately thirty seconds) and then dry the tooth/teeth. The teeth will have a chalky appearance.
5. Prepare the bonding agent according to the manufacturer's directions and apply it to the back of the bracket. Transfer the agent to the dentist for placement on the tooth. Then, pass the bracket. The orthodontist positions it on the tooth. Any excess bonding agent is removed with a scaler or similar instrument from around the bracket.
6. The brackets are held in position on the tooth until the bonding material is set chemically or with a curing light.
7. Remove the cotton rolls and the retractors from the patient's mouth.

Placement of the Arch Wire

The orthodontist selects and shapes the arch wire so the arch wire can be positioned and secured in place. The arch wire is commonly secured into the brackets with elastic or stainless steel ligatures (ties). There is also a bracket that does not require ligature ties; instead, the bracket has a slot that opens for placement and removal of the arch wire. It is called the "Damon SL" (Procedure 17–4).

PROCEDURE

17-4 Placement of the Arch Wire and Ligature Ties

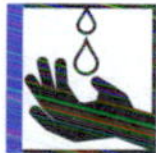
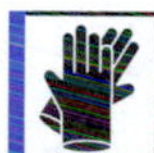
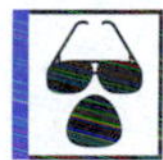
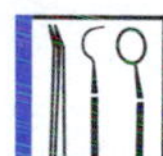
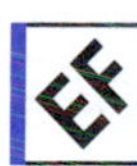

This procedure involves the placement of the arch wire and ligature ties.

EQUIPMENT AND SUPPLIES

- Basic setup: mouth mirror, explorer, and cotton pliers
- Cotton rolls and gauze
- Saliva ejector and HVE
- Selected arch wire
- Weingart pliers
- Bird beak pliers
- Elastics or ligature wire
- Ligature cutting pliers
- Ligature tying pliers
- Distal-end cutting pliers
- Condenser

PROCEDURE STEPS

1. Insert the arch wire into the buccal tubes on the molar bands using the Weingart pliers. If the wire is too long, cut off the ends with the distal-end cutting pliers.
2. The arch wire is placed in the brackets' horizontal slots along the arch. This may be done with plastic rings/elastic ties, ligature wire, or the Damon SL bracket.

Elastic Ties Placement

3. The elastic ties are slipped over the brackets using ligature tying pliers or a hemostat. The ring ties are spread and placed on the gingival extensions of the brackets, pulled over the arch wire, and then wrapped around the occlusal extensions of the brackets.

Ligature Wire Ties Placement

4. Hold the ligature wire between the thumb and the index finger. Wrap the wire around the occlusal and gingival wings of the bracket in a distal-mesial direction. Cross the ends of the wire together. Using a hemostat or ligature tying pliers, twist the ends of the wire together for several rotations. Repeat the process to secure the arch wire (Figure 17–4A).

(continued)

PROCEDURE 17-4 *continued*

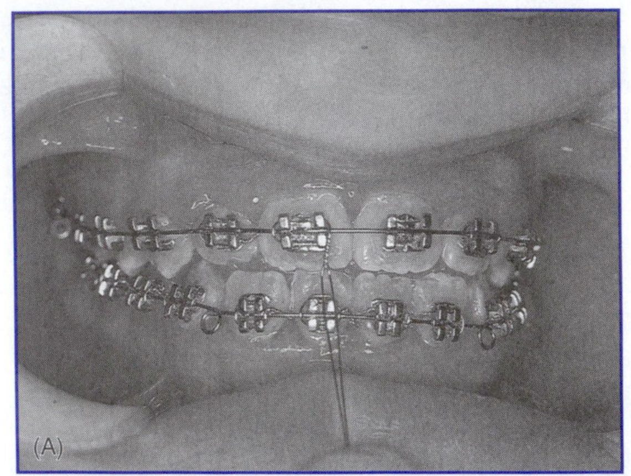

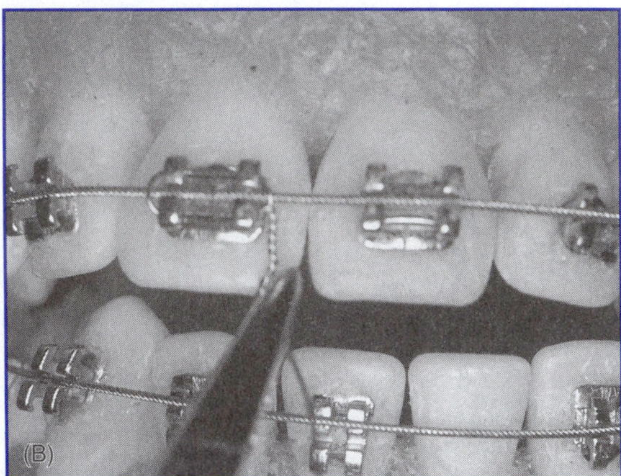

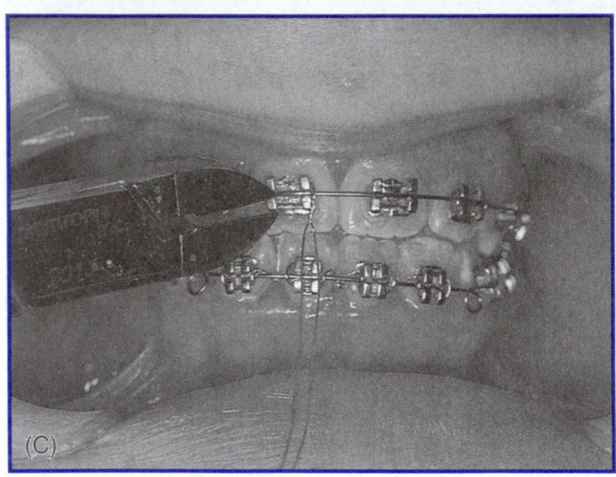

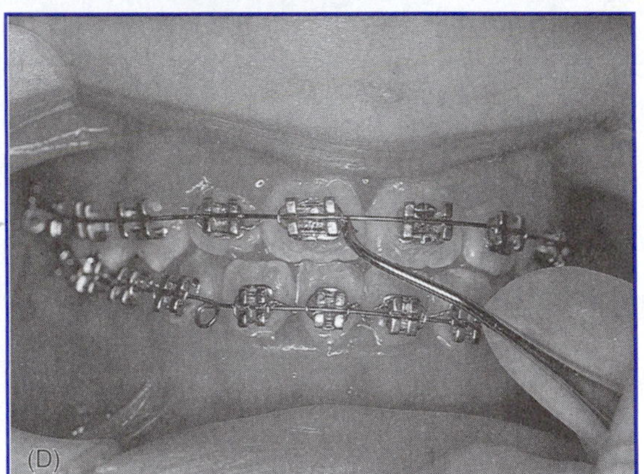

FIGURE 17–4 (A) Ligature wire being looped around the brackets. (B) Ligature wire is twisted. (C) Ligature wire is cut with cutting pliers. (D) and tucked into the embrasure space. *(Courtesy of Rita Johnson, RDH, and Dr. Vincent DeAngelis)*

5. The twisted ends of the ligature wire, called the "pigtail," are cut with ligature wire cutting pliers to 3 to 4 mm (Figure 17–4B and C).
6. The pigtail is bent into the embrasure space with a condenser (Figure 17–4D).
7. After all the pigtail ends have been tucked into place, run a finger over the area to check for sharp ends.
8. Check the distal ends of the arch wire. Cut any excess with distal-end cutting pliers.
9. If the patient's treatment requires rubber elastic bands, they are placed at this appointment. The patient is shown how to place and remove them. The rubber bands stretch with time, so the orthodontist will give instructions on how often to change the rubber bands. The patient is given a sufficient number of elastics with instructions to call the office for more, if needed.

Completion Appointment

Once the teeth have moved into position and the orthodontist is satisfied with the treatment, the braces are removed. The patient receives a coronal polish and an impression is taken for construction of a retainer or positioner to hold the teeth in position (See Procedure 17–5).

PROCEDURE

17-5 Completion Appointment

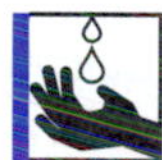 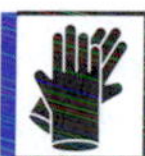 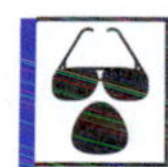 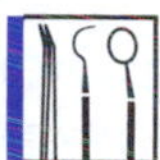 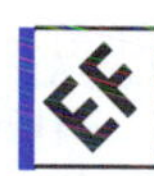

When the orthodontist determines that the patient's teeth have moved to the desired positions, the appliances are removed.

EQUIPMENT AND SUPPLIES

- Basic setup: mouth mirror, explorer, and cotton pliers
- Cotton rolls and gauze
- Scaler
- Ligature wire cutting pliers
- Hemostat
- Bracket and adhesive removing pliers
- Posterior band remover
- Ultrasonic scaler (optional)
- Prophy angle, cups, and prophy paste
- Alginate impression material and selected tray

PROCEDURE STEPS *(Follow aseptic procedures)*

1. The ligature ties are removed first. They are loosened with a scaler or an explorer and then cut with the ligature wire cutting pliers.

Elastic Bands

2. Elastic ties are removed with a scaler.
3. The tip of the scaler explorer is placed under the elastic and rolled over the bracket wings until the elastic is released (Figure 17–5).

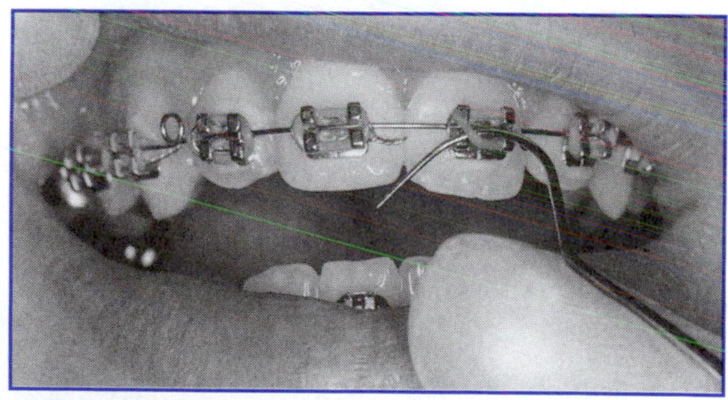

FIGURE 17–5 Removal of the elastic rings. Insert the end of a scaler explorer under the elastic and roll the elastic rings over the wings of the bracket. *(Courtesy of Rita Johnson, RDH, and Dr. Vincent DeAngelis)*

(continued)

PROCEDURE 17-5 *continued*

Ligature Wire Ties

4. Place the beaks of the ligature wire cutting pliers where the wire is exposed and cut the wire.

5. Carefully remove the wire from the wings of the bracket. Repeat on each tooth until all the ligature wires are removed.

6. Using a hemostat, remove the arch wire from the brackets. Pull the arch wire from the buccal tube on one side. Then, hold it securely to prevent injury to the patient while removing the opposite end.

7. To remove the anterior brackets, use a bracket and adhesive-removing pliers. The lower beak of the pliers, with a very sharp edge, is placed from the gingival edge of the bracket; the upper beak, with a nylon tip, is placed on the occlusal edge of the bracket. When the pliers are squeezed together, the sharp lower beak breaks the bond and removes some cement.

8. To remove the posterior bands, band-removing pliers are placed with the cushioned end on the buccal cusp. The end with the blade is placed against the gingival edge of the band. The band is gently lifted toward the occlusal surface.

9. This process is repeated on the lingual surfaces until the band is free.

10. Cement and direct bonding materials are removed from the tooth surface with a hand scaler, an ultrasonic scaler, and/or a finishing bur.

11. A rubber cup polish is completed. Photographs may be taken.

12. An alginate impression is taken of both arches. The impressions are sent to the lab to be used in the construction of the retainer.

13. The patient is reappointed for later that day or for the next day. The retainer or positioner is then placed.

14. The patient is given instructions on placement and removal of the removable appliance and the wearing schedule.

CHAPTER 18

Pediatric Dentistry

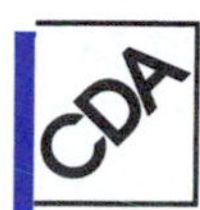

OBJECTIVES

The student should strive to meet the following objectives and demonstrate an understanding of the facts and principles presented in this chapter:

1. Define pediatric dentistry as a specialty.
2. Identify common procedures in pediatric dentistry.
3. Identify the equipment unique to pediatric dentistry.

KEY TERMS

apexogenesis (p. 314)
avulsed tooth (p. 318)
direct pulp capping (DPC) (p. 313)
fluoride application (p. 311)
indirect pulp treatment (IPT) (p. 313)
mouth guards (p. 311)
pedodontics (p. 310)
pit and fissure sealants (p. 311)
pulpectomy (p. 314)
pulpotomy (p. 313)
space maintainers (p. 311)
spot-welded matrix bands (p. 311)
stainless steel crowns (p. 314)
T-band matrix (p. 311)
tongue thrusting (p. 311)
traumatic intrusion (p. 317)

Introduction

The pediatric dental practice provides dental care for children and is often referred to as **pedodontics**. The pediatric specialist treats children from birth through the eruption of their second permanent molars. The pediatric practice sometimes treats medically, mentally, or emotionally compromised adults. The scope of the pediatric treatment for child patients includes restoring and maintaining the primary, mixed, and permanent dentition and applying preventive measures for dental caries, periodontal disease, and malocclusion. Although there has been a decrease in the number of dental caries in children, the restorative aspect is still a comprehensive part of the practice. The primary focus of the pediatric dental practice is preventive treatment and dealing with the compromised adult patient.

The Dental Assistant's Role in Pediatric Dentistry

The role of the dental assistant in the pediatric practice varies depending on the areas of responsibility. Skills the assistant performs at chairside vary in every office and from state to state depending on the state Dental Practice Act.

In many offices, the assistant plays the dominant role in greeting the child, escorting him or her to the treatment area and preparing him or her for treatment. When the pediatric dentist enters the room, the assistant transfers the attention and control to him or her. The assistant's role during treatment is to support the dentist in a manner that the assistant and the dentist have discussed.

The dental assistant is also an educator of both the child and the parents. Topics that might be discussed include oral hygiene techniques, dental nutrition, tooth eruption, and application of fluoride and sealants.

Procedures in Pediatric Dentistry

The first appointment with the pediatric dentist may be for a routine examination followed by treatment, or it may be an emergency appointment due to an injury or pain. Dental care for children involves both the primary and permanent dentition.

The Examination

The examination of a child patient is similar to that of an adult. The gingiva, supporting tissues, and oral mucosa are checked. The surfaces of the teeth are examined with a mouth mirror and an explorer. Radiographs are exposed to show the conditions of the primary teeth and the positions and development of the permanent teeth.

Preventive Procedures

Preventive procedures in pediatric dentistry include educating both the child and parent regarding diet suggestions, oral hygiene techniques, the use of fluorides, pit and fissure sealants, use of mouth guards for sport activities, and preventive orthodontic treatment.

Coronal Polish. Coronal polish followed by **fluoride application** and **pit and fissure sealants** are routine procedures the child receives during examination appointments.

Mouth Guards. Children who are actively involved in contact sports should be fitted for **mouth guards**. The guards offer protection from premature loss of the teeth or from fractures.

Preventive and Interceptive Orthodontic Treatment. Two common procedures are placing space maintainers and correcting oral habits.

Space Maintainers. **Space maintainers** are designed to maintain a space until the permanent tooth erupts. The space is the result of the premature loss of a primary tooth. A space maintainer may be a *fixed* or *removable appliance*.

Oral Habits. **Oral habits** such as thumb sucking and tongue thrusting may need intervention because they can lead to abnormal muscle function, distorted growth of the jaw, malocclusion, changed facial contour, and problems with speech.

Most dentists begin some form of treatment if the child continues to suck his or her thumb at age five. Treatment includes counseling with the child and the parents, "gentle persuasion," and behavior modification techniques.

Tongue thrusting is a habit in which the child's tongue pushes against the anterior teeth during swallowing, causing an anterior open bite. Treatment for this habit includes myofunctional exercises (therapy) or the use of appliances.

Restorative Procedures

Restorative procedures are similar to those performed on adult patients. The materials used in pediatric dentistry are the same materials used in the restoration of permanent teeth. Amalgam is used most frequently for posterior teeth; composite resins are used on anterior teeth and some posterior teeth. Badly decayed teeth are protected with stainless steel crowns permanently cemented in place.

The difference between pediatric and adult restorative procedures is the size of the instruments. Examples of instruments and materials that are reduced in size include the dental high-speed handpiece and burs, dental dam material, and dental dam clamps.

Pedodontic Matrices. The **dental matrices** used in restorative procedures are adapted to the sizes and shapes of the teeth. The tofflemire matrix is used in pediatrics, however custom matrices are more common. Two custom matrices are the **T-band matrix** and **spot-welded matrix bands** (Procedures 18–1 and 18–2).

PROCEDURE

18-1 T-Band Placement

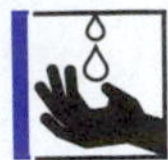 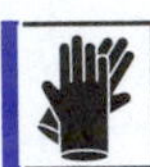 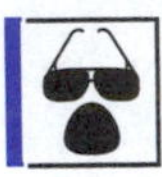 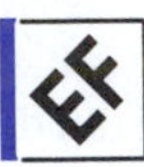

For this procedure, the tooth has been prepared and a matrix is assembled and placed on the tooth. The dentist places the T-band unless the state Dental Practice Act allows the dental assistant to perform this skill.

EQUIPMENT AND SUPPLIES

- T-band assortment
- Burnisher
- Cotton pliers or hemostat
- Crown and collar scissors

PROCEDURE STEPS *(Follow aseptic procedures)*

1. Prepare the T-band ahead of time by selecting the appropriate band size.
2. Loop the band to shape the approximate diameter of the tooth.
3. Fold the "T" ends over the band loop, leaving a circle with long tail or end.
4. The band is placed on the tooth, into the interproximal space covering the margins of the preparation.
5. The portion of the band where the "T" is folded is placed on the buccal surface, away from the margins of the preparation.
6. The band is tightened by pulling on the free end (tail) until the band is tight around the tooth.
7. The free end is bent back toward the "T" to secure the band. The excess band is removed with scissors.
8. The band is burnished and a wedge is placed as needed.
9. To remove the T-band, fold back the overlapping section of band to loosen the band. Use cotton pliers to remove the band from the tooth.

The T-bands are designed for and used on primary teeth. They are often made of brass strips "crossed" at one end. They are supplied in various designs and sizes.

Spot-welded matrix bands also are used for primary teeth. The matrix material is supplied in rolls of one-quarter to three-sixteenths-inch widths and 0.002 gauge thickness. This custom matrix does not require a retainer; however, a spot-welding machine is required. This band is made quickly at chairside.

Pulp Therapy in Primary and Young Permanent Teeth

Caries or traumatic injuries can damage both primary and permanent teeth. The teeth are assessed to determine the status of the pulp. The clinical assessment includes a visual examination and radiographs. The extent of the

PROCEDURE

18-2 Spot-Welded Matrix Band Placement

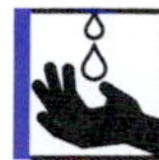 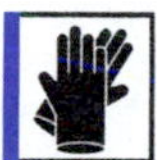 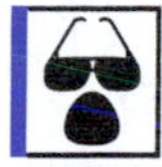 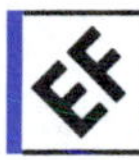

For this procedure, the tooth has been prepared for a restoration and the spot-welded matrix band is prepared by the dental assistant at chairside.

EQUIPMENT AND SUPPLIES

- Spot-welded matrix band material
- Crown and collar scissors
- Cotton pliers, hemostat, or Howe pliers
- Burnisher
- Spot-welding unit

PROCEDURE STEPS *(Follow aseptic procedures)*

1. Cut an approximate length of matrix band material. Turn on the spot-welding unit to warm it up.
2. Loop the matrix material around the tooth, bringing the ends of the material together on the buccal surface.
3. Pinch the band tightly together with a hemostat, cotton pliers, or Howe pliers.
4. Bend the excess material to one side.
5. Take the band to the spot-welding unit and spot weld the band together to form a circle the diameter of the tooth.
6. Trim off the excess and sharp edges of the band.
7. Replace the band on the tooth with the welded area on the buccal surface. Place wedges in the interproximal and contour.
8. To remove the band after the amalgam has been placed, cut the lingual aspect of the band and pull the band in an occlusal/buccal direction with cotton pliers.

lesion is determined by the following: if there is a fistula (pathway from an abscess to the mucosa), if the tooth is mobile, if there is swelling, and/or if there is sensitivity to heat or percussion.

Vital Pulp Therapy. Vital pulp therapy involves the removal of tissue that is potentially infected and focuses on the reparative ability of the pulp. There are three choices in treatment depending on the status of the pulp: **indirect pulp treatment (IPT), direct pulp capping (DPC)**, or a **pulpotomy**.

If the pulp is not yet exposed, indirect pulp treatment (IPT), also known as indirect pulp capping, is indicated. In this case, the pulp has not yet been exposed, but there is a chance that the pulp will be exposed while removing the caries. The technique involves:

1. Leaving a thin layer of sound or carious dentin with no evidence of pulp exposure (Figure 18–1A)

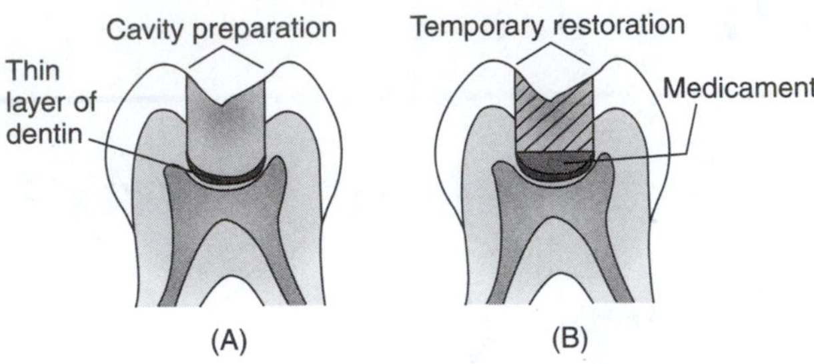

FIGURE 18–1 Indirect pulp treatment.

2. Placing a medicament and a temporary restoration that seals completely (Figure 18–1B)
3. Leaving the medicament and restoration for six to eight weeks
4. Opening the tooth and removing the remaining caries
5. Placing a restoration

If the pulp has been exposed through mechanical or traumatic means but there is a chance for a favorable response, a direct pulp capping (DPC) procedure is indicated. It may be successful and the pulp will heal, or the infection may continue and the tooth will abscess. In the case of an abscess, root canal treatment may be required. The DPC procedure involves placing a medicament, often calcium hydroxide, directly over the exposed pulp. The tooth is then restored or a temporary restoration is placed.

If the pulp of a primary or young permanent tooth has been exposed, a pulpotomy procedure may be indicated to remove a portion of the pulp (Procedure 18–3). For primary teeth, a pulpotomy keeps the pulp vital with no prolonged adverse signs, no internal resorption, and no harm to succedaneous teeth. For the young permanent teeth, a pulpotomy maintains the pulp vitality and allows enough time for the root end to develop and close (in these cases, the treatment is referred to as **apexogenesis**).

Nonvital Pulp Therapy. Nonvital pulp therapy may be indicated for both primary and newly erupted permanent teeth. The tooth is extracted or a **pulpectomy** is indicated. This procedure involves the complete removal of the dental pulp.

Stainless Steel Crowns

Stainless steel crowns are used on both primary and permanent teeth (See Procedure 18-4). On primary teeth, stainless steel crowns are placed until the permanent dentition erupts. On permanent teeth, stainless steel crowns are

P R O C E D U R E

18-3 Pulpotomy

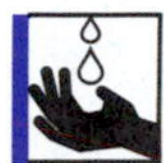 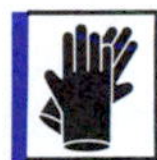 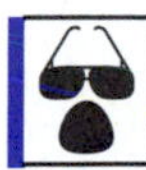

This procedure is performed by the pediatric dentist with the help of a dental assistant. The dental assistant prepares the treatment room, patient, equipment, and supplies. The tooth is opened and treated before a temporary restoration is placed.

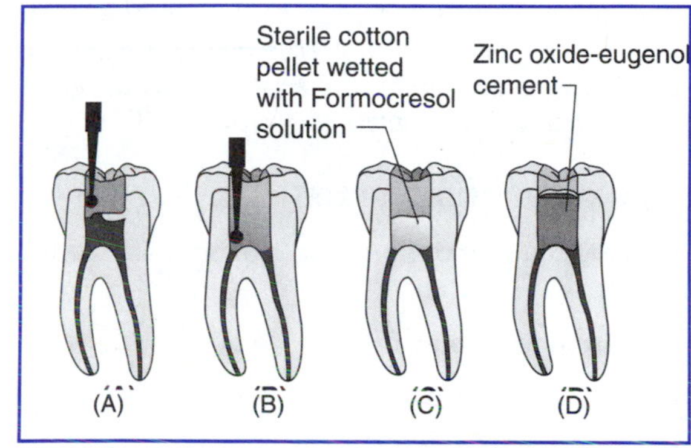

FIGURE 18–2 Pulpotomy procedure.

EQUIPMENT AND SUPPLIES

- Amalgam setup
- Formocresol
- Sterile round burs
- Zinc oxide-eugenol cement (ZOE or IRM)

PROCEDURE STEPS *(Follow aseptic procedures)*

1. Anesthetic is administered.
2. Place the dental dam.
3. Using the high-speed handpiece, a large opening is made in the occlusal surface of the tooth, exposing the coronal portion of the pulp (Figure 18–2A).
4. The coronal portion of the pulp is then removed with a spoon excavator or round bur (Figure 18–2B).
5. Prepare a sterile cotton pellet by wetting it in a Formocresol solution. The dentist places the pellet in the chamber for five minutes. (Formocresol is bactericidal—It preserves a thin layer of the remaining pulp tissue to control hemorrhage) (Figure 18–2C).
6. After the hemorrhage is controlled, the cotton pellet is removed and the pulp chamber is rinsed and dried.
7. Mix zinc oxide-eugenol to a base consistency and transfer it to the dentist. A layer of zinc oxide base is placed in the chamber over the remaining pulp (Figure 18–2D).
8. Place the restoration, such as amalgam, remove the dental dam, and check the occlusion. Stainless steel crowns also are used if there is little tooth structure remaining. Sometimes, the dentist will choose to place a temporary restoration instead of a final restoration.

PROCEDURE

18-4 Stainless Steel Crown Placement

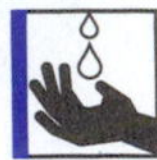 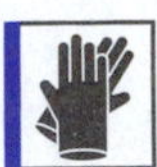 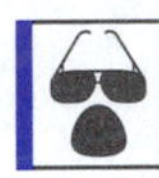 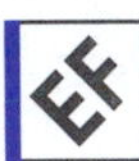

This procedure is performed by the dentist with the help of the dental assistant. The assistant maintains the operating field, mixes materials, and assists in the preparation of the stainless steel crown.

EQUIPMENT AND SUPPLIES

- Basic setup: mouth mirror, explorer, and cotton pliers
- Cotton rolls and gauze
- HVE and saliva ejector
- High-speed handpiece with selected burs
- Low-speed handpiece with green stone and rubber abrasive wheel
- Spoon excavator
- Selection of stainless steel crowns
- Crown and collar scissors
- Contouring and crimping pliers
- Mixing spatula, paper pad, and permanent cement
- Articulating forceps and paper
- Dental floss

PROCEDURE STEPS *(Follow aseptic procedures)*

1. Local anesthetic is administered and the tooth is prepared similar to the preparation for a cast gold crown. The high-speed handpiece with tapered diamonds is commonly used. Transfer instruments and evacuate during the preparation of the tooth.
2. The circumference and height of the tooth are reduced.
3. Decay is removed in the conventional methods and cavity medications are placed.
4. A stainless steel crown is selected from the kit, and it is tried on the tooth. The crown must fit around the circumference of the prepared tooth and contact the adjacent teeth, mesially and distally. Assist the dentist in the selection of the crown. (Some states do not allow dental assistants to perform the function of fitting the crown.)
5. Once the crown is selected, the crown and collar scissors are used to adjust the occlusal-gingival height (Figure 18–3). The gingival margin of the crown should extend one millimeter beyond the margin of the tooth preparation.
6. A green stone is used to smooth the rough edges of the crown. This area is polished with a rubber abrasive wheel.

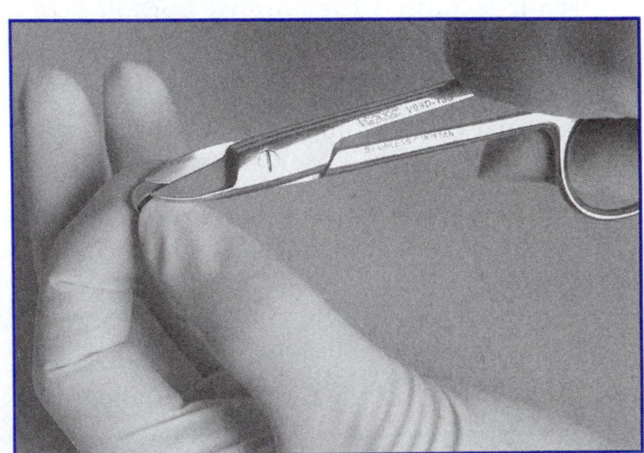

FIGURE 18–3 Stainless steel crown selected and trimmed with crown and collar scissors.

7. Place the crown on the tooth and check the patient's occlusion with articulating paper. Make adjustments, if necessary. Use dental floss to check the contacts. Prepare the articulating paper, dry the tooth, and transfer the paper. Receive the articulating forceps and paper and prepare the handpiece, if necessary.
8. Using contouring and crimping pliers, contour the crown, and then crimp the cervical margins of the crown in toward the tooth.
9. The crown is removed and the tooth is dried thoroughly.
10. The cement is mixed and placed in the crown and on the tooth. Mix the cement and place it in the crown. Transfer the crown to the dentist for placement.
11. Remove the excess cement from around the crown.
12. Rinse the patient's mouth and then dismiss the patient.

placed until an individual can have them replaced with cast gold or porcelain fused to metal crowns. Indications for use of a stainless steel crown include:

- Extensive carious lesions
- Hypoplastic or hypocalcified teeth
- Treatment following a pulpotomy or pulpectomy procedure
- Primary tooth is used as an abutment tooth for space maintainer
- Temporary restoration of fractured teeth

Emergency Treatment for Traumatic Injuries

Fractured Teeth

Fractured teeth are a common emergency in the pediatric practice. The anterior teeth are most often involved. The child should be seen by the dentist as soon as possible after the accident. The dentist examines the teeth, documents the history of the accident, performs vitality tests, and takes radiographs. Treatment is determined by the extent of the injury and the vitality of the pulp.

Traumatic Intrusion

Traumatic intrusion occurs when the teeth are forcibly driven into the alveolus so that only a portion of the crown is visible. The treatment for intrusion is to allow the teeth to re-erupt on their own, or the pediatric dentist will reposition the teeth and splint adjacent teeth to hold position. These teeth may become non-vital and later require endodontic treatment.

Avulsed Teeth

An **avulsed tooth** has been completely removed from the mouth. Primary avulsed teeth are not replaced because infection or ankylosis (**ANG**-kill-loh-sis) may occur. Ankylosis is the fusion of bone and cementum. Permanent teeth that have been avulsed should be replaced as soon as possible after the injury. Instruct the parents to reimplant the tooth immediately. The success rate is relatively high when this is done. If the tooth cannot be reimplanted, instruct the parent to place the tooth in milk, saliva, saline, or water and transport the patient and tooth to the dental office immediately.

Replacing an Avulsed Tooth

1. The tooth is kept moist and the site in the mouth is examined.
2. Local anesthetic is administered.
3. X-rays are taken.
4. The blood clot is removed from the alveolus.
5. The avulsed tooth is cleaned off in a saline solution and then inserted into the alveolus.
6. A splint is placed to retain the tooth in position.
7. Antibiotics, analgesics, and chlorhexidine rinses are prescribed.
8. Endodontic treatment may be required later.

CHAPTER 19

Periodontics

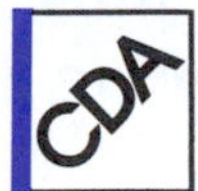

OBJECTIVES

The student should strive to meet the following objectives and demonstrate an understanding of the facts and principles presented in this chapter:

1. Describe the scope of periodontics.
2. Explain the diagnostic procedures involved in a patient's first visit to the periodontal office.
3. Identify and describe periodontal instruments and their uses.
4. Describe nonsurgical procedures and the dental assistant's role in each procedure.
5. Explain surgical procedures and the dental assistant's responsibilities.
6. Identify the types of periodontal dressings and how they are prepared, placed, and removed.

KEY TERMS

coronal polish (p. 326)
curette (p. 323)
electrosurgery (p. 325)
furcation (p. 321)
gingivectomy (p. 328)
gingivitis (p. 321)
gingivoplasty (p. 330)
hoe scaler (p. 324)
interdental knives (p. 325)
osseous surgery (p. 330)
ostectomy (p. 330)
osteoplasty (p. 330)
periodontal dressing (p. 330)
periodontal flap surgery (p. 330)
periodontal knives (p. 324)
periodontal pocket (p. 322)
periodontal probe (p. 323)

periodontal probing (p. 322)
periodontitis (p. 321)
periodontium (p. 320)
periosteal elevators (p. 325)
plaque (p. 322)
pocket marking pliers (p. 325)
prophylaxis (p. 326)
recession (p. 322)
root planing (p. 328)
scaling (p. 325)
sickle scalers (p. 323)
surgical scalpel (p. 325)
tooth mobility (p. 322)
ultrasonic instruments (p. 324)

Introduction

The periodontist specializes in diseases of the tissues around the root of the tooth. This specialty addresses symptoms, probable causes, diagnosis, and treatment of periodontal disease.

The Periodontal Dental Assistant

The team in a periodontal office includes the periodontist, dental assistants, dental hygienists, and business office staff.

The dental assistant performs chairside assisting duties and the expanded functions allowed by state Dental Practice Acts, including placing and removing periodontal dressing, removing sutures, and performing coronal polish. The dental assistant takes radiographs, makes impressions for study models, places sealants, and administers fluoride treatments. The dental assistant also gives pre- and postoperative instructions and prepares the treatment room for oral surgery. These functions are in addition to treatment room preparation and maintenance and sterilization procedures. The dental assistant educates and motivates the patient throughout the treatment. In some offices, the dental assistant also may perform laboratory tasks, such as pouring study models or making periodontal splints.

Periodontal Disease

According to the American Academy of Periodontology, three of four adults will experience, to some degree, periodontal problems at some time in their lives. Periodontal disease occurs in children and adolescents with marginal gingivitis and gingival recession.

Periodontal disease involves the **periodontium,** the tissues that support the teeth, and includes the following:

- **Gingiva**—Tissues that surround the teeth.
- **Epithelial attachment**—Area at the bottom of the sulcus where the gingiva attaches to the tooth.

- **Sulcus**—Space between the tooth and the free gingiva. In healthy mouths, the sulcus is 1 to 3 mm deep.
- **Periodontal ligaments or membranes**—Fibers of connective tissue that surround the root of the tooth and attach the cementum to the bone.
- **Cementum**—Hard surface that covers the dentin on the root of the tooth.
- **Alveolar bone**—Bone that forms the socket that encases the root of the tooth.

Symptoms of Periodontal Disease

The symptoms of periodontal disease include bleeding gingiva, loose teeth (mobility), inflamed gingiva, abnormal contour of the gingiva, periodontal pocket formation, malocclusion, halitosis, pain and tenderness, and recession and discoloration.

Types of Periodontal Disease

There are two main classifications of periodontal disease: **gingivitis** and **periodontitis**.

Gingivitis. Gingivitis is inflammation of the gingival tissues. It is common in all ages. Causes may include buildup of plaque and calculus, poor-fitting appliances, and poor occlusion; the condition may occur in association with certain systemic diseases (scurvy), hormonal changes (pregnancy), or prolonged drug therapy (phenytoin, which is an anticonvulsant). The tissues become reddish in color, interdental papilla may be swollen and bulbous, and tissues may bleed after brushing and flossing. Gingivitis precedes periodontitis but does not always progress to it. Proper brushing and flossing can reverse this condition in some cases by removing the plaque.

Periodontitis. Periodontitis involves the formation of periodontal pockets. This occurs when margins of the gingiva and periodontal fibers recede and the supporting bone becomes inflamed and destroyed. Tooth mobility may increase as the pockets become deeper; and there may be **furcation** (area where the roots divide) involvement in multi-rooted teeth.

Periodontal Diagnostic Procedures

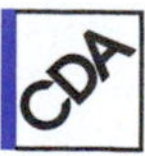

The first appointment with the periodontist is often an information-gathering appointment. After completing the medical dental history, the patient is seated in the treatment room for an extraoral and intraoral examination. Radiographs and impressions are taken and a periodontal screening is completed. Information to share with each patient includes following oral hygiene instructions, diet suggestions and modifications, personal habit changes, and the importance of routine office visits.

Clinical Examination

Clinical examination includes an extraoral examination of the face and neck; an intraoral examination of the tongue, palate, buccal mucosa, the teeth, the oropharynx area; and the periodontal examination.

Periodontal Examination. The periodontal examination is a thorough evaluation of the periodontium. The periodontal chart depicts the condition of the patient's periodontal tissues. Charting is completed either manually or on a computer. The oral cavity is examined, and information is gathered by the operator while the dental assistant records the information on the periodontal chart.

- **Patient oral hygiene** is evaluated and the amount of **plaque** and calculus present is determined. This evaluation includes both *supragingival* and *subgingival* deposits.
- **Periodontal probing** measures the depth of the **periodontal pocket** with a periodontal probe. A normal sulcus is 3 mm deep or less. When the depth is greater than 3 mm, it is termed a periodontal pocket. To determine the sulcus depth, six sites are probed and recorded on each tooth. There are three sites on the facial, including mesiofacial, midfacial, and distofacial, and three sites on the lingual, including mesiolingual, midlingual, and distolingual. The periodontal probe is inserted into the sulcus until the operator feels resistance. Tactile sensation indicates the level of the epithelium attachment. The calibrations on the probe measure the depth of the pocket. These are recorded on the chart.
- **Tooth mobility** measures movement of the tooth within the socket. The mobility test is done by pushing the tooth in a buccolingual direction using the handle ends of two instruments or by using the automatic device for assessing mobility.
- **Furcation involvement** measures destruction of interradicular bone in the furcation area of multi-rooted teeth.
- **Appearance of the gingiva** is evaluated in terms of color, size, shape, texture, position, consistency, bleeding, and amount of exudate (pus).
- **Bleeding** is the amount of blood present during probing. It is a major indicator of inflamed gingiva.
- **Recession** is the loss of the gingival tissue exposing the underlying cementum/dentin, usually seen on the facial surface.
- **Occlusion** is evaluated and described. The occlusal bite relationship is checked with articulating paper or wax to identify areas that show excessive biting or chewing force.

Radiographic Interpretation

Radiographs are useful when evaluating the periodontium for periodontal disease. Radiographs show the teeth and the level and position of the alveolar bone.

Periapical x-rays supplemented with bite-wing radiographs are most commonly taken, and the x-rays must be as dimensionally accurate as possible. Usually, a full-mouth series is taken for comparisons throughout the mouth.

Presentation of the Treatment Plan

After gathering all the periodontal diagnostic information, the periodontist determines the appropriate treatment plan for the patient. The patient is scheduled for a consultation appointment. During this appointment, the prognosis (anticipated outcome) of the patient's condition and the treatment sequence are explained. Charts, radiographs, study models, and photographs are used to educate the patient.

Periodontal Instruments

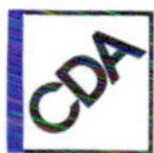

Periodontal instruments are designed to probe, scrape, file, and cut the hard surfaces of the teeth, alveolar bone, and soft tissues of the gingiva. These instruments must be kept sharp. Usually, the hygienist or a specially trained assistant is responsible for maintaining periodontal hand instruments.

Periodontal Probes

The **periodontal probe** is the primary instrument used in the periodontal examination. This is a **calibrated instrument** used to measure the depth of periodontal pockets. The probe is also used to measure areas of recession, bleeding, or exudate. The calibrations on the periodontal probe are in millimeters and vary depending on the manufacturer and the operator's preference.

Sickle Scalers

Sickle scalers are sharp hand instruments that are used to remove hard deposits such as supragingival (above the gingiva) and subgingival (below the gingiva) calculus from the teeth. Scalers are supplied in a variety of shapes and angulations to access all surfaces of the teeth. The working end of a scaler has two sharp edges that come to a point.

Curettes

The **curette** is a hand instrument used to remove subgingival calculus, smoothing the root surface, and to remove the soft tissue lining of the periodontal pocket. The working end has a cutting edge on one or both sides of the blade and the end is rounded, not pointed like the scaler (Figure 19–1). The curette is a finer instrument that is designed to adapt to the curves of the root surfaces.

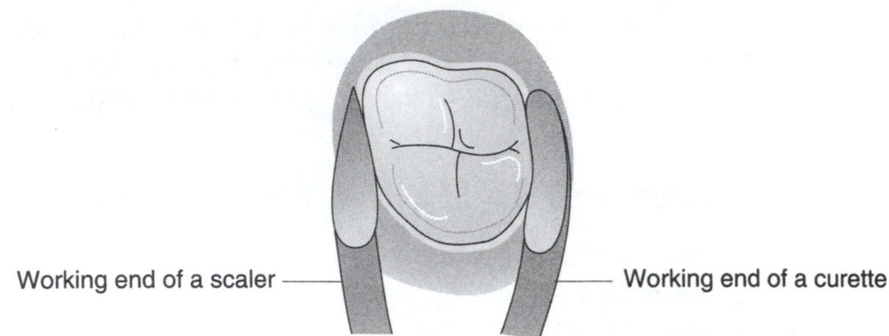

FIGURE 19–1 Cross section of a scaler and a curette.

Hoe Scalers

The **hoe scaler** has a blade bent at a 90° angle at the end of the working end. The hoe scaler is placed in the periodontal pocket to the base and then pulled toward the crown of the tooth with even pressure to plane and smooth the root surface.

Chisel Scalers

Chisel scalers are used most often in the anterior sextant of the mouth. The blade of the chisel is slightly curved and the cutting edge is beveled.

Files

Periodontal files are used in a pulling motion interproximally to remove calculus and for root planing. Files are also used to remove overhanging margins of dental restorations.

Ultrasonic Instruments

Ultrasonic instruments are used to remove hard deposits, stains, and debris during scaling, curettage, and root planing procedures. Ultrasonic units generate high-power vibrations to a handpiece using a variety of tips. These vibrations cause the calculus to fracture and be dislodged. Because ultrasonic vibrations cause heat, the units have cooling systems that circulate water through the handpieces and out openings near the tips.

Periodontal Knives

Periodontal knives or gingivectomy knives are used to remove gingival tissue during periodontal surgery. The knives most commonly used are the broad-bladed Kirkland knives. These knives are kidney shaped and sharp around the entire periphery of the blade.

Interdental Knives

Periodontal knives that are used to remove soft tissue interproximally are called **interdental knives**. The Orban No. 1 and 2 are spear-shaped knives with long, narrow blades and cutting edges on both sides of the blade.

Surgical Scalpel

The **surgical scalpel** is used for periodontal surgical procedures to remove gingival tissue. The surgical scalpel is also known as the Bard-Parker scalpel. The blades are supplied in different shapes and sizes. Disposable scalpels are also available.

Electrosurgery

The **electrosurgery** setup consists of a control box, foot-operated on-off controls, one terminal plate placed behind the patient's back or shoulders, and another terminal that is a probe with various cutting tips that the dentist uses for the surgery. The electrosurgery unit uses tiny electrical currents to incise the gingival tissue and also coagulate the blood during the procedure.

Pocket Marking Pliers

Pocket marking pliers are used to transfer the measurement of the pocket to the outside of the tissue so the operator can see the depth level of the pocket. Pocket marking pliers have one straight, thin beak that is placed in the pocket and another that is bent at a right angle at the tip. When the beaks are pinched together, the gingival tissue is perforated, leaving small, pinpoint markings.

Periosteal Elevators

Periosteal elevators are used to reflect soft tissue away from the bone. The elevators are usually double ended, with one long, tapered end and one round, bladed end.

NONSURGICAL PROCEDURES

Occlusal Adjustment

Occlusal adjustment or equilibration is a procedure that involves adjustment of the occlusal surface to eliminate detrimental forces and to provide functional forces for stimulation of a healthy periodontium (Procedure 19–1).

Scaling and Polishing

The purpose of **scaling** is to remove plaque, calculus, and stains from the surfaces of the teeth. The deposits above the gingival margin, supragingival deposits, and those just below the gingival margin, subgingival deposits, are

PROCEDURE

19-1 Occlusal Adjustment

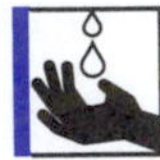
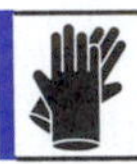
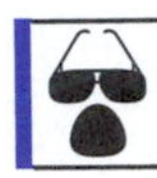
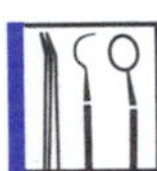

This procedure is performed by the periodontist. It involves marking the patient's bite and adjusting the occlusal surfaces of the teeth. The dental assistant prepares the articulating paper or wax; maintains the operating field; and changes burs, discs, and stones in the handpiece.

EQUIPMENT AND SUPPLIES *(Figure 19–2)*

- Basic setup: mouth mirror, explorer, and cotton pliers
- Cotton rolls and 2 × 2 gauze sponges
- Saliva ejector, HVE tip, air-water syringe tip
- Articulation forceps and articulating paper and/or occlusal wax

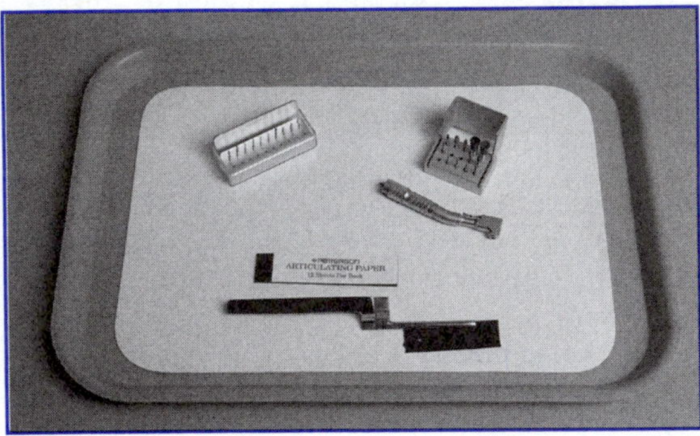

FIGURE 19–2 Occlusal equilibration armamentarium.

- Low-speed handpiece
- Diamond burs, various discs and stones
- Polishing wheels and discs

PROCEDURE STEPS *(Follow aseptic procedures)*

1. Seat and prepare the patient for the occlusal adjustment procedure.
2. Prepare the articulating forceps with paper, or prepare to transfer the wax. Dry the quadrant with the air syringe or a gauze sponge.
3. The periodontist places the articulating paper over the occlusal surfaces and instructs the patient to bite down and grind the teeth side to side.
4. The articulating paper is removed, and the colored marks left by the paper are evaluated. The markings indicate how teeth in the maxillary and mandibular arches occlude.
5. Change burs, discs, and stones as requested by the periodontist. Transfer the handpiece to the periodontist, and use the air-water syringe and the evacuator to keep the area clean and clear during the adjustments procedure.
6. This process is repeated until the teeth occlude evenly over the quadrant.
7. Each quadrant is evaluated and adjusted.

removed with scalers and curettes. Next, the coronal surfaces of the teeth are polished with rubber cups, brushes, an abrasive, porte polishers, and dental tape. This procedure is called a **prophylaxis**. Depending on the state Dental Practice Act, dental assistants can remove supragingival deposits and/or perform the **coronal polish**.

PROCEDURE

19-2 Scaling, Prophylaxis, and Polishing

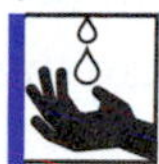
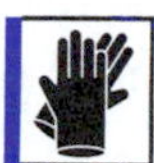
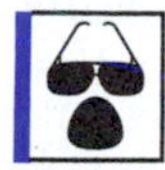
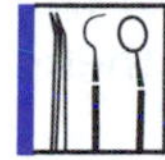
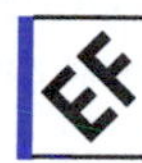

This procedure is done by the periodontist or the dental hygienist. A dental hygiene assistant assists during this procedure. Responsibilities include instrument transfer, rinsing the oral cavity, evacuation with the HVE, removing debris from instruments, retraction, and maintaining patient comfort.

EQUIPMENT AND SUPPLIES *(Figure 19–3)*

- Basic setup: mouth mirror, explorer, and cotton pliers
- Saliva ejector, HVE tip, and air-water syringe tip
- Cotton rolls and gauze sponges
- Periodontal probe
- Scalers: Jacque and Shepherd's hook
- Curettes: Universal and Gracey
- Dental floss and dental tape
- Prophy angle—rubber cups and brushes
- Prophy paste
- Optional—disclosing solution or tablets

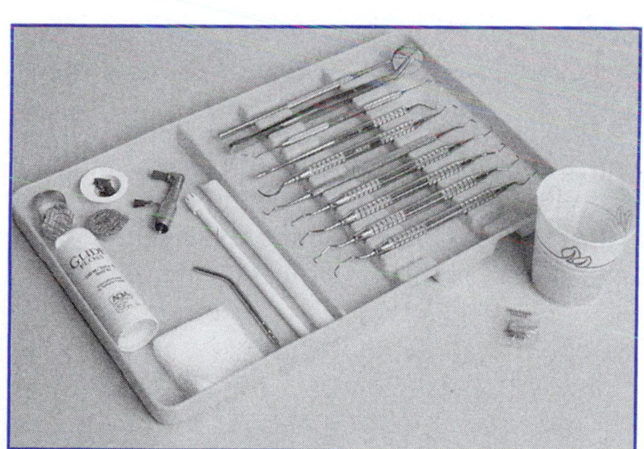

FIGURE 19–3 Scale and polish (prophylaxis) tray setup.

PROCEDURE STEPS *(Follow aseptic procedures)*

1. The operator examines the oral cavity.
2. The operator uses scalers and curettes to remove calculus and debris from around the teeth. Often, the operator cleans all surfaces of the teeth in one quadrant before moving to the next quadrant.
3. After all the calculus has been removed, the operator polishes the teeth with prophy paste, rubber cup, and brush.

NOTE: Some practices use a prophy jet (spray saltwater) as an alternative to the rubber cup polish.

4. The operator uses dental tape and prophy paste to clean the interproximal areas. Then, the entire mouth is flossed and rinsed.

In a routine prophylaxis, deposits from above and just slightly below the gingival margins are removed. In a periodontal scaling, the subgingival deposits are more extensive and involve removal of irritants from deep pockets and smoothing of the root surface (Procedure 19–2).

Root Planing

After the plaque and calculus are removed from the periodontal pocket and the root surface, the cementum is often rough and irregular. This provides a surface ideal for accumulation of plaque and calculus formation. The roughness is removed by **root planing**. This is a process of planing or shaving the root surface with curettes and other periodontal instruments to leave a smooth root surface. For the patient's comfort, anesthetic is administered during this procedure.

Gingival Curettage

Gingival curettage, also known as soft tissue curettage, is a procedure that involves scraping the inner gingival walls of the periodontal pockets to remove inflamed tissue and debris. This is accomplished with curettes and ideally is performed after the scaling and root planing of the tooth.

SURGICAL PERIODONTAL PROCEDURES

The accepted rationale for periodontal surgery is to arrest the disease process, reduce the periodontium to a level that is easier for the patient to keep clean, and perform effective scaling and root planing procedures.

Gingivectomy

A **gingivectomy** is the surgical removal of diseased gingival tissue that forms the periodontal pocket. This surgical procedure reduces the height of the gingival tissue, which provides visibility and access to remove irritants and smooth the root surface (Procedure 19–3). This promotes the healing process and makes it easier for the patient to access the area during cleaning.

PROCEDURE

19-3 Gingivectomy

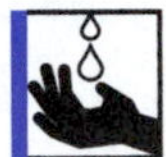
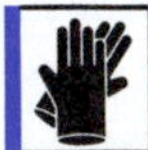
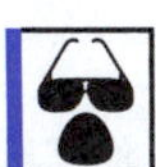
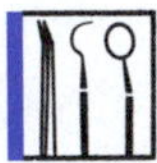

This procedure is performed by the periodontist to remove diseased gingiva and clean the periodontal pockets. The dental assistant prepares the instruments and materials, prepares the patient, and performs assisting responsibilities during the procedure. According to state Dental Practice Acts, the dental assistant may place and remove the periodontal dressing.

EQUIPMENT AND SUPPLIES

- Basic setup: mouth mirror, explorer, cotton pliers
- Periodontal probe
- Cotton rolls and gauze sponges
- Saliva ejector, HVE tip, air-water syringe tip, surgical aspirator tip
- Anesthetic setup
- Pocket marker
- Periodontal knives—broad bladed and interproximal
- Scalpel, blades, and diamond burs
- Scalers and curettes
- Soft tissue rongeurs and surgical scissors
- Hemostat
- Suture needle and thread
- Periodontal dressing materials

PROCEDURE STEPS *(Follow aseptic procedures)*

1. The anesthetic is administered to anesthetize the tissues and reduce the blood flow to the area.
2. The periodontist examines the patient's periodontal chart, then the area is examined with a periodontal probe.
3. The depths of the pockets are marked with pocket markers (Figures 19–4A and B).
4. The broad-bladed knife or scalpel is used to incise the marked gingiva. Evacuate the area and transfer instruments (Figure 19–4C).
5. Interdental knives are used to remove interproximal tissue. Scissors, rongeurs, and burs are used to remove tissue tags. Have gauze ready to receive any tissue from instruments and to clean the area of debris.
6. After the tissue is removed, the periodontist scales and planes the root surfaces. Irritants are removed and the surfaces are smoothed to promote healing. Continue to pass instruments and evacuate the area. A sterile saline solution may be used to irrigate the area.
7. If sutures are needed, they are placed at this time. Prepare the suture needle and thread and have them positioned in a hemostat, ready to pass to the dentist. Retract tissue as needed.
8. After the sutures are placed and the area is irrigated with the sterile saline solution, a periodontal dressing is prepared and placed. Assist the periodontist with the suture placement, evacuate the area, and prepare the periodontal dressing.
9. After the placement of the dressing is completed, the patient is given postoperative instructions and dismissed. Make sure the patient does not have any debris on his or her face, give postoperative instructions, and dismiss the patient.

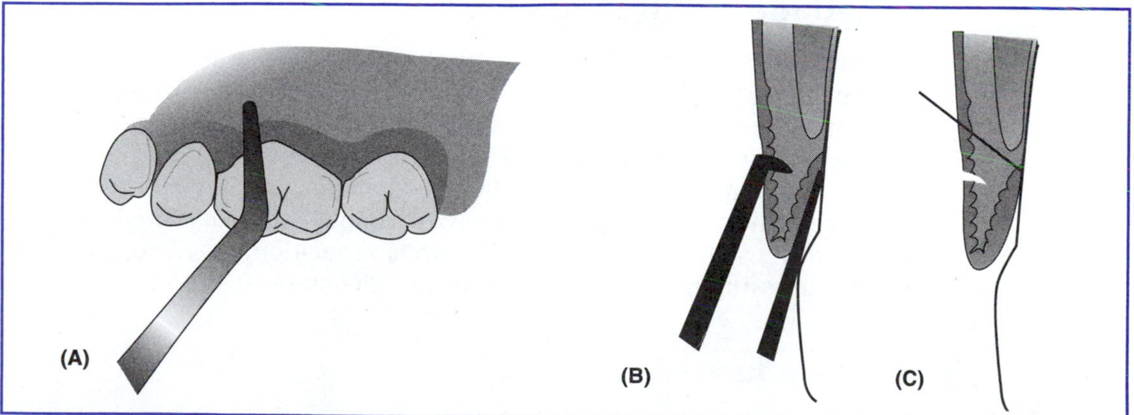

FIGURE 19–4 A gingivectomy procedure. (A) and (B) Marking the pocket depth with the pocket marker. (C) Incising the marked tissue with periodontal knives.

Gingivoplasty

Gingivoplasty is reshaping the gingival tissue to remove deformities such as clefts, craters, and enlargements. A gingivoplasty does not involve the removal of periodontal pockets; it is completed to recontour the gingiva and often immediately follows a gingivectomy. A gingivoplasty is performed with periodontal knives, a scalpel, rongeurs, rotary diamonds, curettes, and surgical scissors. The gingival margin is tapered and thinned, creating a scalloped edge. Interdental grooves are contoured.

Postoperative Treatment Following Surgery

- **Oral hygiene.** Normal brushing and flossing should be completed in areas not involved in the surgery. Brush only the biting surfaces of the teeth involved in surgery. Gently rinse the mouth with warm saltwater after twenty-four hours.
- **Diet.** Avoid hot, spicy foods and citrus foods; eat soft foods; and chew on the healthy side of the mouth so that the periodontal dressing is not disturbed.
- **Pain.** The patient may expect mild to moderate discomfort, and medication should be prescribed.
- **Swelling and bleeding.** Some swelling may occur. Place an ice pack over the area for ten minutes and remove for ten minutes. Repeat as needed. Some seepage and bleeding may occur and is normal; however, if it persists, call the periodontist.

Periodontal Flap Surgery

Periodontal flap surgery involves surgically separating the gingiva from the underlying tissue. The gingiva is incised with a scalpel and then separated with a periosteal elevator. Once the tissue is retracted, the periodontist has good visibility and access to bone, tooth, and the tooth roots.

When the flap is retracted, the diseased tissue and debris are removed, the roots are planed, and the alveolar bone is trimmed and contoured. The area is rinsed with a saline solution and the flap is repositioned and sutured. A **periodontal dressing** may be applied to protect the surgical site.

Osseous Surgery

Osseous surgery removes defects/deformities in the bone caused by periodontal disease and other related conditions. Two types of bone surgeries that correct the deformities are **osteoplasty**, reshaping the bone, and **ostectomy**, removal of bone (Procedure 19–4).

PROCEDURE

19-4 Osseous Surgery

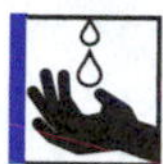 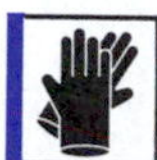 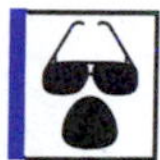 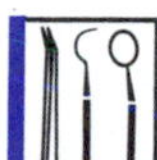

This procedure is performed by the periodontist. It involves removing and recontouring diseased and defective bone tissue. The extent of the periodontal disease process determines the amount and type of surgery performed.

EQUIPMENT AND SUPPLIES

- Basic setup: mouth mirror, explorer, cotton pliers
- Periodontal probe
- Cotton rolls and gauze sponges
- Saliva ejector, HVE tip, air-water syringe tip, surgical aspirator tip
- Anesthetic setup
- Scalpel and blades
- Periodontal knives—broad bladed and interproximal
- Tissue retractor
- Periosteal elevator
- Diamond burs and stones
- Rongeurs, chisels, and files
- Scalers and curettes
- Hemostat and surgical scissors
- Suture setup
- Periodontal dressing materials

PROCEDURE STEPS *(Follow aseptic procedures)*

In osseous surgery, a flap of soft tissue is incised and reflected to expose the bone for reshaping and/or removal. This procedure is performed by the periodontist.

1. After the anesthetic is administered, the soft tissue is incised and loosened from the underlying bone. Transfer instruments and maintain good visibility for the operator.
2. The tissue flap is reflected and stabilized with tissue retractors. Retract and hold the tissue.
3. Once the bone is exposed, the diseased bone tissue is excised. Scalers and curettes are used to remove calculus and diseased tissue and the roots are planed. Transfer instruments, rinse the area with a sterile saline solution as needed, evacuate, and keep the instruments clean by removing debris from instruments with the gauze sponge.
4. The bone is shaped and contoured using diamond burs and stones, rongeurs, chisels, and files.
5. The tissue flap is replaced and positioned over the alveolar bone, then sutured in place. Prepare the suture and stabilize the tissue with tissue forceps during the suturing procedure.
6. Prepare the periodontal dressing materials and assist the operator in the placement. In some states, the dental assistant is allowed to place and remove the periodontal dressing.
7. Remove any debris from the patient's face, give postoperative instructions, and dismiss the patient.

Periodontal Dressing

Periodontal dressings or packs are placed after periodontal surgical procedures (Procedures 19–5 and 19–6). The dressings are bandages used to protect the tissue during the healing process.

PROCEDURE

19-5 Preparation and Placement of Non-Eugenol Periodontal Dressing

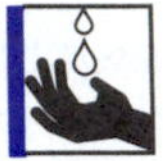 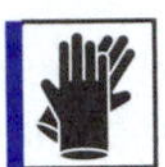 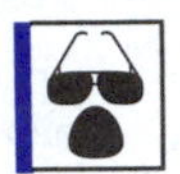 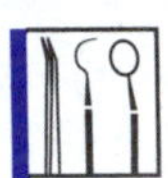 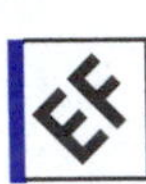

The periodontist routinely places the dressing, however in some states the dental assistant is allowed to place and remove the periodontal dressing. The dressing is placed after the surgery to protect the tissues and promote the healing process.

EQUIPMENT AND SUPPLIES

- Basic setup: mouth mirror, explorer, and cotton pliers
- Gauze sponges
- Non-eugenol periodontal dressing material (base and accelerator)
- Paper pad and tongue depressor
- Lubricant
- Instrument to contour dressing (spoon excavator, sickle scaler)

PROCEDURE STEPS *(Follow aseptic procedures)*

1. After the hemorrhaging is controlled, the patient's lips are coated lightly with Vaseline.
2. The dressing materials are dispensed into equal lengths and mixed with a tongue blade until homogeneous. (Using a paper pad and tongue blade make cleanup easier). The material is allowed to set for two to three minutes until the tackiness is gone.
3. Lubricate gloved fingers with Vaseline so the putty-like material can be handled easily.
4. The dressing comes with a retardant to slow the setting time, if necessary; it can be molded easily for three to five minutes and worked for fifteen to twenty minutes.
5. The dressing is molded into a thin strip slightly longer than the length of the surgical site. Divide the strip into two equal lengths, one for the facial surface and one for the lingual surface.
6. To begin the placement, form the end of one strip into a hook shape. Wrap this hook around the distal of the most posterior tooth (Figure 19–5).
7. Adapt the remainder of the strip along the facial surface, gently pressing the pack into the interproximal areas.
8. The second strip is applied to the lingual surface in the same manner. The pack is wrapped around the last posterior tooth and then adapted to the lingual surface, moving toward the midline.
9. The pack should cover the gingiva evenly without interfering with occlusion or the tongue movements.
10. Check the dressing for overextensions. These areas are removed with a spoon excavator or

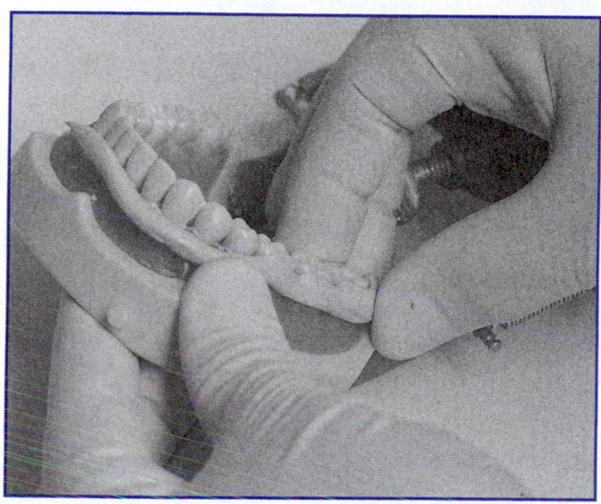

FIGURE 19–5 Placing the dressing on the tissue.

scaler. Gently press the instrument into the dressing to detach the extra material. Smooth the pack and evaluate it for an even thickness.

11. Ask the patient how the pack feels. Instruct the patient to move his or her tongue, cheeks, and lips to mold the pack. Make any adjustments to ensure that the dressing is securely in place, trimmed, and contoured.
12. Give the patient instructions about the periodontal dressing, including:
    - The pack is kept on for one week after surgery.
    - The pack will harden in a few hours and then withstand normal chewing stresses.
    - The pack may chip and break off during the week but should remain intact as long as possible. If there is pain when pieces of the pack come off or the pack becomes rough, the patient should call the office.
    - The patient should brush the occlusal surface of the teeth involved in the surgery and continue to brush and floss the rest of the teeth as normal.

PROCEDURE

19-6 Removal of the Periodontal Dressing

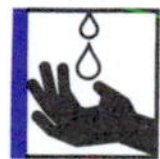 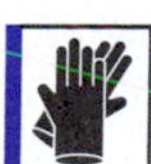 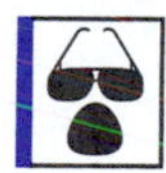 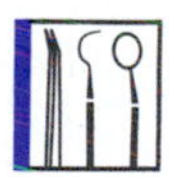 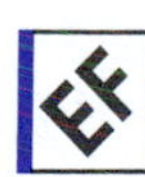

This procedure is performed by the periodontist or the dental assistant. The patient has worn the dressing for a week to ten days. The patient's mouth is examined before removing the dressing to check for areas where the dressing may have come loose or come off completely.

EQUIPMENT AND SUPPLIES

- Basic setup: mouth mirror, explorer, and cotton pliers
- Saliva ejector, HVE tip, air-water syringe tip
- Gauze sponges and tissue
- Instruments to remove the dressing (spoon excavator, sickle explorer, surgical hoe)

PROCEDURE STEPS *(Follow aseptic procedures)*

1. After seating the patient, the surgical site is evaluated and the dressing is removed.
2. A surgical hoe or a spoon excavator is inserted along the margin. Lateral pressure is applied to pry the dressing away from the tissue.
3. The pack may come off in large pieces and then scalers and floss can be used to remove any particles from the interproximal areas and tooth surfaces. Cotton pliers are used to remove particles of dressing that are embedded in the surgical site.
4. Gently rinse the entire area with warm water to remove any debris. The air-water syringe can be used carefully.

The purposes of the periodontal dressing include:

- Minimizing postoperative infection and hemorrhage
- Protecting the tissues during mastication
- Covering the surgical site in order to reduce pain due to trauma or irritation
- Providing support for teeth that are mobile

CHAPTER 20

Fixed Prosthodontics

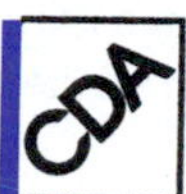

OBJECTIVES

The student should strive to meet the following objectives and demonstrate an understanding of the facts and principles presented in this chapter:

1. Define the scope of fixed prosthodontics.
2. Describe various types of fixed prostheses and their functions.
3. Describe dental materials used in fixed prostheses.
4. Explain the involvement of the laboratory technician in the fabrication of fixed prostheses.
5. Describe the role of the dental assistant in all phases of fixed prosthodontic treatment.
6. Explain techniques for retaining the prosthesis when there is little or no crown on the tooth.
7. Describe implant retainer prostheses.

KEY TERMS

bite registration (p. 341)
dental casting alloy (p. 339)
full-cast crown (p. 336)
inlays (p. 336)
onlays (p. 336)
partial crown (p. 336)
porcelain-fused-to-metal crowns (p. 339)
post-retained cores (p. 345)
prostheses (p. 336)
retention core (p. 345)
retention pins (p. 345)
shade guide (p. 341)
veneers (p. 337)

Introduction

Fixed prosthodontics is the specialty that deals with replacement of missing teeth or parts of teeth with extensive restorations. The restorations or **prostheses** (artificial parts for missing tissues) are fabricated in a dental laboratory from detailed impressions taken in the dental office. When finished, the prostheses are cemented permanently in the patient's mouth.

Patient Considerations

When a patient needs fixed prosthodontic treatment, the dentist performs an examination that includes:

- A medical and dental history
- Examination of the intra- and extraoral tissues
- Radiographs
- Impressions for study models (diagnostic casts)
- Intraoral photographs
- Extraoral photographs

Types of Fixed Prostheses

Fixed prostheses are **indirect restorations,** meaning they cannot be placed directly in the mouth after the tooth is prepared, such as amalgam or composite restorations, which are **direct restorations.** Instead, impressions are taken and then the fixed prostheses are fabricated in a dental laboratory. The indirect restorations are designed to replace missing tooth structure including full crowns, partial crowns, inlays, onlays, bridges, and veneers.

Crowns

Crowns cover teeth with extensive decay or breakdown. The tooth may require a full crown, which is often referred to as a **full-cast crown**. A full crown covers the entire coronal surface of the tooth.

A **partial crown** is a cast restoration that covers three or more, but not all, surfaces of a tooth.

Inlays and Onlays

Inlays and onlays are restorations that replace missing tooth structure within the tooth. **Inlays** cover the area between the cusps in the middle of the tooth and the proximal surfaces that are involved. **Onlays** are like inlays except they include the cusp ridges of the tooth. Inlays and onlays are also cast restorations that are made of porcelain or gold.

Bridges

A bridge is a restoration that spans the space of a missing tooth or teeth. The bridge is divided into units, and each unit of a bridge represents a tooth. A bridge may replace one or more adjacent teeth in the same arch.

Veneers

Veneers are thin layers of tooth-colored material that cover the facial surface. They are used to cover badly stained teeth and to reshape the anatomy of teeth. Veneers improve appearance with very little removal of tooth structure.

There are many types of veneers, materials used, and techniques. Direct resin veneers, indirect resin veneers, and porcelain veneers are three types.

Direct Resin Veneers. **Direct resin veneers** are made in the dental office directly on the patient's tooth. This procedure requires one appointment. In preparation for the veneer procedure, little, if any, tooth structure is removed. The tooth is etched, adhesive is applied, and opaquers and body shade are placed. The veneers are contoured and finished. These materials are light cured and require polishing and periodic maintenance.

Indirect Resin Veneers. **Indirect resin veneers** require two appointments. At the first appointment, the tooth is prepared and an impression is taken. The impression is sent to the laboratory for fabrication of the veneer. During the second appointment, the veneer is bonded in place.

Porcelain Veneers. **Porcelain veneers** are similar to indirect resin veneers in that they require two appointments and are fabricated in the dental laboratory. Porcelain veneers are natural in appearance and are durable. The technique for the porcelain veneer is sensitive to shade selection and gingival margin adaption for the veneer to look natural and adapt well (Procedure 20–1).

P R O C E D U R E

20-1 Porcelain Veneers

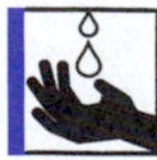 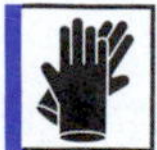 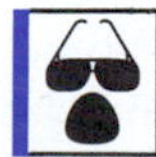 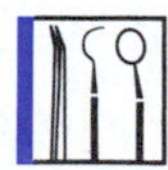

This procedure is performed by the prosthodontist and is completed in two appointments. During the first appointment, the tooth is prepared and impressions are taken; at the second appointment, the porcelain veneer is applied. Between appointments, the impressions are sent to a dental laboratory, where the porcelain veneer is fabricated.

(continued)

PROCEDURE 20-1 *continued*

EQUIPMENT AND SUPPLIES
(For the preparation appointment)

- Basic setup: mouth mirror, explorer, and cotton pliers
- Cotton rolls, 2 × 2 gauze
- HVE tip, air-water syringe tip
- Anesthetic setup
- High-speed handpiece and assorted burs
- Shade guide
- Spoon excavator
- Low-speed handpiece with prophy angle, rubber cup, and pumice
- Retraction cord and placement instrument
- Bite registration materials
- Alginate impression materials for model of opposing arch
- Final impression materials (polysiloxane or polyether)
- Temporary veneer (optional)
- Laboratory prescription form

PROCEDURE STEPS *(Follow aseptic procedures)*

Preparation Appointment (First Appointment)

1. A bite registration and an opposing arch impression are taken.
2. The teeth are cleaned with a rubber cup and pumice to remove extrinsic stains. A shade is selected by the dentist to determine how light the patient wants the veneers and to estimate how light the finished shade will be.
3. The teeth are prepared according to the design of the veneer. The incisal edge and the cervical margin are prepared carefully so the finished veneer is even with the gingival crest or just slightly subgingival.
4. The retraction cord is placed to achieve hemostasis and to ensure visualization of the margins.
5. A final impression is taken with a dimensionally stable material such as polysiloxane or polyether.
6. Temporary veneers are placed if necessary, although most patients do not require them.
7. The retraction cord is removed after the temporary veneers are placed.
8. The patient is informed that the gums will be tender for several days.
9. The patient is dismissed.

Laboratory Fabrication

1. The impressions are sent to the dental laboratory with a laboratory prescription.
2. The laboratory technician follows the dentist's prescription regarding length of veneer, shade, thickness, and texture. (Color photos of the patient are helpful in the designing and shading process.)
3. The laboratory technician fabricates the veneers and returns them to the office.

EQUIPMENT AND SUPPLIES
(For the cementation appointment)

- Basic setup: mouth mirror, explorer, and cotton pliers
- Cotton rolls, 2 × 2 gauze, cheek and lip retractors
- Saliva ejector, HVE tip, air-water syringe tip
- Porcelain veneers from the laboratory
- Low-speed handpiece with prophy angle, rubber cup, and pumice
- Silane coupling agent and small applicator (brush)
- Retraction cord and placement instrument
- Chlorhexidine soap
- Plastic or ultrathin metal strips
- Etchant and applicator
- Bonding agent and curing light

Cementation Appointment (Second Appointment)

1. The second appointment should be scheduled as close as possible to the first appointment because the patient is often without temporary coverage. The laboratory should be scheduled ahead of time so the turnaround time is minimal.
2. Complete a preliminary cleaning of the teeth with pumice to remove plaque and stains.
3. The veneers are tried on the tooth and adjustments are made with finishing diamonds. (The veneers are very fragile and require careful handling.)
4. Once all adjustments are completed, clean and dry the inside of the veneers thoroughly. Acid etchant is used to clean and decontaminate the inside surface of the veneer.
5. Apply a thin layer of silane coupling agent (this material allows bonding to porcelain).
6. Place the light-cured bonding agent in the veneers. Make sure there are no air bubbles. The material fills the veneer and is spread evenly. The veneers are then placed in a light-protected area or box until the teeth are prepared.
7. Prepare the teeth for bonding by placing a retraction cord on the facial surface. Clean the facial surface with chlorhexidine soap and a prophy cup or brush.
8. Isolate the teeth being bonded with cotton rolls, cheek and lip retractors, a saliva ejector, and plastic or ultrathin metal strips.
9. Etch the teeth to be bonded, following the directions of the specific adhesive system.
10. Apply the adhesive to the teeth being bonded.
11. Seat each veneer in the correct position.
12. In some cases, the veneer is spot-cured and excess cement is removed.
13. Light cure each veneer in place.
14. Remove excess cement with a scalpel.
15. Contour and refine the margins with finishing diamonds or burs.
16. Polish the veneers with rubber wheels, cups, and polishing paste.

Types of Materials Used for Fixed Prostheses

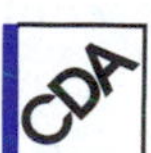

The materials used for the construction of fixed crowns, bridges, inlay, onlays, and veneers depends, among other considerations, on their locations in the mouth, the strength required, the amount of tooth structure, and esthetics.

Gold Casting Alloys

Gold used in crowns, inlays, and onlays is not pure gold but a combination of metals. When two or more metals are combined, they form an **alloy.** Pure gold is too soft for use in cast restorations, so other metals, such as platinum and palladium, are added, along with iron, tin, or zinc, to form **dental casting alloy**.

Restorations made of gold alloy include full gold crowns, inlays, and onlays. These are fabricated mainly for the posterior teeth where they are not as visible. Gold crowns are also fabricated with tooth-colored veneers. The veneers may cover the entire crown or just the facial surface. Crowns that have veneers are known as **porcelain-fused-to-metal crowns**, or ceramometal crowns (Procedure 20–2).

P R O C E D U R E

20-2 Preparation for a Porcelain-Fused-to-Metal Crown

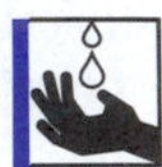

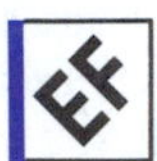
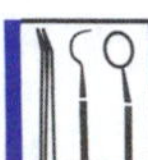

This procedure is performed by the prosthodontist and the dental assistant. Like the porcelain veneer procedure, this process involves two appointments. The following procedure includes the steps in the preparation appointment, including retention procedures, and the steps in the cementation appointment.

EQUIPMENT AND SUPPLIES *(Figure 20–1)*

- Basic setup: mouth mirror, explorer, and cotton pliers
- Cotton rolls, gauze, dental floss, articulating paper, and forceps
- HVE tip, saliva ejector, and three-way syringe tip
- Anesthetic setup
- Dental dam setup (optional)
- High-speed handpiece with a selection of diamonds, discs, and burs

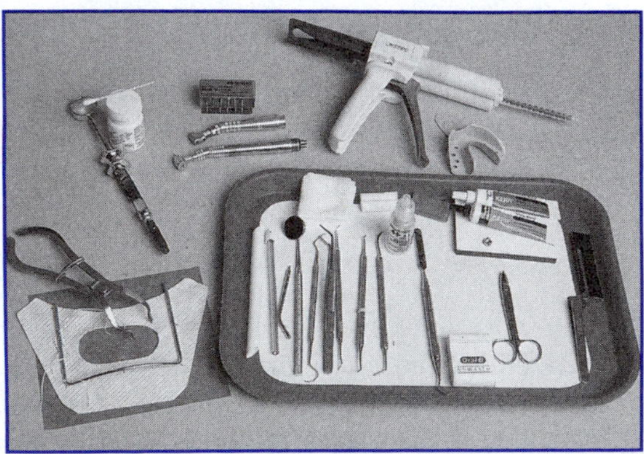

FIGURE 20–1 Tray setup for the preparation appointment (armamentarium).

- Irreversible hydrocolloid (alginate) impression materials
- Spoon excavator, scaler, plastic filling instrument, and cement spatula
- Tooth shade guide (optional)
- Retention materials depending on the amount of tooth structure retained—core buildup materials and postretention pins (optional)
- Gingival retraction cord and placement instrument
- Final impression materials and tray (stock or custom tray)
- Bite registration materials
- Crown and collar scissors
- Provisional (temporary) coverage materials
- Low-speed handpiece with burs, discs, and stones
- Laboratory prescription and container for impressions (off-tray item)

PROCEDURE STEPS *(Follow aseptic procedures)*

1. The patient is administered local anesthetic. Prepare the syringe, transfer the syringe to the prosthodontist and, during the administration of the anesthetic, observe the patient.
2. Alginate impressions are taken for fabrication of certain types of temporaries and also for a model of the opposing arch. Select the trays, mix the irreversible hydrocolloid, and take the impressions. The impressions are stored properly until needed and/or poured in plaster or stone.

3. While waiting for the anesthetic to take effect before the tooth is prepared, the tooth shade is selected. A **shade guide** is used to match the natural teeth.

NOTE: This is a very important step for the esthetics of the crown and the appearance of the patient. The shade guide includes a variety of shades, and the shades can be variegated to match the varying shading of the patient's natural teeth.

Moisten the shade guide and hold it close to the natural teeth under natural light. Record the information on the patient's chart and on the laboratory prescription.

4. Crowns are prepared with the high-speed handpiece and diamond burs. (The tooth must be reduced to accommodate the thickness of the metal and porcelain materials and to have enough strength.)

5. The margins of the preparation are either finished in a **chamfer** or **shoulder** preparation. The chamfer provides adequate bulk and extends easily into the gingival sulcus. The shoulder provides a ledge that is sometimes beveled. Prepare and transfer the high-speed handpiece, then evacuate and maintain the operating field with the air-water syringe. Retract and exchange instruments as needed.

The abutment teeth are prepared for full crowns by tapering margins of the preparation to the crown of the tooth. This preparation design allows for the placement and withdrawal of the finished restoration.

6. Once the tooth is prepared, the gingival tissue is retracted from the preparation so that a detailed impression can be made of the margins. The margins of the preparation must be detailed in the impressions so the finished crown fits snugly and securely on the tooth. The retraction cord is placed around the prepared tooth and pushed into the sulcus with a plastic filling instrument or a retraction cord-condensing instrument. In some states, the dental assistant is permitted to place the gingival retraction cord. Transfer a piece of retraction cord in cotton pliers to the prosthodontist. Then, transfer the appropriate cord-condensing instrument. The retraction cord remains in place for five minutes.

7. The prosthodontist selects the tray and impression material to be used. There are a variety of materials that are suitable for final impressions. The tray and syringe are selected and prepared and the materials are mixed.

8. Transfer cotton pliers to remove the retraction cord. Transfer the syringe material and receive the cotton pliers and cord. The prosthodontist removes the retraction cord, receives the syringe, and dispenses the material around the margins of the preparation. During this time, mix and load the heavier material into the tray. The prosthodontist places and holds the tray with the impression material in the patient's mouth. Once the prosthodontist has seated the tray, move the light from the patient's face and clean up the impression materials. The final impression is rinsed, disinfected, and placed in a plastic laboratory container.

9. The **bite registration**, also called the occlusal registration, is taken after the final impression is completed. The purpose of the bite registration is to record the way the patient occludes the maxillary and mandibular teeth. There are many types of materials that can be used to record the bite of the patient, including wax and vinyl polysiloxane materials. Prepare the materials and transfer them to the prosthodontist, who places the tray and takes the bite impression. In some states, the dental assistant legally can take the bite impression. After the bite registration is taken, rinse the patient's mouth. The materials are rinsed, disinfected, and placed in a plastic laboratory container.

The provisional (temporary) restoration is very important in crown and bridge construction. The temporary retains the teeth in the same position so that the adjacent and opposing teeth do not shift position. The

(continued)

PROCEDURE 20-2 *continued*

temporary protects the prepared tooth so the patient can function normally. Between appointments, the temporary should look natural and be acceptable to the patient.

There are many types of temporary techniques and materials available. Some temporary crown forms are preformed, while others are custom made for each patient. The provisional must be fitted to the tooth to protect the margins, maintain the space, and be esthetically pleasing.

10. After trimming and contouring the temporary, it is polished and cemented with temporary cement. The dental assistant either assists the prosthodontist or makes the temporary restoration, depending on the expanded functions laws. When assisting with the temporary, prepare the materials and trays as dictated by the technique. Some temporaries require crown and bridge scissors and crimping and contour pliers, while others need burs, discs, and stones to contour and finish. Transfer and receive the instruments and keep the area rinsed and dried. Once the temporary is completed, mix the temporary cement and place some in the crown. Transfer the bite stick for the patient to bite on, then transfer a 2 × 2 gauze sponge to wipe off any excess.
11. Once the cement is dried, the bite stick is removed and a scaler is used to remove excess dry cement. Transfer dental floss to check the interproximal contacts.
12. Hold articulating paper in articulating forceps for the patient to bite on to test the bite. If adjustments are needed, transfer the low-speed handpiece with finishing burs. The patient's mouth is rinsed and evacuated before the patient is dismissed.
13. After the patient has been dismissed, the patient's impressions and models are disinfected and the laboratory prescription is ready for the laboratory pickup. The following information is usually included on the laboratory prescription:
    - Patient's name
    - Description of the prosthesis
    - Types of materials the prosthodontist wants the prosthesis to be constructed from
    - The shade or shading desired
    - The prosthodontist's name, license number, address, telephone number, fax number, and signature
    - The date when the case must be back in the dental office

These porcelain-fused-to-metal crowns are very popular and are commonly used where strength and esthetics are needed. They resist fracture, abrasion, and discoloration (Procedure 20–3).

Role of the Dental Assistant

The dental assistant is involved in all stages of fixed prosthodontic treatment. The dental assistant explains the steps of the procedure to the patient, answers questions, and gives postoperative and home-care instructions.

The dental assistant is responsible for preparation of equipment and supplies needed for both appointments. Each tray setup is arranged according to the sequence of the procedure, with auxiliary instruments and materials close

P R O C E D U R E

20-3 Cementation of Porcelain-Fused-to-Metal Crown

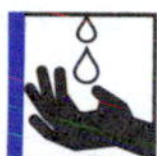
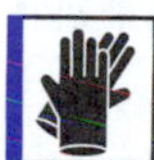
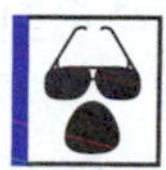
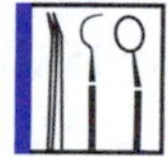
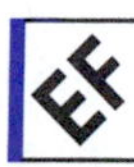

The following procedure is performed by the prosthodontist and the dental assistant. The temporary is removed, the permanent prosthesis is evaluated, and the final cementation is completed.

EQUIPMENT AND SUPPLIES *(Figure 20–2)*

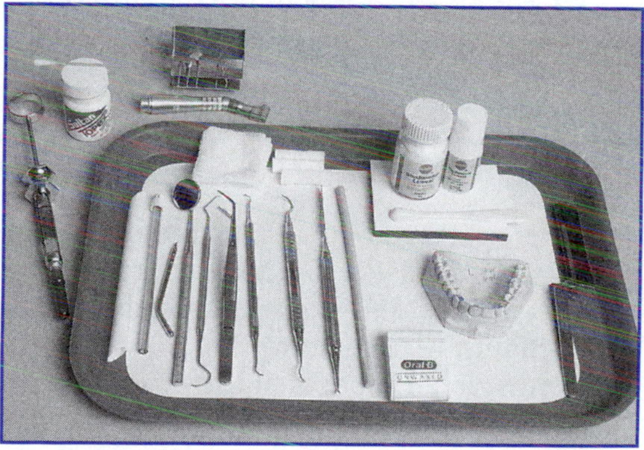

FIGURE 20–2 Tray setup for the cementation appointment.

- Basic setup: mouth mirror, explorer, and cotton pliers
- Cotton rolls, gauze, dental floss, articulating paper, and forceps
- HVE tip, saliva ejector, and air-water syringe tip
- Low-speed handpiece with finishing burs, discs, and stones
- Anesthetic setup (optional)
- Spoon excavator and scaler
- Plastic filling instrument (PFI)
- Orangewood bite stick (crown remover, crown seater, and mallet are optional)
- Final cementation materials (glass ionomer cement, polycarboxylate cement, resin cements, or zinc phosphate cement)
- Porcelain-fused-to-metal crown from laboratory

PROCEDURE STEPS *(Follow aseptic procedures)*

1. The day before the patient's appointment, make sure the laboratory has completed the crown and that it is in the office.
2. Once the patient arrives for the appointment, prepare him or her and explain the treatment. Prepare the topical and local anesthetic, then transfer the syringe and observe the patient. Once the anesthetic is placed, rinse and evacuate the mouth. (Step 2 may be optional for some patients.)
3. The provisional coverage is removed with a crown remover, scaler, and other instruments that fit under the margin of the temporary.
4. Once the temporary is removed, the excess cement is removed. The dental assistant either assists during this stage of the procedure by transferring instruments and keeping the area clean and free of debris or removes the temporary and excess cement as part of the expanded functions. Once the temporary is removed, rinse and dry the area and prepare the crown.
5. The cast crown is positioned on the preparation. A bite stick and/or mallet may be used. The occlusion, the margins, and contacts are all evaluated and adjustments are made, if

(continued)

PROCEDURE 20-3 *continued*

necessary. If the porcelain is adjusted, it is sent back to the laboratory to be refinished. Transfer instruments, dental floss, and articulating paper and forceps. Keep the area clean and dry and transfer the low-speed handpiece with finishing burs, discs, and stones. If the casting has to be returned to the laboratory, disinfect the crown and prepare it for return to the laboratory.

6. Before cementing the crown, the area is isolated with cotton rolls and protective liners and/or a cavity varnish is placed.
7. The permanent cement is mixed according to manufacturer's directions and placed in the crown and on the prepared tooth.
8. Once the crown is seated on the tooth, the patient bites on a bite stick or crown seater until the cement hardens. Prepare the permanent cement when the prosthodontist is ready and place some cement inside the crown. Pass the plastic filling instrument and place cement on the preparation. Receive the PFI and transfer the crown and the bite stick for the patient to bite down on.
9. After the cement has hardened, it is removed with a scaler, excavator, or an explorer. The patient's mouth is rinsed and evacuated. Dental floss is used to remove excess cement interproximally.
10. The patient is given instructions for brushing and flossing the area and told to call the office if there are any questions or problems. Document the procedure and dismiss the patient.

at hand. Procedures require many different types of dental materials, including alginate, bite registration materials, final impression materials, retraction cord, temporization materials, and final cements. The dental assistant prepares and/or utilizes these materials throughout the procedure.

The dental assistant assists the dentist in all aspects of the procedure, from selecting the shade of the tooth to general chairside assisting. In some states, the qualified dental assistant can perform procedures such as placing the retraction cord, placing and removing temporaries, taking preliminary impressions, and removing excess cement. The dental assistant also coordinates the patient's appointments and the laboratory schedule. In some offices, the dental assistant may perform some laboratory functions, such as making custom trays and pouring study models.

RETENTION TECHNIQUES

Often, the teeth being restored with a fixed prosthesis have substantial loss of tooth structure due to decay, fractures, or large, deteriorated restorations. Root canal therapy may be required in some teeth before the crowns and bridges are made.

The dentist improves the retentive capability of the tooth if the tooth being restored will not retain the restoration alone. There are several options for building up the tooth including core build-ups, retention pins, and post-retained cores.

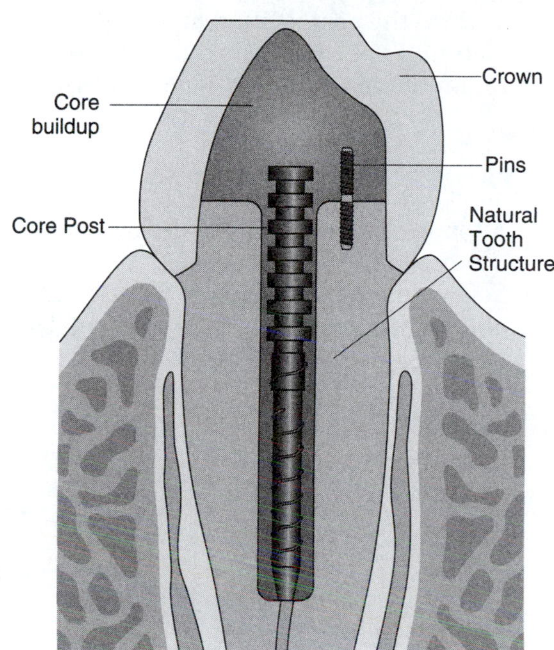

FIGURE 20–3 Tooth with core post, core buildup, and pins.

Core Buildups

A core buildup is treatment performed for vital teeth that have very little crown structure. For this procedure, the dentist removes any decay and defective restoration and then builds a core that supports and provides more retention for the cast restoration.

The core buildup or **retention core** is made of amalgam, composite, or a silver alloy/glass ionomer combination (Figure 20–3).

Retention Pins

The dentist often places **retention pins** for additional retention of the core buildup. The pins are placed strategically depending on the amount of buildup needed and the type of restoration. Pins are placed before the core material. The core buildup material surrounds the pins (Figure 20–3).

Post-Retained Cores

Post-retained cores are often the treatment of choice when the tooth is nonvital and has had root canal therapy. A portion of the root canal filling is removed and a post is fitted in the canal and cemented in place.

Once the post is fitted in the root canal, it is cemented in place. Core buildup materials are then placed around the post. The tooth is then ready for preparation of the prosthesis (Figure 20–3).

IMPLANT RETAINER PROSTHESIS

After several months, the dental implants have been in place long enough for the osseointegration process to be substantial. A fixed prosthesis stage can begin. Retainers that cover the implant may be a crown or part of a bridge. The abutments are fabricated in the dental laboratory and are either screw-retained or cement-retained (Figure 20–4).

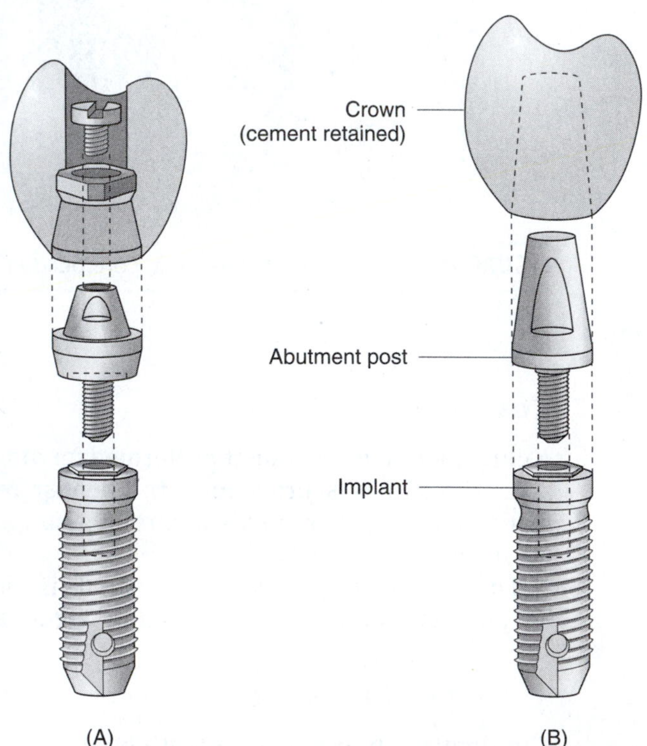

FIGURE 20–4 (A) Screw-retained implant prosthesis. (B) Cement-retained implant prosthesis.

CHAPTER 21

Removable Prosthodontics

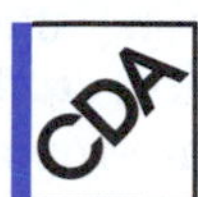

OBJECTIVES

The student should strive to meet the following objectives and demonstrate an understanding of the facts and principles presented in this chapter:

1. Define removable prostheses and list the reasons for using them.
2. Outline the steps of the diagnostic appointment and list the materials needed.
3. Describe the consultation appointment and the materials required for the case presentation.
4. Describe the partial denture components, and the appointment schedule.
5. Describe the complete denture, patient considerations, and the appointment schedule.
6. Explain the steps of denture reline procedures.
7. List the steps to polish a removable prosthetic appliance.

KEY TERMS

abutment (p. 349)
border molding (p. 355)
centric occlusion (p. 356)
connectors (p. 349)
denture base (p. 350)
framework (p.349)
muscle trimming (p. 355)
partial dentures (p. 348)
prostheses (p. 348)
relined (p. 359)
rests (p. 349)
retainer (p. 350)

INTRODUCTION

Removable prosthodontics, like fixed prosthodontics, refers to the replacement of missing teeth and tissues with artificial structures, or **prostheses**. The difference is the prosthesis can be removed from the mouth by the patient for cleaning, examination, and repair. Removable prosthodontics involve two types of prostheses: **partial dentures** and **complete (full) dentures.**

The partial denture replaces one or more teeth in one arch and is retained and supported by the underlying tissues and remaining teeth.

The complete denture replaces all the teeth in one arch. A full denture is retained and supported by the underlying tissues of the gingiva and oral mucosa, the alveolar ridges, and/or the hard palate. In some cases, teeth are retained in the arch or implants are placed to support the denture.

THE DENTAL ASSISTANT'S ROLE

The dental assistant's functions are to prepare materials, record measurements and details for the fabrication of the denture, give patient education and support, and perform some laboratory procedures. The procedures in removable prosthodontics do not require many instrument exchanges, and the dental assistant does not continually maintain the oral cavity throughout the appointment with the air-water syringe and the HVE.

DIAGNOSIS AND TREATMENT PLANNING

The first appointment for a removable prosthesis is to examine the patient. A medical history is taken or reviewed to determine the patient's state of health. The dentist examines the patient's remaining teeth and tissues.

After a prophylaxis (if natural teeth remain), preliminary impressions for study models and working casts are taken. Radiographic films are exposed and processed by the dental assistant as part of the diagnostic aids. Photographs are taken of the patient, including full face, frontal view, profile view, and a close-up. The patient is then scheduled for a consultation appointment in a few days.

THE CONSULTATION APPOINTMENT

The dental assistant has all of the items prepared so that the dentist can explain the diagnosis, the proposed treatment plan, and the prognosis to the patient. The treatment plan may involve restorative dentistry, periodontal treatment, endodontic treatment, or surgical procedures. These procedures must be completed and the patient must be completely healed before prosthodontic preparation can begin.

THE REMOVABLE PARTIAL DENTURE

Partial dentures are designed to restore missing teeth and to preserve the remaining hard and soft tissues of the arches. The partial denture distributes the forces of mastication between the abutment teeth and the alveolar mucosa. The **abutment** is a natural tooth that becomes part of the support for the partial. The abutment teeth must be in good condition or be restored to withstand the stresses of chewing with a partial denture.

Components of a Removable Partial Denture

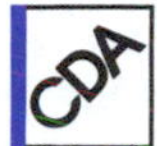

The components of the removable partial denture are the metal framework, rests, connectors, retainers, denture base, and artificial teeth.

The Metal Framework. The metal **framework** is the skeleton of the removable partial (Figure 21–1A) to which the remaining units (such as the rests, connectors, and retainers) are attached. Part of the framework is a mesh or loop area that is designed to retain the acrylic base material. The acrylic portion of the partial denture surrounds the framework.

The Rests. The **rests** are the part of the removable partial denture that contacts a tooth to provide vertical and horizontal support. The rests control the position of the partial in relationship to the supporting structures. These rests are positioned on the occlusal, incisal, or cingulum (lingual) surfaces (Figures 21–1A, B, and C).

The Connectors. The **connectors** unite the various parts of the partial into one unit, hold the working parts in the proper position, and distribute the stresses. They are divided into major and minor connectors.

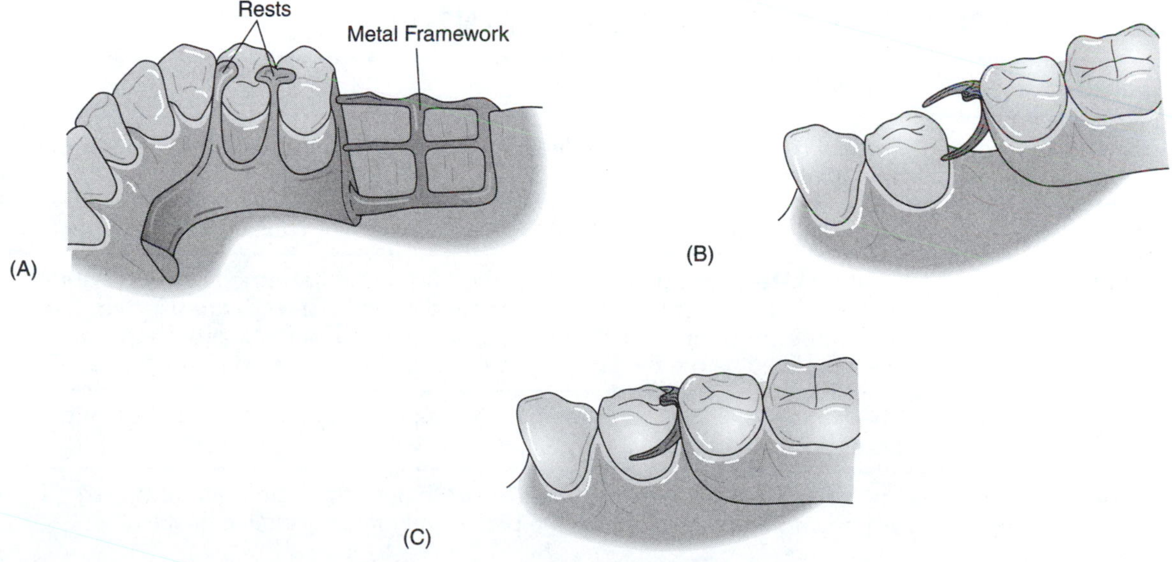

FIGURE 21–1 Partial denture with: (A) metal framework, (B) Placement of clasp with rest on the tooth. (C) Partial in place.

The Retainer. The **retainer** is sometimes called a clasp. The retainer contacts the abutment teeth and prevents the partial from moving. The position of the prosthesis is controlled by the retainer and its relationship to the remaining teeth and supporting structures.

Denture Base. The **denture base** is most often made of acrylic resin with fibers to give a natural appearance. It rests upon the oral mucosa, providing coverage and stability.

Artificial Teeth. The artificial teeth are made of either acrylic resin or porcelain. They are supplied in a variety of shapes (molds), sizes, and shades.

Partial Denture

The abutment teeth where the metal framework of the partial rests must be prepared before the final impressions are taken. The occlusal surfaces of the teeth are reduced to allow for clearance of the metal framework of the partial between the arches.

After the abutment teeth have been prepared, the dentist takes final impressions and a bite registration. These are sent to the dental laboratory with a laboratory prescription form. The dental laboratory follows the dentist's instructions and constructs an appliance that consists of the cast framework and the denture teeth set in the wax bite rim. The partial denture is **articulated** on the models to simulate how the appliance will occlude and mesh in various jaw positions. The laboratory then sends the partial to the dental office for the try-in and any adjustments. See Table 21–1 for the appointments for a partial denture.

TABLE 21–1 APPOINTMENTS FOR A PARTIAL DENTURE

Appointment	Procedure
Examination	Prophylaxis is completed, preliminary impressions are taken, and radiographs and photographs are taken.
Consultation	Treatment is explained to the patient and treatment choice is decided.
Final impressions	Abutment teeth are prepared, final impressions are taken, bite or occlusal registration is taken, and the shade and mold of artificial teeth are selected. **Note:** Sometimes restorative, periodontal, endodontic, or surgical procedures must be completed before the final impressions can be completed (Procedure 21–1).
Try-in and adjustment	The framework is placed in the patient's mouth and adjustments are made accordingly (Procedure 21–2).
Delivery	The partial is seated in the patient's mouth and instructions are given regarding how to place and remove the partial and oral hygiene techniques (Procedure 21–3).
Adjustment	As needed, the adjustments are made.

P R O C E D U R E

21-1 Final Impressions for a Partial Denture

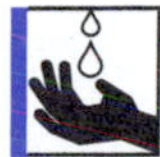 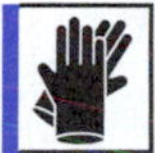 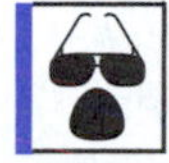 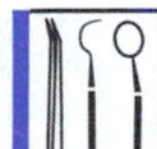

This procedure is performed by the dentist or prosthodontist. After preparing the materials needed for the final impressions, the dental assistant greets and seats the patient. A protective drape is placed on the patient and the procedure is explained to him or her.

EQUIPMENT AND SUPPLIES

- Basic setup: mouth mirror, explorer, and cotton pliers
- Mouthwash
- Custom tray or stock tray
- Contouring wax for the impression trays
- Impression materials—spatula and mixing pad or dispensing gun and tips
- Wax or silicone bite registration materials
- Tooth shade and mold guides
- Laboratory prescription form
- Disinfectant and container for impressions and bite registration

PROCEDURE STEPS *(Follow aseptic procedures)*

1. The dentist examines the oral cavity and tries the custom or stock tray in the patient's mouth. Sometimes, wax is placed on the borders of the tray to secure a contoured fit. Once the tray is prepared, an adhesive is painted on the inside of the tray.
2. The final impression material is prepared and placed in the tray according to the manufacturer's directions.
3. Once the final impressions are completed, receive the final impressions and either disinfect them right away or set them aside to disinfect after the procedure is completed.
4. The occlusal or bite registration is taken. When completed, it is also disinfected in preparation for the laboratory. Prepare the materials being used for the bite registration. Soften the wax in warm water and then fold it several times before placing it in the patient's mouth. Mix other materials on a paper pad and place them on a quadrant tray. Then, place them in the patient's mouth or dispense them directly into the oral cavity with a dispensing gun and tip. After the bite materials set and they are removed from the mouth, disinfect them and put them with the final impressions.
5. The shade of the artificial teeth is taken with a moistened shade guide under natural light. This can be completed at any point in the appointment sequence. Once the shade is determined, record it on the laboratory prescription and the patient's chart. Assist the dentist in the shade determination and the recording.
6. The dentist or prosthodontist completes the laboratory prescription with the details of the partial denture design. Make sure the patient's face is clean of impression materials and debris and then dismiss him or her.

PROCEDURE

21-2 Try-In Appointment for a Partial Denture

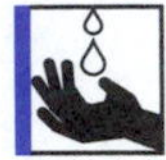 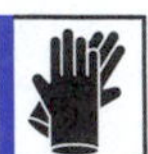 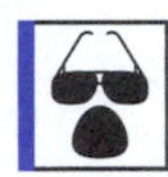 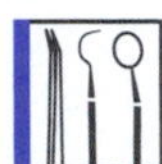

This procedure is performed by the dentist or prosthodontist. The dental assistant prepares the materials and the patient.

EQUIPMENT AND SUPPLIES

- Basic setup: mouth mirror, explorer, and cotton pliers
- Hand mirror for patient viewing
- Articulating paper and forceps
- Adjusting instruments, including wax spatula, pliers, and a heat source
- Low-speed handpiece with burs, discs, and stones
- Contour pliers
- Partial denture from the laboratory

PROCEDURE STEPS *(Follow aseptic procedures)*

1. The appliance is placed in the patient's mouth and adjustments are made accordingly. If adjustments are made to the denture base and/or the position of the teeth, prepare the spatula by warming it in the heat source (alcohol torch or Bunsen burner) and transfer it to the dentist. Transfer the articulating paper and evaluate the occlusion. If adjustments are needed, transfer the handpiece and burs.
2. The patient is given a hand mirror for viewing. Dismiss the patient and disinfect the partial to prepare it for the laboratory.

THE COMPLETE DENTURE

The complete denture is also called the full denture. When all the natural teeth are lost, a denture is fabricated to restore function and improve esthetics for the patient. (A person is said to be **edentulous** when he or she has no teeth remaining.) The denture is supported by the alveolar bone and the oral mucosa.

Components of the Complete Denture

The denture has two basic components: the **base** and the **denture teeth.**

Denture Base. The base is made of denture acrylic and may have a metal mesh embedded in the acrylic for additional strength. The acrylic resins are pigmented to shade the base to resemble the normal gingiva; often, fibers are part of the acrylic to give the denture a natural appearance. The base covers the alveolar ridge and gingival tissues.

PROCEDURE

21-3 The Delivery Appointment for a Partial Denture

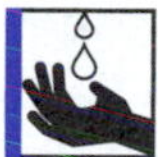
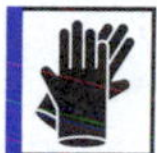
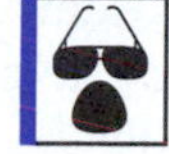
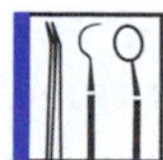

This procedure is performed by the dentist or prosthodontist with the assistance of the dental assistant. The partial denture will be returned from the laboratory in a sealed container.

EQUIPMENT AND SUPPLIES

- Basic setup: mouth mirror, explorer, and cotton pliers
- Partial denture
- Articulating paper and forceps
- Low-speed handpiece and acrylic burs and finishing burs

PROCEDURE STEPS *(Follow aseptic procedures)*

1. The preparations for the patient are completed.
2. The materials and equipment are similar to the try-in appointment with the exception of the wax adjustment instruments.
3. The patient is seated. If the patient has an old appliance, it is removed and placed in a cup with water.
4. The dentist seats the new partial denture and makes any necessary adjustments. Rinse the partial denture and hand it to the dentist for insertion. Articulating paper is used to check the patient's occlusion. If adjustments are needed, transfer the low-speed handpiece with finishing or acrylic burs. Transfer contouring pliers for adjustments to the metal clasps.
5. The dentist instructs the patient on how to insert and remove the partial denture. Explain the care of the partial and the supporting teeth. Also explain that it may take several days to adjust to the partial and sore spots that may appear. If the patient has any problems or questions, instruct him or her to call the office for an appointment.

Denture Teeth. The denture teeth used in construction of the denture are made of porcelain or acrylic resin.

Immediate Dentures

The sequence of the appointments for the complete denture depends on whether the patient is edentulous or has remaining teeth. When the patient is edentulous, he or she may already have complete dentures. These dentures may have to be replaced with new dentures for better fit and retention, or the dentures may have broken or been lost.

When the patient has remaining teeth, he or she will need to have the teeth extracted before receiving the denture. In this situation, there are two treatment sequences:

1. The patient can have all remaining teeth extracted and the alveolar bone shaped and contoured (alveoplasty). The patient waits for four to six months for the tissues and the alveolar bone to heal before the denture construction begins.
2. In the second treatment sequence, the patient has only the posterior teeth extracted (the anterior teeth remain). The construction of the denture begins as soon as the hard and soft tissues of the posterior areas have healed completely. When the dentures are completed, the anterior teeth are extracted and the denture is inserted. This is called an **immediate denture.**

The following sequence of appointments takes into consideration when the patient is having the surgery appointments. Most patients elect to have the immediate denture sequence, and those additional appointments are noted in the procedure descriptions. For a brief overview of the appointments for a complete denture, see Table 21–2.

TABLE 21-2 APPOINTMENTS FOR A COMPLETE DENTURE (BRIEF OVERVIEW)

Appointment	Procedure
Examination	An oral exam is completed. Preliminary impressions and radiographs are taken. The patient is asked to bring photos for the next appointment.
Consultation	Treatment is explained to the patient. Discussion of the treatment includes both the dentist's and the patient's responsibilities.
Oral surgery	During the appointment, the posterior teeth are removed and the alveolar bone is contoured.
Final impressions	When the healing of the posterior extractions are complete, the patient returns to the dental office and final impressions are taken (Procedure 21–4).
Jaw relationships	The jaw relationship is determined with baseplates and bite rims (Procedure 21–5).
Try-in	Denture teeth are mounted in the wax bite rim according to the dentist's directions. During the try-in appointment the dentist or prosthodontist can alter teeth to the desired position (Procedure 21–6).
Denture delivery	The patient is scheduled for surgery to have the anterior teeth extracted and the immediate denture seated (Procedure 21–7).
First follow-up (scheduled several days after the patient receives the denture)	With the immediate denture, the patient is seen the next day in the dental office.
Adjustments	As needed, adjustments are made.

PROCEDURE

21-4 Final Impression Appointment

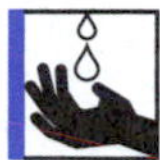
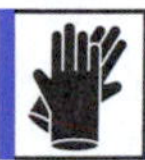
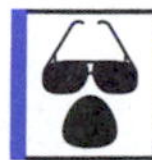
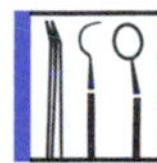

This procedure is performed by the dentist or prosthodontist. Materials are prepared and transferred to the dentist by the dental assistant.

EQUIPMENT AND SUPPLIES *(Figure 21–2)*

- Basic setup: mouth mirror, explorer, cotton pliers
- HVE tip, air-water syringe tip
- Cotton rolls and gauze
- Mouthwash for patient to rinse with prior to impressions being taken
- Custom tray
- Compound wax and Bunsen burner for border molding the rims of the trays
- Laboratory knife to trim border molding
- Impression materials—spatulas and mixing pads or dispensing gun and tips
- Laboratory prescription form

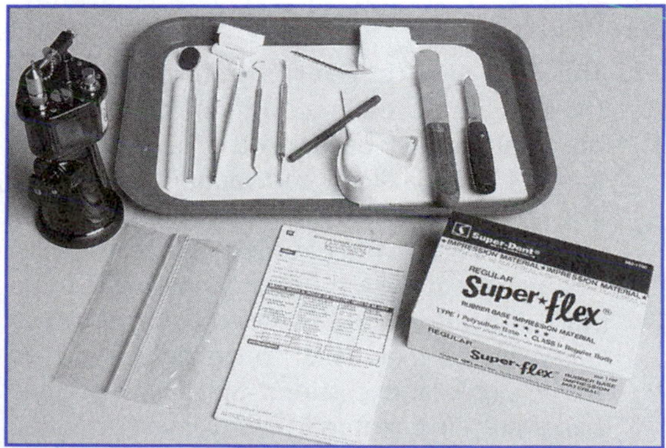

FIGURE 21–2 Tray setup for final impressions for a complete denture with custom trays.

- Disinfectant and container for impressions and bite registration

PROCEDURE STEPS *(Follow aseptic procedures)*

1. The final impressions are taken after custom trays have been fabricated from the casts taken at the examination appointment. The custom trays are inserted into the patient's mouth and evaluated for fit.
2. The impression compound is heated and placed along the borders of the custom tray. The tray is cooled and then placed in the patient's mouth. With the tray in the patient's mouth, the lips, cheeks, and tongue are moved to establish accurate length for the periphery and adjacent tissues to be included in the final impression. This is called **border molding** or **muscle trimming**.
3. Final impression materials are prepared and placed in the custom trays. The maxillary impression must include the tuberosities, frenum attachments, and other landmarks of the arch. The mandibular impression must include retromolar pads, oblique ridge, mylohyoid ridge, and frenum attachments.
4. Once the material has set, it is removed from the patient's mouth. The mouth is then rinsed thoroughly.
5. This procedure is repeated with the opposing arch if a full denture is being fabricated for both arches.
6. The impressions are disinfected and sent to the dental laboratory with the prescription form.
7. After the impressions have been taken, the patient is dismissed.

PROCEDURE

21-5 Jaw Relationship Appointment

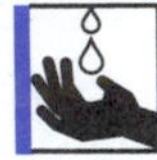 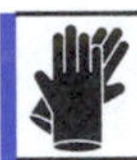 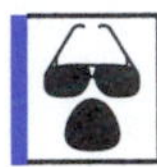 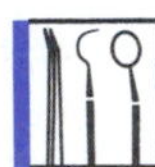

This procedure is performed by the dentist or prosthodontist. During this appointment, the measurements, shape, and shade of the denture are determined. The dental assistant prepares equipment and materials and assists the dentist throughout the procedure.

EQUIPMENT AND SUPPLIES *(Figure 21–3)*

- Basic setup: mouth mirror, explorer, and cotton pliers
- HVE tip and air-water syringe tip
- Hand mirror
- Laboratory knife, #7 wax spatula, Bunsen burner
- Shade guide
- Millimeter ruler and boley gauge

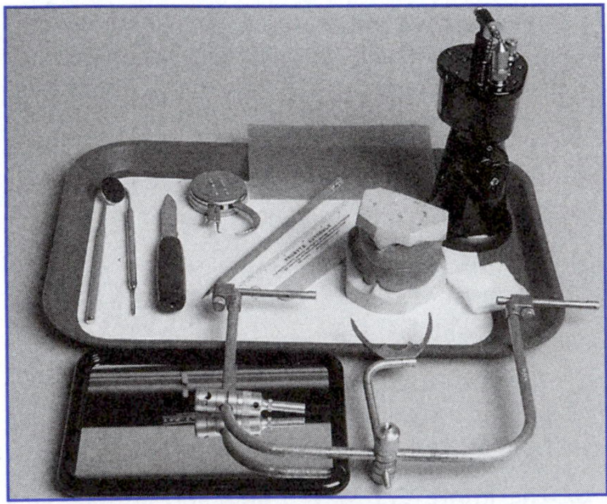

FIGURE 21–3 Tray setup for a jaw relationship appointment.

- Baseplates and bite rims
- Face bow
- Photographs of the patient, showing the shapes and shades of the teeth
- Laboratory prescription form
- Disinfectant

PROCEDURE STEPS *(Follow aseptic procedures)*

1. The baseplates and bite rims are inserted into the patient's mouth. The dentist determines and marks the midline of the maxillary and mandibular arches.
2. The bite rims represent the teeth and give the vertical dimension. The dentist adjusts the wax bite rims with the laboratory knife and wax spatula until the patient has a natural lip drape and the correct amount of tooth and gingiva is visible when the patient is talking and smiling and the lips are in a resting position. The cuspid lines are determined to position cuspids at the corners of the mouth.
3. The **centric occlusion** is determined when the jaws are closed in a position that produces maximal contact between the occluding surfaces of the maxillary and mandibular arches. The jaw relationships are determined by evaluating how the mandible relates to the maxilla. The patient moves the mandible as far backward (retrusion) and forward (protrusion) as possible, and then as far to the right and then the left (lateral excursion). Specially designed baseplates and materials assist in determining these measurements. Once determined, the information is used to articulate the casts to duplicate the normal motions of the patient.

4. After the jaw relationships are determined, the denture teeth are selected and the arrangement of the anterior teeth are discussed with the patient. The proper shade is determined using the shade guide and natural light. The shade guide is compared with the patient's complexion and remaining natural teeth or photographs to achieve a natural look. Usually, the age of the patient indicates the shade range (the teeth stain and become darker with age). The shape (mold) of the teeth is determined by evaluating the remaining natural teeth or from photographs. Sometimes, the shape of the patient's face also is used to guide the selection.
5. Because patients are concerned about the natural appearance of the teeth, some patients want to duplicate the arrangement of the teeth, including spaces, overlapping, and so on. Other patients want to correct the alignment of the natural teeth in the new denture. Spending a little more time at this point and having clear communication with the patient to determine what's the expected outcome often pays off when the patient receives the denture and is pleased with the appearance.

PROCEDURE

21-6 The Try-In Appointment

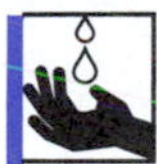 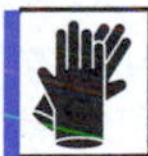 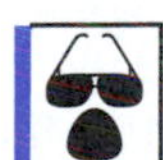 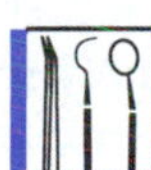

This procedure is performed by the dentist or prosthodontist. The dental assistant prepares the patient, the instruments, and materials and coordinates with the dental laboratory.

EQUIPMENT AND SUPPLIES

The equipment and supplies are the same for the try-in appointment as they are for the jaw relations and measurement appointment.

PROCEDURE STEPS *(Follow aseptic procedures)*

1. The try-in denture is disinfected before being placed in the patient's mouth.
2. The patient is seated and the denture is inserted into the patient's mouth. The dentist or prosthodontist and/or the dental assistant spends a few minutes talking with the patient. This allows the patient time to adjust to the denture.
3. The denture is evaluated for esthetics, retention, and comfort. The occlusion is checked with articulating paper.
4. The dentist makes adjustments to the position of the teeth. The shade can be changed by the dental laboratory technician in the dental laboratory, if necessary.
5. Once the dentist and the patient are satisfied with the denture, it is disinfected and placed back on the articulator to be returned to the laboratory.

PROCEDURE

21-7 The Delivery Appointment for the Complete Denture

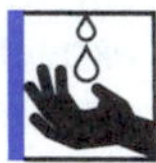 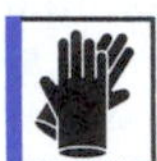 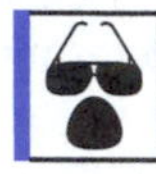 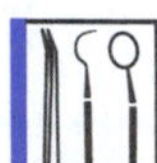

This procedure is performed by the dentist or prosthodontist. The dental assistant prepares the patient and coordinates with the dental laboratory. The dentures come back from the laboratory in a container that keeps them moist.

EQUIPMENT AND SUPPLIES *(Figure 21–4)*

- Basic setup: mouth mirror, explorer, and cotton pliers
- HVE tip and air-water syringe tip
- Dentures from the laboratory
- Hand mirror
- Articulating forceps and paper
- High-speed handpiece and diamond and finishing burs
- Low-speed handpiece and assorted acrylic burs and discs
- Home-care instructions pamphlet, denture brush and container to place dentures in when they are not in the patient's mouth

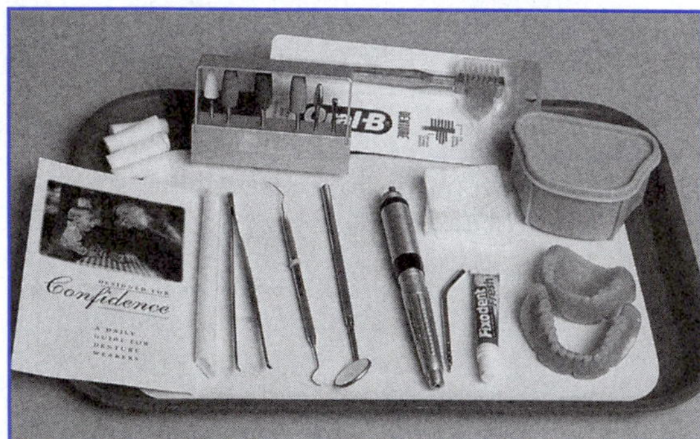

FIGURE 21–4 Tray setup for seating completed dentures.

PROCEDURE STEPS *(Follow aseptic procedures)*

1. The patient is seated and the appliances are removed and placed in a container to keep them moist.
2. If the patient is receiving an immediate denture, the denture is inserted after the extractions and alveoplasty. If there are more than simple extractions, the patient is scheduled with an oral maxillofacial surgeon. The dental laboratory sends the denture to the surgeon's office instead of to the dentist's office before the patient's surgery.
3. The new denture is inserted into the patient's mouth and the patient is given a few minutes to adjust. Then, the dentist begins the examination.
4. The patient's occlusion is evaluated and, if adjustment is needed, burs and discs are used. The denture is removed from the patient's mouth and the dentist uses a low-speed handpiece and acrylic burs to reduce any high spots on the inside of the base (the part of the denture that is against the tissues) of the denture. Sometimes after the adjustments, the denture needs to be polished in the laboratory. If this process is necessary, the denture must be disinfected before replacing it in the patient's mouth.

5. The dentist or prosthodontist evaluates the retention of the denture and the jaw relationships by having the patient demonstrate various facial expressions, swallowing, chewing actions, and speaking.
6. The patient learns to insert and remove the denture and daily maintenance of the denture (see Table 21–3).
7. The patient is given instructions to call the office with any questions or problems and is scheduled for an adjustment appointment in a few days. The patient is dismissed. As a courtesy, often the dentist or dental assistant calls the patient the following day to check on the patient's progress with the new denture.

TABLE 21-3 HOME-CARE INSTRUCTIONS

Keep the denture moist when not wearing it to prevent dimensional change.
Do not use abrasive dentifrice on the acrylic because it is easily abraded.
Do not clean acrylic dentures in hot water, because the acrylic can be deformed and distorted when exposed to high temperatures.
Dentures have low thermal conductivity, so the patient will notice a decrease in thermal changes to the tissues under the acrylic denture base.
Rinse thoroughly twice a day and after eating, if possible.
Use a soft denture brush and toothpaste designed for partials and dentures.
Remove the denture and rinse the oral cavity daily.
Denture adhesives are not needed with a well-fitting denture. As the tissues change and the denture does not adapt as well, adhesives will fill in the spaces so retention is increased.
Commercial cleaners are available for overnight soaking. Use warm water with these products.
The patient may want to fill the sink with water or place a washcloth in the sink in case the denture or partial is dropped.

Denture Reline

The tissue side of the denture bases may need to be **relined** to improve the fit of the denture and the comfort of the patient. Over time, the supporting tissues often shrink and change in size because of the pressure put on them by the complete or the partial denture. The denture relining adds a new layer of acrylic to the inside of the denture. This procedure can be done in the dental office (chairside) or sent to the dental laboratory (Procedure 21–8).

PROCEDURE

21-8 Denture Relining

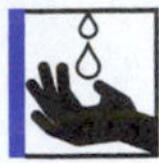 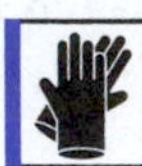 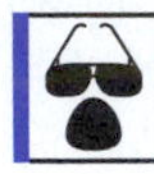 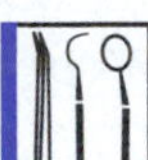

This procedure is performed by the dentist or prosthodontist. The dental assistant prepares the patient and the materials. The reline materials are available in either hard or semi-soft materials. There is a variety to choose from, depending on the dentist's preference.

EQUIPMENT AND SUPPLIES

- Basic setup: mouth mirror, explorer, and cotton pliers
- Low-speed handpiece with acrylic burs
- Chairside reline materials
- Mouth rinse

Chairside Relining

PROCEDURE STEPS *(Follow aseptic procedures)*

1. Clean the denture by placing it in an ultrasonic unit for several minutes.
2. The dentist or prosthodontist uses acrylic burs to roughen the tissue side of the denture.
3. The material is mixed according to manufacturer's directions and then placed in the clean denture, covering the entire tissue surface. The materials have low thermal reaction and cure directly in the patient's mouth.
4. The patient rinses with mouthwash to clean saliva and debris from the tissues.
5. The denture is inserted into the patient's mouth and the patient is asked to bite until the material reaches the initial set stage. Explain to the patient that sometimes the tissue will have a slight burning sensation from the acrylic material during the setting time.
6. The denture is removed to complete the setting process.
7. Excess material is trimmed away and the denture is polished. Follow routine disinfecting before the denture is inserted into the patient's mouth.

Laboratory Relining

The patient's denture is prepared in the same manner as it is for the chairside relining procedure. The following are the impression and laboratory steps. The tray setup is the same as that in the chairside relining, except for the type of materials used. Often, the denture or partial is used as the tray for the impression materials. A variety of impression materials, including polysulfides, polyethers, and silicone, are used to take the impression.

PROCEDURE STEPS *(Follow aseptic procedures)*

1. The impression material is mixed and placed in the denture (tray) according to the manufacturer's directions. The material should cover the entire tissue surface of the denture evenly and without excess.
2. The denture is inserted into the patient's mouth and positioned firmly. The patient should occlude and hold until the material is set.
3. After the material sets, the denture is removed from the patient's mouth, disinfected, and prepared to be sent to the dental laboratory. The laboratory prescription is completed and the patient is dismissed.
4. The dental laboratory processes the impression materials into an acrylic resin base that is fused to the denture.

5. The patient returns to the dental office as soon as the laboratory can process the denture. The turnaround time varies from hours to several days. The procedure is scheduled with the laboratory to minimize the time the patient is without the denture.
6. When the patient returns to the office, the denture is seated and adjustments are made as needed.

Polishing the Removable Prosthesis

After the dentist has adjusted the tissue surface of the removable prosthesis with acrylic burs, discs, and stones, it may need to be polished to smooth the surface. Polishing can be accomplished on a dental lathe with rag wheels, pumice slurry, and various other polishing agents, such as Tripole or a paste of tin oxide and water (Figure 21–5). Care must be taken not to overheat the denture, because the denture base has a relatively low heat-transfer temperature. If the denture is overheated, it may be distorted, which affects fit and appearance. Also, plastic teeth should be protected because they will abrade easily. Once the polish is complete, the prosthesis is washed in soap and water, disinfected, and stored in water until it is delivered to the patient. Separate burs, rag wheels, and pumice should be used for each patient to maintain infection control. Burs and rag wheels can be sterilized. The pumice is mixed with a disinfectant and green soap mixture and should be changed daily or after each use, if possible.

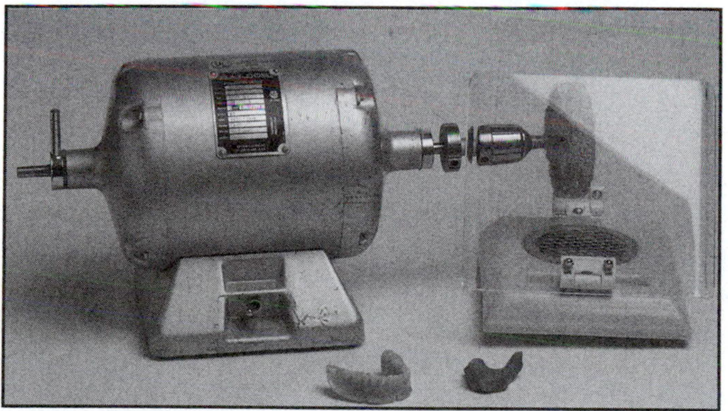

FIGURE 21–5 Dental lathe, rag wheel, and tripole to polish prosthesis.

SECTION 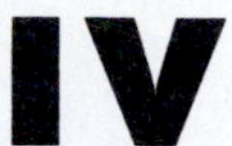

Advanced Functions

CHAPTER 22

Pit and Fissure Sealants, and Bleaching Techniques

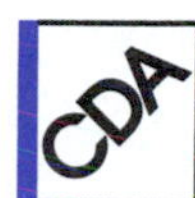

OBJECTIVES

The student should strive to meet the following objectives and demonstrate an understanding of the facts and principles presented in this chapter:

1. Define coronal polish.
2. List the types of abrasives commonly used.
3. List and explain the types of equipment and materials used to perform a coronal polish.
4. Describe the steps in a coronal polish procedure.
5. Explain the purpose of using pit and fissure sealants and where they are placed.
6. Describe the types of sealant materials.
7. List and describe the steps of sealant application.
8. Explain the benefits of the bleaching process used in dentistry.
9. Describe the procedures for dental office bleaching of vital and nonvital teeth and for home bleaching.
10. Explain information given to the patient concerning outcomes, procedures, responsibilities, and precautions related to bleaching.

KEY TERMS

abrasives (p. 366)
acid etched (p. 379)
assisted bleaching (p. 386)
axial walls (p. 376)
carbamide peroxide (p. 382)
cavity liners (p. 376)
cavity preparation (p. 374)
cavity varnish (p. 376)
cement bases (p. 376)
chemically cured (p. 378)
clinical crown (p. 366)
dental composites (BIS-GMA) (p. 376)
direct pulp capping (p. 375)
extrinsic stains (p. 366)
hard deposits (p. 366)
high-strength bases (p. 376)
indirect pulp capping (p. 375)
light cured (p. 378)
low-strength bases (p. 376)
mechanical bond (p. 379)
occlusal (p. 370)
oral prophylaxis (p. 366)
polishing (p. 366)
polymerization (p. 378)
power bleaching (p. 382)
proximal (p. 372)
soft deposits (p. 366)
walking bleach technique (p. 382)

INTRODUCTION

The oral prophylaxis procedure is twofold. First, the hard deposits (scaling) are removed by the dentist or dental hygienist. Second, the teeth are polished with a rubber cup. In some states, a registered or an expanded-function dental assistant can do this part of the prophylaxis.

Coronal Polish Defined

The **coronal polish** procedure involves removing soft deposits and extrinsic stains (stains on the tooth surface) of the teeth and restorations. This is accomplished with an abrasive, a dental handpiece, a rubber cup (sometimes this procedure is called a "rubber cup" polish), a brush, dental tape, and floss. The coronal polish is the polishing of the clinical crown, which may involve both enamel and exposed dentin that is visible in the mouth. Often, exposed dentin is not polished because of the possibility of increased sensitivity. Composite restorations, acrylic veneers, and porcelain-filled surfaces are also not polished because of the possibility of removing the finish and decreasing surface hardness. Different abrasives are used on each surface.

ABRASIVES AND POLISHING AGENTS

Abrasives and polishing agents are available to remove deposits and stains. Abrasives are materials that cut or grind the surface, leaving grooves and a rough surface, while polishing produces a smooth, glossy surface with fine abrasive materials. Abrasives remove small amounts of enamel during the polishing procedure; therefore, it is best to follow the coronal polish procedure with a fluoride treatment and/or to use a fluoride prophy agent.

Abrasives

Abrasives are materials composed of particles that are supplied as powders or pastes. They are selected according to the amount of stain and soft deposits to be removed. Abrasives should always be as moist as possible yet easy to use without dripping or spattering. These particles have characteristics that affect their abrasiveness.

Rate of Abrasion. The rate of abrasion is the time it takes to remove stains and deposits from a surface. This depends on several factors:

- By *increasing the speed of the handpiece,* the rate of abrasion is increased; this also increases the heat production.
- The *pressure* can control the rate of abrasion. The firmer the pressure, the more abrasive; the rate of frictional heat increases also.
- The *amount of abrasive* material used affects the rate of abrasion. The more material used, the faster the abrasive works.
- The *type of abrasive* used determines the rate of abrasion. The larger and harder the particles, the faster the abrasion; the rate of heat production also increases.
- The *dryer the abrasive* material, the more abrasive it is.

EQUIPMENT AND SUPPLIES

The tray setup for the coronal polish includes patient safety glasses, hand mirror, mouth mirror, explorer, cotton pliers, cotton swabs (Q-tips), 2 × 2 gauze, cotton rolls, saliva ejector, evacuator, air-water syringe tip, low-speed handpiece, rubber cups, brushes, prophy paste, tongue depressor, dental floss, dental tape, disclosing solution, and dappen dish for disclosing solution (Figure 22–1). Barriers are placed on the dental unit, and the dental assistant follows OSHA guidelines and wears PPE.

Use of the Dental Handpiece for the Coronal Polish

For the coronal polish procedure, a low-speed dental handpiece is used with a prophy angle attachment (right angle). The handpiece is held in a modified pen grasp. The fingers should close up on the prophy angle attachment, and the body of the handpiece should rest in the "v" of the hand. This gives the operator control and prevents fatigue.

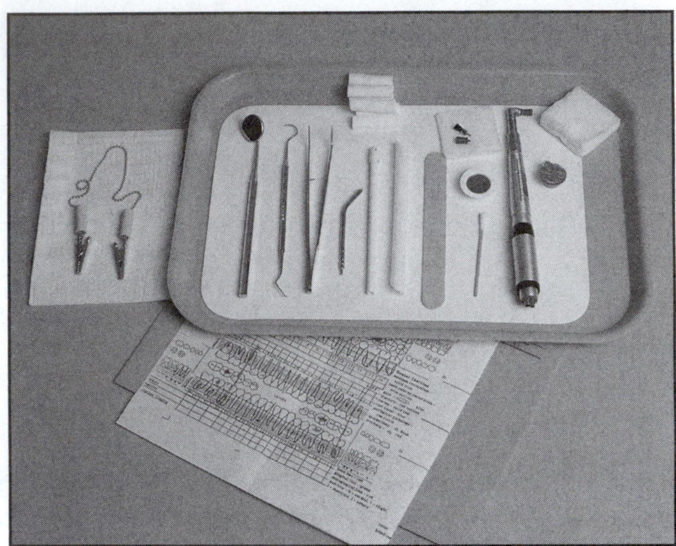

FIGURE 22–1 Tray setup for the coronal polish procedure.

Points for Using the Dental Handpiece

- Use a slow, even speed.
- Use a light to moderate pressure.
- Always use a fulcrum.
- Start and stop the handpiece inside the patient's mouth to minimize splatter.

Use of the Rubber Prophy Cup

The **rubber prophy cup** is used with abrasive agent to polish the teeth and dental appliances (Procedure 22–1). Rubber prophy cups are available in several designs to fit the prophy angles. Disposable prophy angles with attached prophy cups and brushes are also available.

The rubber cup should be soft and flexible to adapt to the contours of the teeth. Edges should not be rough or frayed as this could irritate the tissues. The edge of the cup is the part that actually does the polishing. The center of the cup holds and transports the abrasive agent. The cup is flexed to adapt to the tooth surface by applying slight pressure to one edge. The cup is most efficient on the facial and lingual surfaces of the teeth and fixed appliances, along the gingival margin, and 1 to 2 mm into the sulcus.

22-1 Polishing with a Rubber Cup

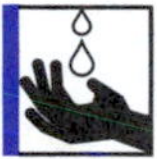
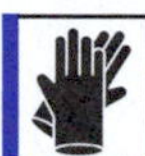
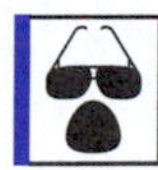
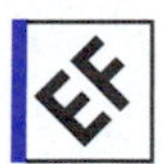
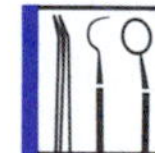

This procedure is performed by the dental assistant, hygienist, or dentist. The following procedure for polishing with the rubber cup explains the positioning techniques and the action of the rubber cup.

EQUIPMENT AND SUPPLIES

- Basic setup: mouth mirror, explorer/periodontal probe, and cotton pliers
- Saliva ejector, HVE tip, air-water syringe tip
- 2 × 2 gauze sponges, cotton tip applicator
- Dappen dish
- Lip lubricant
- Disclosing solution (optional)
- Low-speed handpiece
- Prophy angle attachment
- Assortment of rubber cups and brushes
- Prophy paste in different grits
- Finger rings to hold prophy paste cup
- Dental tape and dental floss

PROCEDURE STEPS *(Follow aseptic procedures)*

1. The patient is seated and prepared for the coronal polish procedure. Sometimes, lip lubricant is offered for the patient's comfort. The dental assistant reviews the patient's medical history and inspects the oral cavity. The amount of extrinsic stain determines the grit of the abrasive to be used.
2. The dental assistant may dry the teeth and place disclosing solution on the teeth for easier detection of plaque.
3. After the teeth are dry, a cotton tip applicator is used to place the solution on all surfaces of the teeth. This is done one quadrant, one arch, or one side at a time.
4. After placing abrasive polishing agent in the cup, place the cup near the gingival sulcus and as far into the mesial or distal surface as possible. Establish a fulcrum as close to the tooth being polished as possible.
5. Apply light pressure to flex the cup and flare it into the sulcus 1 to 2 mm.
6. Sweep the rubber cup toward the incisal or occlusal edge. If the crown of the tooth is long, lift the cup halfway up the tooth and make a second stroke toward the occlusal (Figure 22–2).
7. At the incisal or occlusal edge, lift the cup slightly off the tooth and replace it near the gingiva to repeat the stroke, moving toward the opposite side of the tooth.
8. Repeat the stroke, overlapping each time, until the entire tooth surface is polished.
9. When finished with one tooth, move to the adjacent tooth using the same steps until the surfaces of all teeth have been polished.
10. For the patient's comfort, rinse the mouth frequently, at least after polishing each quadrant.
11. When all the teeth have been polished, rinse and evacuate the patient's mouth thoroughly, removing all debris.

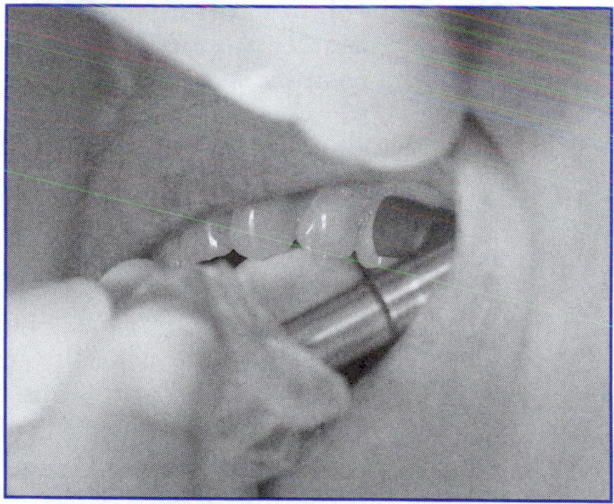

FIGURE 22–2 Maxillary left posterior: Buccal surfaces, lingual surface. Retract cheek to position prophy angle and have patient close slightly. Fulcrum on same arch.

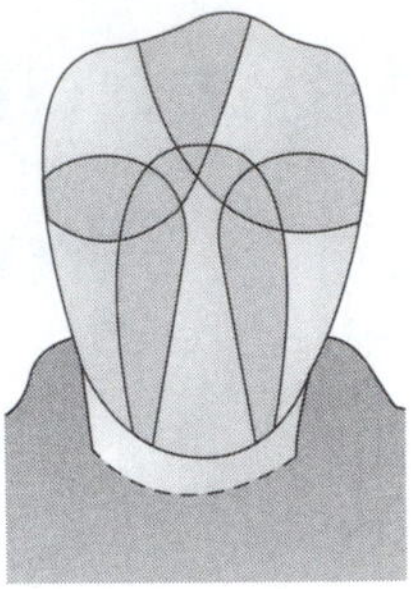
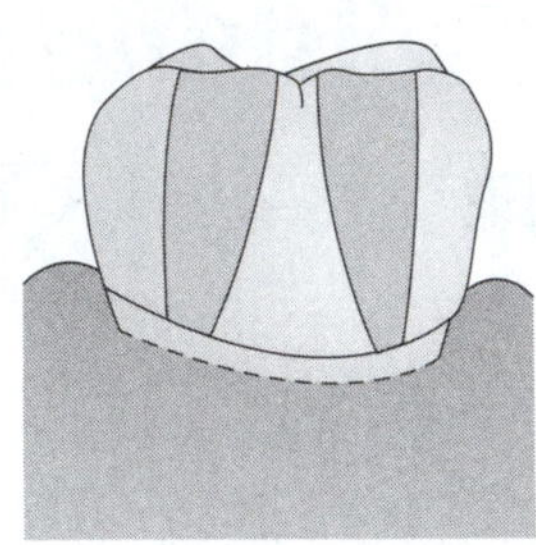

FIGURE 22–3 Examples of the polishing stroke.

A short, intermittent, overlapping stroke is used with a slow-revolving rubber cup. This stroke covers the tooth, leaves no unpolished surfaces, and minimizes the frictional heat produced (Figure 22–3).

The Prophy Brush

The **prophy brushes** used for the coronal polish procedure are supplied in several styles. Like the rubber cup, they are either "snap on" or "screw on," depending upon which prophy angle they are used with. For the coronal polish, a soft, flexible brush is used. Softening can be accomplished by soaking the brush in hot water before using it.

Prophy brushes are used on the **occlusal** surfaces to effectively clean the deep pits and fissures and also on the lingual of the anteriors, however, the bristles should *never* contact the gingival tissues and should be positioned only above the gingival third of the tooth. The prophy brush is used only on the enamel surface. The brush is used in the same manner as the cup: flexed in the central fossa with a light, intermittent, and overlapping stroke. With the lingual surfaces, the brush is placed in the lingual pit and moved toward the incisal edge (Procedure 22–2).

Dental Tape and Dental Floss

Dental tape is used on the interproximal surfaces of the teeth with an abrasive agent. Care must be used not to damage the interdental papilla or free gingival margins when using the tape. After all the interproximal surfaces have been polished with dental tape and abrasive, the teeth must be flossed to remove any particles of abrasive left after rinsing. **Dental floss** is placed interproximally, wrapped around the tooth, and moved in an up-and-down motion (Procedure 22–3).

> **Note:** If fluoride is to be applied as the next step of this procedure, unwaxed floss should be used instead of waxed floss. (Waxed floss coats the teeth, preventing the fluoride from being absorbed by the teeth.)

PROCEDURE

22-2 Polishing with a Prophy Brush

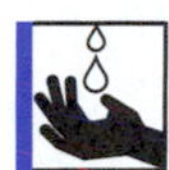 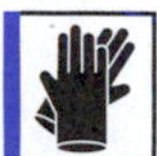 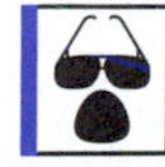 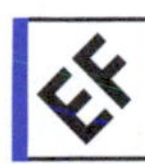

This procedure is performed by the dental assistant, hygienist, or dentist. The prophy brush procedure follows the rubber cup polish. It includes the techniques used to manipulate and position the brush.

EQUIPMENT AND SUPPLIES

- Refer to Procedure 22–1, Polishing with a Rubber Cup.

PROCEDURE STEPS *(Follow aseptic procedures)*

1. Place the softened brush on the prophy angle and apply prophy paste to the brush.
2. Establish a fulcrum close to the posterior tooth to be polished.
3. Move the brush bristles toward the mesial buccal cusp tip and continue until the brush comes off the occlusal surface.
4. Replace the brush bristles in the central fossa.
5. Apply slight pressure again, and move the brush up toward the distal buccal cusp until the brush comes off the occlusal surface.
6. Repeat this procedure on the occlusal surface of each posterior tooth until all of the occlusal surfaces are cleaned.
7. Repeat this process on the occlusal surfaces of all teeth.
8. For the lingual surfaces of the anterior teeth, place the prophy brush in the lingual pit, above the cingulum.
9. Apply light pressure to flex and spread the bristles of the brush.
10. Move the brush toward the incisal edge to polish the lingual surface.
11. Repeat on all lingual surfaces that have deep pits and grooves.
12. When finished with the brush, rinse and evacuate the oral cavity thoroughly.

CORONAL POLISH PROCEDURE

The coronal polish procedure involves using the rubber cup, brush, and dental tape and floss (Procedure 22–4). This procedure is completed after all hard deposits have been removed from the surfaces of the teeth. The dental assistant becomes the operator for this procedure and should be positioned on the side of the chair that is most comfortable. Usually a right-handed assistant is on the right side of the patient.

During the procedure the dental assistant is responsible to keep the patient's mouth free of excess saliva and debris, direct the dental light for optimal visual access, and keep the patient comfortable.

PROCEDURE

22-3 Polishing with Dental Tape and Dental Floss

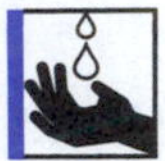 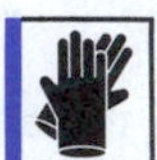 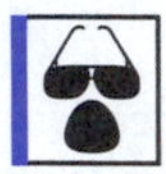 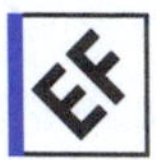 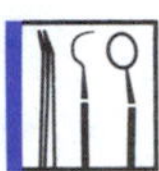

This procedure is part of the coronal polish. After the rubber cup and brush have been used, the interproximal surfaces of the teeth are cleaned with dental tape; then dental floss is used.

EQUIPMENT AND SUPPLIES

- Refer to Procedure 22–1, Polishing with a Rubber Cup.

PROCEDURE STEPS *(Follow aseptic procedures)*

1. Cut off a piece of dental tape twelve to eighteen inches long.
2. Wipe some abrasive agent into the interproximal contact areas of the teeth in a quadrant with a cotton tip or finger.
3. Wrap the tape around the middle fingers of both hands, leaving a length of tape just long enough to wrap around the tooth while maintaining control.
4. Take the tape through the contact at an oblique angle (\ ) in a back-and-forth motion, using gentle pressure and holding the tape against the tooth. (This helps prevent the tape from snapping through the contact and damaging the gingiva.)
5. Wrap the tape around the tooth to cover the line angles of the tooth on both the buccal and the lingual.
6. When the **proximal** surface of one tooth is complete, lift the tape up and over the interdental papilla without removing the tape through the contact; readapt the tape on the proximal surface of the adjacent tooth.
7. Polish this surface with the tape and abrasive and then remove the tape up through the contact. If the tape is pulled through the embrasure area, be careful not to injure the gingival tissues.
8. Continue around each tooth in both arches until all proximal surfaces have been polished, including the most distal surface of each quadrant. Use different areas of the tape as needed, and rinse areas thoroughly and evacuate all debris.
9. Follow by using dental floss to remove debris left. Floss all areas and rinse thoroughly.

CAVITY LINERS, VARNISHES, AND CEMENT BASES

The dental assistant should be familiar with and knowledgeable about the properties and preparation of cavity liners, varnishes, and cement bases. Cavity preparation and terminology also should be familiar so the dental assistant can plan ahead to prepare and place the materials the dentist asks for; however not all states allow dental assistants to place bases, liners, and cavity varnish; but the dental assistant can assist the dentist during this step of restorative procedures.

PROCEDURE

22-4 Coronal Polish

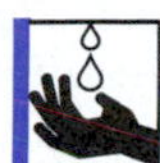 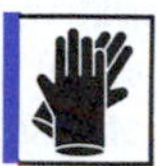 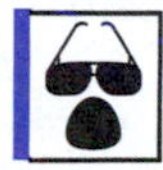 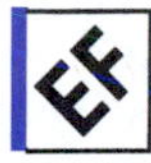 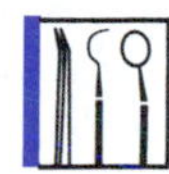

This procedure is performed routinely by the dental assistant and the dental hygienist. This procedure describes the protocol for performing a coronal polish, including preparation of materials and the patient, positioning of the operator and the patient, sequence of procedure, and evaluating the procedure.

EQUIPMENT AND SUPPLIES

- Basic three setup: mouth mirror, explorer, and cotton pliers
- Saliva ejector, HVE tip, air-water syringe tip
- 2 × 2 gauze sponges, cotton tip applicators, tongue blade, and cotton rolls
- Lip lubricant and disclosing solution in dappen dish
- Low-speed handpiece with prophy angle attachment
- Prophy cups and brushes (dappen dish with warm water to soak brushes in)
- Prophy pastes, with a variety of grits and finger ring holder
- Dental tape and dental floss
- Auxiliary aids as needed

The following items are needed off the tray:

- Patient's chart
- Red/blue pencil, lead pencil, and pen
- Barriers for the dental unit
- Patient napkin and napkin chain
- Patient safety glasses
- Patient hand mirror

PROCEDURE STEPS *(Follow aseptic procedures)*

1. After gathering the preceding equipment and materials, prepare the operatory for the patient.
2. Prepare the patient.
   - Following the established procedure, seat the patient and review and update the patient's records.
   - Explain the procedure to the patient.
   - Follow aseptic procedures to prepare the patient for the coronal polish.
   - Evaluate the patient's condition by performing an oral inspection.
   - Select abrasive agents to be used after examining the teeth. Depending on the amount and type of stain, abrasives are selected.
   - Lubricate the patient's lips, dry the teeth, and apply the disclosing agent with the cotton tip applicator.
   - Adjust the dental unit light for good vision.
3. Position the operator and the patient. When the operator is polishing the maxillary and mandibular right facial and the maxillary and mandibular left lingual, the patient's head is turned away from the operator. When the operator is polishing the maxillary and mandibular right lingual and the maxillary and mandibular left facial, the patient's head is turned toward the operator.
4. Begin the sequence of the procedure.
   - Begin the polish on the quadrant or arch according to the predetermined, established routine.

(continued)

PROCEDURE 17-2 *continued*

- Follow criteria previously discussed regarding the use of abrasives and the rubber cup, prophy brush, tape, and floss.
- Rinse the patient's mouth after each quadrant is polished, or as needed.

5. Evaluate the coronal polish.
   - Once all steps of the coronal polish have been completed, rinse the patient's mouth thoroughly with the spray from the air-water syringe and the evacuator.
   - Apply disclosing solution to detect any areas of plaque or stain that were missed.
   - Using the mouth mirror and the air syringe, inspect each surface for any remaining soft deposits and/or stains. Note these areas on the patient's chart for future reference.
   - Polish the areas missed with a prophy cup and/or brush.
   - Rinse the patient's mouth to remove all the abrasive agent.
   - Inspect the teeth for a lustrous shine showing no debris or extrinsic stains. The soft tissues should be free of abrasion or trauma. The patient is ready for a fluoride treatment. The dentist may want to examine the patient before he or she is dismissed.
6. Chart the coronal polish. It is the dental assistant's responsibility to record the coronal polish completely and accurately on the patient's dental chart. The entry is recorded in ink, dated, and signed or entered into the computer system. Include any comments about the condition of the patient's mouth and the type(s) of material(s) used.

Cavity Preparation/Pulpal Involvement

The **cavity preparation** for a restoration depends on the amount of decay, the location of the decay, and the type of materials used to restore the tooth. If the dental assistant is placing the liners, base, or varnish, he or she should examine the cavity preparation to assess pulpal involvement.

Treatment of Cavity Preparations

The treatment of cavity preparations varies with the amount of enamel and dentin removed and how near the prep is to the pulp.

1. Treatment of the ideal cavity preparation:
   - A base is not required because only a minimal amount of enamel and dentin has been removed. Some dentists place only the restoration, while others prefer to place a fluoride-releasing liner. If an amalgam restoration is going to be placed, two thin layers of cavity varnish are often placed over the dentin.
   - If a composite restoration is to be used, a glass ionomer liner or calcium hydroxide is placed over the exposed dentin.

2. Treatment of the beyond-ideal cavity preparation:
   - With a beyond-ideal preparation, the level of the dentin is restored with a cement base.
   - With an amalgam restoration, there are several options. One option is to place two thin layers of varnish to seal the dentinal tubules and then place a layer of a cement base, such as zinc phosphate.
   - Another option is a reinforced ZOE base, which has a soothing effect on the pulp. Varnish is not used with this material.
   - Other options include polycarboxylate or glass ionomer base, which also do not require varnish.
   - Under composite restorative materials, use a glass ionomer base or calcium hydroxide.
3. Treatment of the near-exposure cavity preparation:
   - The closer the cavity preparation comes to the pulp, the more precautions that are needed. There are also several options for treatment of the near-exposure preparation.
   - With preparations that are going to be restored with amalgam, a liner of calcium hydroxide, glass ionomer, or ZOE is placed first over the deepest portion of the prep in the dentin. Once this layer is placed, two thin layers of varnish are inserted over the exposed dentin. Then, a layer of cement base is applied. Zinc phosphate, polycarboxylate, or glass ionomer cements can be used for this layer.
   - Another option for amalgam restorations is to place a liner over the deepest portion of the preparation, then a layer of reinforced ZOE, polycarboxylate, or glass ionomer cement. This is then sealed with cavity varnish.
   - With some preparations, the dentist may choose not to place cavity varnish.
   - When composite materials are to be used to restore the tooth, a liner is placed first, then a layer of either polycarboxylate or glass ionomer cement. Varnish is not placed and a ZOE base liner is not used because they inhibit the setting of the composite.
   - When a cavity liner is placed on a near exposure, the procedure is often referred to as an **indirect pulp capping**.
4. Treatment of the exposed-pulp cavity preparation:
   - In an exposed pulp, the dentist must decide whether endodontic treatment is indicated or attempt to save the vitality of the tooth. If the treatment of choice is to save the pulp, a procedure called a **direct pulp capping** is performed.

- One treatment involves the placement of calcium hydroxide or glass ionomer liner and then reinforced ZOE as a temporary restoration. This gives the dentist time to see whether the pulp is going to heal.
- Another treatment involves the placement of a liner, followed by a layer of ZOE cement, two thin layers of varnish, and a cement base.
- Some dentists prefer to place a liner and then a layer of polycarboxylate or glass ionomer cement base.

Cavity Liners

Cavity liners are placed in the deepest portion of the cavity preparation on the **axial walls** or pulpal walls. After the liners are hardened, they form a cement layer with minimum strength. They are placed on the dentin or on an exposed pulp and protect the pulp from chemical irritations and also provide a therapeutic effect to the tooth. Examples of cavity liners are calcium hydroxide, zinc oxide eugenol, and glass ionomer. Liners also are often called **low-strength bases** (Procedure 22–5).

Cavity Varnish

Cavity varnish is used to seal the dentinal tubules to prevent acids, saliva, and debris from reaching the pulp. Cavity varnish is used under amalgam restorations to prevent microleakage and under zinc phosphate cements to prevent penetration of acids to the pulp. If cavity liners or medicated bases are used, varnish is placed after or on top of these materials (Procedure 22–6).

Cement Bases

Cement bases are mixed to a thick putty consistency and placed in the cavity preparation to protect the pulp and provide mechanical support for the restoration. These cement bases are placed on the floor of the cavity preparation to raise the level of the floor of the preparation to the ideal height. Several different types of cements can be used for bases. These include: glass ionomers, hybrid ionomers, reinforced zinc oxide eugenol, zinc phosphate, and polycarboxylate. The preparation, sensitivity of the pulp, and type of restoration indicate which cement to use. These materials are often referred to as **high-strength bases** (Procedure 22–7).

Pit and Fissure Sealant Materials

Several materials have been used as sealants for pits and fissures, but the most commonly used are **dental composites (BIS-GMA)** that have been diluted to be less viscous to enhance the flow characteristically needed with sealants. These materials are clear, opaque, or lightly tinted colors.

PROCEDURE

22-5 Placing Cavity Liners

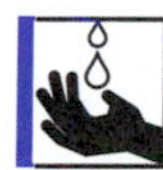
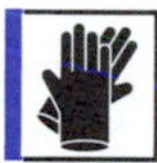
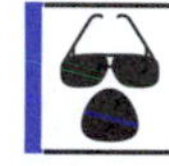
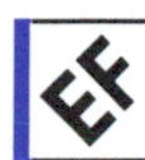

This procedure is performed by the dentist or an expanded-function dental assistant. The preparation of the cavity has been completed, and this procedure begins the restorative process.

EQUIPMENT AND SUPPLIES

- Cavity liner (calcium hydroxide, glass ionomer, or zinc oxide eugenol)
- Application instrument—small, ball-shaped instrument or explorer
- Gauze sponges and cotton rolls
- Mixing pad and spatula, if material is mixed
- Curing light (if material is light cured)

PROCEDURE STEPS *(Follow aseptic procedures)*

1. Examine the cavity preparation. Determine the deepest portion of the cavity preparation and access to that area.
2. Clean and dry the cavity preparation. Remove debris from the cavity preparation. Wash and dry the area with the air-water syringe.
3. Prepare the liner to be used. Dispense and mix according to directions.

Note: Usually, light-cured materials do not have to be mixed but are placed directly in the preparation.

4. Place the liner in the cavity preparation. Using a small, ball-ended instrument, place the material in the deepest portion of the cavity preparation in a thin layer. Be careful not to touch the instrument to the sides of the preparation. The material will flow into the area and can be spread in the direction desired with the small ball of the instrument.
5. Complete placement. Remove the instrument, wipe it clean with a gauze, and repeat this procedure until the liner covers the deepest portion of the cavity preparation (Figure 22–4).
6. If the liner is self-curing, the mix must be allowed to harden. If the liner is light curing, the light is held over the tooth and activated to cure the material for the appropriate time (usually ten to twenty seconds).
7. Examine the cavity preparation. After the liner has cured, examine the preparation. If any material is on the enamel walls, remove it with an explorer.

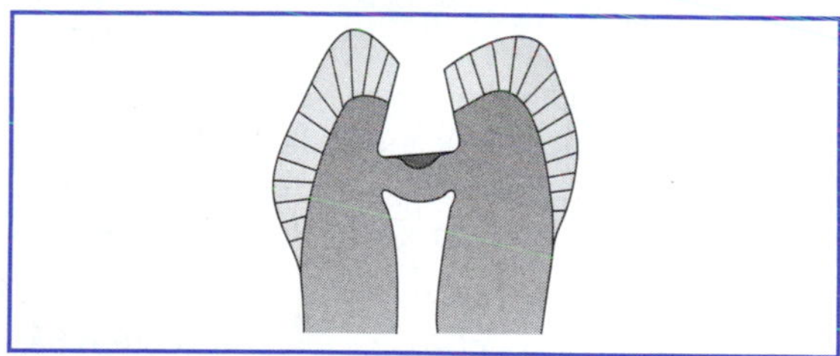

FIGURE 22–4 Placement of cavity liner in preparation.

PROCEDURE

22-6 Placing Cavity Varnish

 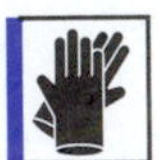 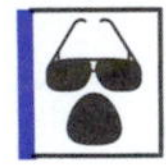 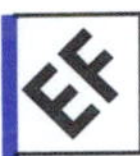

This procedure is performed by the dentist or the expanded-function dental assistant. The preparation of the cavity has been completed, and this procedure is part of preparing the tooth for the restoration.

EQUIPMENT AND SUPPLIES

- Cavity varnish (varnish and solvent)
- Cotton pliers
- Application instruments (cotton balls or cotton pellets, sponge applicators, brush applicators)
- Gauze sponges

PROCEDURE STEPS *(Follow aseptic procedures)*

1. Prepare two very small cotton balls or pellets about 2 mm in size to look like small footballs.
2. Evaluate the cavity preparation to determine access, visibility, and placement of liners or bases.
3. If the tooth has not been washed and dried, do so at this time with the air-water syringe.
4. To prevent contamination of the varnish, pick up both cotton pellets or balls with the sterile cotton pliers and place in the varnish. Then, place the cotton on gauze to remove excess varnish.
5. Using the cotton pliers, pick up one cotton ball or pellet and paint a thin layer of varnish on the dentin in the cavity preparation. A sterile disposable brush or sponge may also be used (Figure 22–5).
6. Allow the cavity to dry for thirty seconds. Place a second coat of varnish. Using the cotton pliers, pick up the second cotton pellet or ball from the gauze and apply a second layer of varnish (this prevents any voids). To prevent contamination, never place an applicator that has been used in the mouth back in the bottle of varnish.
7. Clean up after the procedure. If any excess varnish was placed on the enamel surface, remove it with varnish solvent and a small applicator.

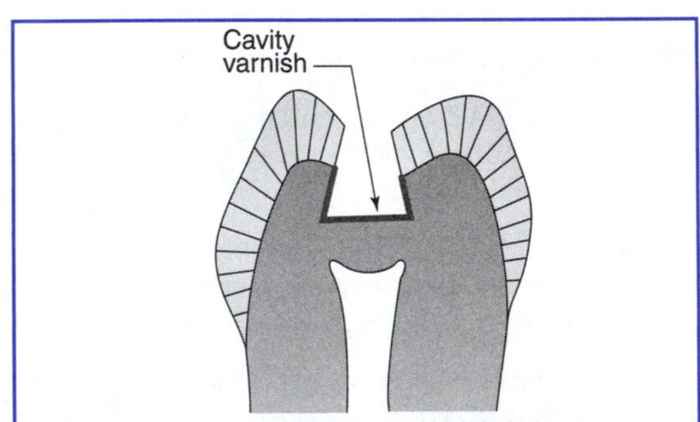

FIGURE 22–5 Placement of cavity varnish in preparation.

The difference in the types of sealant materials is in the curing or hardening process. The two methods of **polymerization** (hardening) are:

1. **Chemically cured**, also known as self-cure or auto-polymerization
2. **Light cured**, the use of curing light to harden materials

PROCEDURE

22-7 Placement of Cement Bases

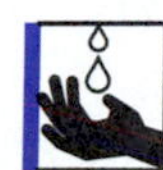
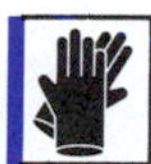
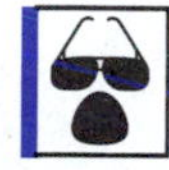
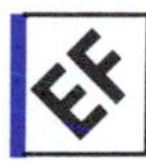

This procedure is performed by the dentist or the expanded-function dental assistant. The preparation of the cavity has been completed, and this procedure is part of preparing the tooth for the restoration.

EQUIPMENT AND SUPPLIES

- Cement base materials
- Mixing pad
- Cement spatula
- Gauze sponges
- Plastic filling instrument
- Explorer or spoon excavator

PROCEDURE STEPS *(Follow aseptic procedures)*

1. Determine the previous treatments and decide where to place the base and the size of area. Evaluate access and visibility.
2. Prepare the preparation area. Remove debris with the air-water syringe and HVE.
3. Prepare the cement base materials according to manufacturer's instructions. Mix the cement base to a thick putty consistency and gather into a small ball.
4. Collect the base on the blade of the plastic filling instrument. Place the base in the cavity preparation.
5. Using the small condensing end of the plastic filling instrument, condense the base into place on the floor of the cavity prep. If the material is sticky, place a small amount of powder on the mixing pad and dip the end of the condenser as needed. Continue until a sufficient base layer is placed.
6. Evaluate the placement. The base should cover the floor of the cavity preparation leave enough room for the restorative materials and should not be on pins or in retentive grooves.
7. Remove any excess materials with a spoon excavator or an explorer.
8. Clean up the mixing materials. Remove cement from the spatula as soon as possible and remove the paper from the pad.

Acid Etching/Conditioning Material

Enamel sealants bond mechanically to the tooth surface (not chemically). The **mechanical bond** is achieved by the sealant flowing into the irregularities of the treated enamel and locking into place. The enamel using surface is **acid etched**, or **conditioned** using a phosphoric acid solution applied to a clean tooth with a brush, syringe, or cotton pledget. The etchant gel or a liquid is applied for thirty to ninety seconds. During that time, the etchant is "dabbed" or flowed over the area, but never rubbed. When the time is complete, the tooth is rinsed thoroughly for the specified time. The tooth surface looks frosted or chalky and appears dull. If the enamel does not appear chalky and white, the procedure must be repeated. If the tooth is contaminated with saliva before the sealant is placed, the etching procedure must be redone. The acid etchant/conditioner is applied on the occlusal surface 2 to 3 mm beyond the area to be sealed. The tooth must be etched beyond the sealant to prevent fracture of the sealant and possible microleakage.

Placement of Pit and Fissure Sealants

The dentist diagnoses which teeth need sealants after a thorough examination, including radiographs. Children with newly erupted molars and premolars that are caries free benefit the most from sealants (Procedure 22–8). Sealants are often placed on one or two quadrants at a time to ensure adequate isolation of the teeth.

PROCEDURE

22-8 Procedure for Placing Enamel Sealants

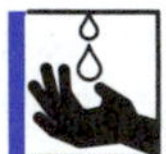
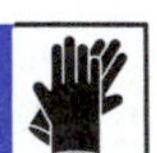
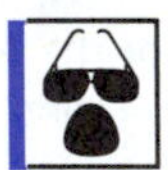
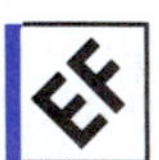

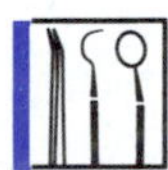

This procedure is performed by the dental assistant, hygienist, or dentist depending on the state dental practice act. Before the sealant is placed, the tooth/teeth is/are polished with a rubber cup. Equipment for the preparation of the tooth/teeth and the sealant procedure are listed.

EQUIPMENT AND SUPPLIES *(Figure 22–6)*

- Basic setup: mouth mirror, explorer, cotton pliers
- Air-water syringe tip, HVE tips, and saliva ejector
- Rubber cup
- Low-speed handpiece with right angle attachment
- Flour of pumice or prophy paste without fluoride
- Dental dam setup or Garmer cotton roll holders and short and long cotton rolls
- Etchant/conditioner

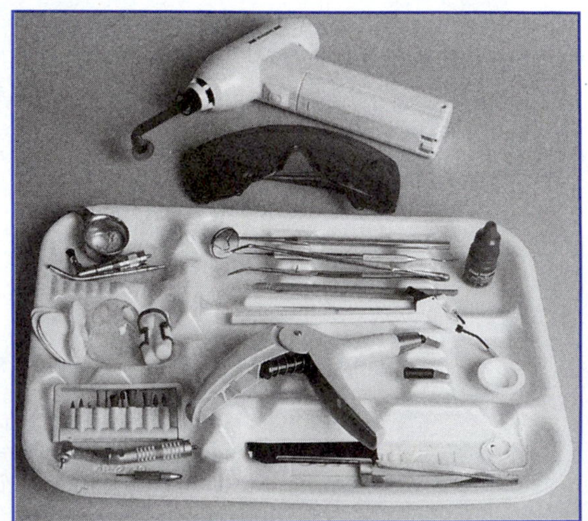

FIGURE 22–6 Equipment for placing pit and fissure sealants.

- Sealant material: base material and catalyst (for self-cure) or base material (for light cure)
- Applicators (brush, small cotton pellets, or syringe) for etchant and sealant
- Sealant dappen dish
- Light-curing unit
- Articulating paper and forceps
- Assorted burs and/or stones
- Floss

PROCEDURE STEPS *(Follow aseptic procedures)*

1. Polish the surfaces of the teeth to receive sealants. Use flour of pumice or a non-fluoride prophy paste with a rubber cup or bristle brush to clean the occlusal surfaces. Once polished, rinse the teeth and dry thoroughly. If the pits and fissures are deep, check them with an explorer and then rinse and dry again.
2. Dental dam isolation is ideal because it keeps the teeth dry and protects the tissues from the acid etchant. Depending on the skill of the operator, the dental dam may be placed on more than one quadrant at a time. Cotton roll isolation is commonly used; however, care must be given to ensure the teeth are kept isolated. Garmer clamps used with long and short cotton rolls are very effective.
3. After the tooth is isolated, completely dry it. Following manufacturer's directions, apply the acid etchant. Using an applicator, apply etchant to the occlusal surface, into the pits and fissures and two-thirds up the cuspid incline. Use a gentle dabbing motion while applying the sealant for the designated time (usually sixty seconds).
4. Rinse the tooth with water, and use the evacuator tip to remove the remaining acid and water. Rinse for twenty to thirty seconds. Reisolate with dry cotton rolls if this method was used.
5. Dry the tooth with the air for twenty to thirty seconds. Examine the etched surface. It should appear dull and chalky white. If the tooth does not have this appearance, etch again for fifteen to thirty seconds.
6. Follow the manufacturer's directions to prepare and apply the sealant material. With the applicator selected, place the sealant so that it flows into the pits and fissures and reaches the desired thickness. The applicator tip or an explorer can be used to move the sealant and prevent air bubbles.
7. Allow the self-curing sealants to set (polymerize) for the time recommended by the manufacturer. For light-cured sealants, hold the curing light 2 mm directly above the occlusal surface and expose for the appropriate time (materials differ, so the curing time can range from twenty to sixty seconds).

NOTE: Use tinted protective eyewear during the curing process.

8. Evaluate the sealant using an explorer, to see whether the sealant is hardened and smooth. If there are irregularities or voids, repeat the process to properly seal those areas. If the surface has been free of saliva, additional sealant can be added without etching the tooth first. However, if saliva has contacted the tooth, then the process must be repeated.
9. After the sealant has set, rinse or wipe the surface with a moist cotton roll/pellet to remove the air-inhibited layer.
10. Remove cotton rolls or the dental dam. Check the contacts with dental floss, and look for any excess use materials. Dry the teeth and articulating to paper evaluate high spots. If the markings are dark, use a bur or stone to reduce them.
11. Apply fluoride to the sealed tooth to cover any areas that were etched but not sealed. Sealants are recorded on the patient's chart. Instruct the patient to check the sealants every six months to a year to ensure that they have been completely retained.

Bleaching Techniques

Cosmetic tooth bleaching has become one of the most requested services provided by the dental profession and is often delegated to a dental assistant. Specific training and clinical experience are required for this person to become confident and competent.

There are two methods of bleaching: One method is done in the dental office, and the other method is done at home. Patients can have one or the other or a combination of both services to meet their needs. Both vital and nonvital teeth are bleached in the office. There are advantages and disadvantages with each method, thus the options should be presented to the patient. Considerations include the amount of stain and its origin, the number of visits to the office versus the amount of time the bleaching trays are worn at home, the expense of the in-office bleaching (which is higher than in-home bleaching), and the amount of instruction and guidance the patient requires.

Nonvital Bleaching

Endodontically treated teeth sometimes turn dark due to blood, pulpal debris, and restorative materials used to fill the canal. These teeth can be lightened by both internal and external bleaching. One of the most common bleaching techniques is the **walking bleach technique**, which uses a thick paste of hydrogen peroxide, sodium perborate, or a combination of the two placed in the coronal portion of the nonvital tooth. With the bleach mixture temporarily sealed in place, the patient can leave the office and return for evaluation and another possible treatment as instructed by the dentist. Sometimes, heat is applied to achieve the results desired (Procedure 22–9).

Vital Bleaching In-Office

Bleaching vital teeth in the office involves the application of bleaching liquids or gels, often with the application of heat and a curing light. This is sometimes called **power bleaching**. The patient's teeth are isolated tightly to prevent irritation to the gingiva from the chemicals; then they are polished with pumice or prophy paste. The actual bleaching steps depend on the type of materials used, but, for most, a fresh mix is applied every ten to fifteen minutes for three to four applications. The bleaching materials are evacuated between applications and then completely when the procedure is finished. Then, rinse thoroughly, remove isolation, and polish with a fluoride prophy paste (Procedure 22–10).

The patient is scheduled for his or her next appointment within one to two weeks. The patient should be told that the teeth may be sensitive. This process usually takes three appointments.

Home Bleaching Techniques

For home bleaching (Procedure 22–11), the patient applies a bleaching agent, usually **carbamide peroxide** or diluted hydrogen peroxide, in a custom-fit tray for specific times. There are multiple materials, and the techniques vary

PROCEDURE

22-9 Nonvital Bleaching

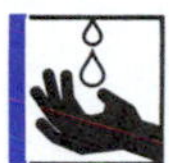 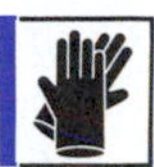 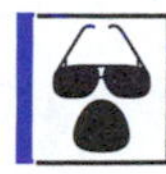 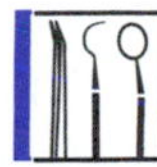

This procedure is performed by the dentist. The patient has received information on the procedure and the possible outcome before the procedure begins. More than one treatment may be necessary.

EQUIPMENT AND SUPPLIES

- Basic setup: mouth mirror, explorer, cotton pliers
- Cotton rolls, gauze sponges, cotton pellets
- HVE tip, air-water syringe tip, saliva ejector
- Dental dam setup
- Protective gel
- Waxed dental floss
- High-speed handpiece and assorted burs
- Low-speed handpiece
- Prophy brush
- Cement base materials
- Bleaching materials
- Heat source
- Temporary coverage and cement
- Finishing burs

PROCEDURE STEPS *(Follow aseptic procedures)*

1. The dentist examines and evaluates the root canal treated tooth.
2. Place the dental dam and ligature of waxed dental floss on the designated tooth or teeth. Once the dam is in place, apply more protective gel to further seal the dam.
3. Remove the access restoration and any debris in the crown. With the crown of the tooth open, some dentists scrub the chamber with a soap solution and a prophy brush or cotton pellet.
4. The root canal is sealed with 2 to 3 mm of a thick base cement or with a light-cured resin ionomer or bonded composite. This is a critical step, because the tooth must be sealed to prevent the bleach from penetrating the root. This can be done using the gel bleach in the office or the walking technique, or a combination of both techniques. If bleaching results are not achieved, heat may be also used with the office bleaching gel technique. Stains caused by endodontic procedure and drugs often need the application of heat with the bleaching agents.
   - Gel bleaching in the office involves the tooth chamber remaining filled for thirty minutes. Change the bleaching gel every ten minutes. Then, place a cotton pellet and temporary in the crown. The patient should be reappointed in three to seven days for evaluation.
   - With walking bleaching, a thick mixture of bleaching agent is placed in the crown and covered with temporary cement. Reappoint the patient in two to five days to remove the cotton pellet.
5. Desired results should be achieved in three appointments, however, if the tooth remains darker than the patient prefers, a veneer should be considered. The shade can be altered slightly with the shade of the restorative materials. The temporary filling is removed, and the chamber is rinsed and evacuated. Etching is applied to the inside of the crown. Rinse. Apply the dental adhesive and then fill the chamber with restorative material and light cure.
6. Polish the restoration with finishing burs and polish.
7. Reappoint the patient in a few days to evaluate the color and whether there is the possible need of a veneer.

PROCEDURE

22-10 In-Office Bleaching of Vital Teeth

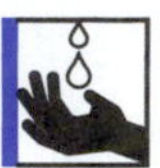
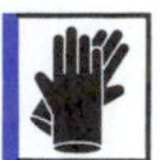
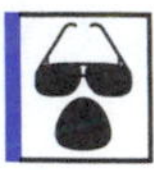

This procedure is performed by the dentist in the office. The procedure is explained to the patient with the possible outcomes.

EQUIPMENT AND SUPPLIES

- Protective gel
- Dental dam, dam napkin, holder
- Scissors
- Waxed dental floss
- High-speed handpiece and assorted burs
- Low-speed handpiece
- Prophy brush
- Cement base materials
- Bleaching materials
- Heat source
- Temporary coverage and cement
- Finishing burs

PROCEDURE STEPS *(Follow aseptic procedures)*

1. The procedure is explained and videos, photos, and pamphlets may be available for the patient. The teeth and surrounding tissues are examined. "Before" photos may be taken of the patient.
2. Cover all surrounding tissues with protective gel. Isolation with a dental dam is the safest method to protect the tissues. Place the dental dam, punching the holes as close as possible to match the tooth. With the dental dam on, place a ligature of waxed floss around each tooth, and pull the floss toward the cervix and secure.
3. Polish the crowns of the teeth to remove plaque and debris that may interfere with the bleaching process. Prophy paste or flour of pumice may be used.
4. Follow the manufacturer's instructions for the specific steps of the materials being used. Materials are mixed to a thick consistency and placed on the facial and lingual surfaces of the tooth or in a tray. Some materials require the use of a bleaching heat and/or light source and are used for approximately thirty minutes. The no-heat materials are applied every ten minutes, with fresh materials mixed each time for three to four applications. Rinse and evacuate between each application to remove the bulk of the bleaching gel.
5. After thoroughly rinsing the area, cut the ligatures and interseptal dental dam and remove these from the patient's mouth. Rinse again, and remove any protective gel with floss and wet gauze.
6. Polish the teeth with a composite resin polishing cup or a fluoride prophy paste. (This step may vary with different types of materials.)
7. Although the bleaching process may take some time before the shade can be evaluated, the patient's tissues are examined and the patient is instructed to avoid substances that may stain the teeth. The patient should also be warned that the teeth may be sensitive following the bleaching procedure. Usually, three appointments one to two weeks apart are required to reach the desired shade.

PROCEDURE

22-11 Home Bleaching

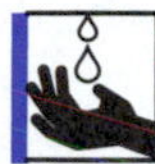 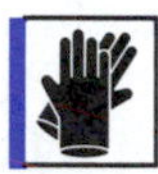 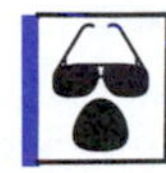 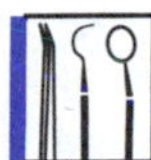

This procedure is performed by the patient at home after an examination by the dentist. The patient is given a bleaching kit and step-by-step instructions from the dentist. This procedure is divided into appointments and steps that occur between appointments.

EQUIPMENT AND SUPPLIES

- Basic setup: mouth mirror, explorer, cotton pliers
- Alginate
- Rubber mixing bowl and spatula
- Impression trays
- Camera
- Custom-fit, vacuum-formed tray
- Home bleaching kit

PROCEDURE STEPS *(Follow aseptic procedures)*

First Appointment

1. The dentist examines the teeth, considering the shade of the teeth, sensitivity, restorations, and areas of abrasion and erosion. General procedures are completed before the bleaching process begins. The bleaching techniques are explained, and the procedure that best meets the patient's needs is selected.
2. Alginate impressions are taken of the arches being bleached. Before photographs are taken.

Between Appointments

1. The alginate impressions are poured in stone and prepared.
2. A custom-fit, vacuum-formed tray is made. This may be done in the office lab by the dental assistant or at a commercial lab.

Second Appointment

1. With the home technique, the patient tries on the trays to ensure a good fit.
2. Instructions are given, including when and for how long to wear the trays, how to prepare the materials, how to place the custom-fit trays, what to do in case the gingiva becomes irritated, and how to handle other side effects.
3. In some cases, the patient receives one bleaching application in the office, before beginning the home bleaching. The teeth are polished, and then the bleaching agent is prepared and placed in the trays. The trays are inserted into the patient's mouth for thirty to sixty minutes, then removed. The teeth are suctioned off and rinsed thoroughly.
4. Some offices schedule an appointment to follow-up with the patient's progress and to examine the tissues. This appointment is usually within two weeks of the second appointment.

greatly. The advantages of the home bleaching techniques include fewer visits to the dental office, less expense, and patients can apply the bleach at their convenience. The disadvantages of these techniques are that the patients must be motivated to following the routine, the time involved for the bleaching process can take several weeks, the bleaching materials can cause nausea and sensitivity to the gingiva, and there is lack of direct monitoring by the dentist. As an alternative, patients can come to the office for a startup, or **assisted bleaching**, appointment and then complete the process with home bleaching. Usually, the two appointments are needed to set up the patient for home bleaching. At the first appointment, the impressions for the custom trays are made. The second appointment is for delivery of the bleaching trays; instructions are also given to the patient.

CHAPTER 23

Dental Dam and Matrix and Wedge Techniques

CDA

OBJECTIVES

The student should strive to meet the following objectives and demonstrate an understanding of the facts and principles presented in this chapter:

1. Explain the purpose of the dental dam.
2. Identify the armamentarium needed for the dental dam procedure and explain the function of each component.
3. Explain how to prepare the patient for the dental dam placement, explain how to determine the isolation area, and describe and demonstrate how dental dam material is prepared.
4. List and demonstrate the steps in placing and removing the dental dam.
5. Define matrix and wedge. List the uses and types of matrices.
6. Describe the functions, parts, placement, and removal of the Tofflemire matrix.
7. Explain and demonstrate placement and removal of the strip matrix.

KEY TERMS

anchor tooth (p. 389)
dental dam clamps (p. 389)
dental dam forceps (p. 390)
dental dam frame (p. 389)
dental dam napkins (p. 389)
dental dam punch (p. 389)
interseptal (p. 391)
inverting (p. 391)
key hole punch (p. 392)
matrix band and retainer (p. 396)
septum (p. 392)
wedge (p. 396)

INTRODUCTION

Dental dam placement is one method used to isolate teeth that are going to be restored. After the patient has received the anesthetic, the dental dam is prepared and placed. The dental assistant assists the dentist in the placement or places the dental dam before the dentist begins to prepare the tooth. The dam can be placed to isolate one tooth or one or more quadrants.

MATERIALS AND EQUIPMENT

The dental dam procedure requires a variety of instruments and materials. The materials and equipment may be on a separate tray (Figure 23–1), stored at the dental unit, or in a tub for easy use. Materials include the dental dam material, dental dam napkin, dental floss, tape, dental dam clamps, forceps, frame, punching guides, and a punch.

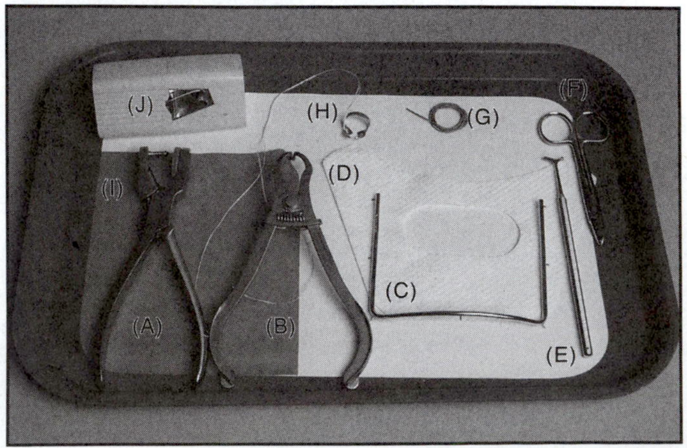

FIGURE 23–1 Dental dam tray setup (labeled). (A) Dental dam punch. (B) Forceps. (C) Frame. (D) Dental dam napkin. (E) Tucking instrument. (F) Scissors. (G) Widgets. (H) Clamp. (I) Dental dam. (J) Floss.

Dental Dam Material

The dental dam is a latex or latex-free material supplied in various sizes, weights, and colors selected according to the operator preference. The most common sizes of the dental dam are the 5 × 5 or the 6 × 6 precut squares. These squares usually come in a box of fifty or more and are lightly powdered on one side to prevent sticking.

Dental dam is available in different weights (thicknesses), including thin, medium, heavy, extra heavy, and special heavy.

Dental dam is available in various colors (shades), from dark gray or green to lighter pastels. The darker shades provide more contrast with the teeth and make it easier for the operator to see.

Dental Dam Napkin

Dental dam napkins are used for patient comfort and to absorb saliva, water, and perspiration. Disposable napkins are made of a soft, absorbent fabric and are precut.

Dental Dam Frame

The **dental dam frame**, or holder, is designed to stretch and secure the dam in place across the patient's face. The frame stabilizes the dental dam and keeps the operating area open. Frames are made of metal or plastic and have small projections around the borders to secure the dental dam.

Dental Dam Punch

The action of the **dental dam punch** is similar to that of the paper punch, although the design is much different. The punch has a handle and a working end. The working end of the punch has a **stylus,** is a sharp projection to punch through the dental dam, and a **punch table** or **plate.** The table has four or five differently sized holes and rotates to facilitate punching holes for the various teeth (Figure 23–2). The punch table should be adjusted so that the hole is centered under the stylus before the punch is made.

Dental Dam Clamps

Dental dam clamps are supplied in numerous designs and sizes to fit around the teeth to stabilize and secure the dental dam material in place. The tooth that the clamp is placed on is called the **anchor tooth**. The anchor tooth is one or two teeth distal to the tooth or teeth being restored (Figure 23–2).

Selecting the Clamp

The tooth to be clamped must be evaluated before the clamp selection is made. The mesiodistal width at the cementoenamel junction (CEJ) of the tooth must be evaluated prior to selecting a clamp. The width on the tooth must be about

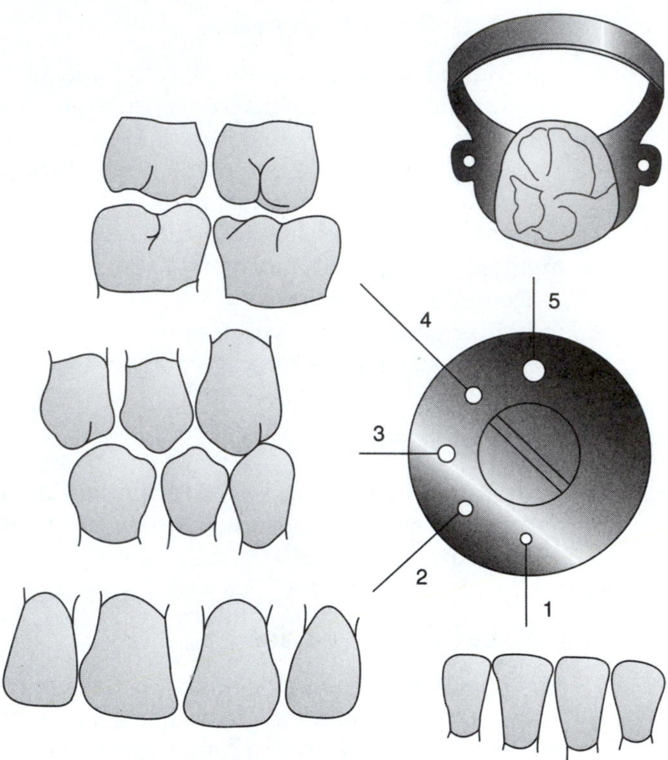

Hole number 5–Molars, and used for anchor tooth
Hole number 4–Molars
Hole number 3–Cuspids and premolars
Hole number 2–Upper incisors
Hole number 1–Lower incisors

FIGURE 23–2 Punch table with corresponding teeth and tooth with clamp in position.

the same as the width between the points of the jaws of the clamp. The faciolingual width at the CEJ of the tooth must also be estimated to ensure the clamp fits tightly. To place the clamp, the jaws are opened wide enough to clear the height of contour, which is the widest part of the tooth. Then, the jaws are closed slowly on the tooth to fit tightly at the CEJ.

Dental Dam Forceps

Dental dam forceps are used to place and remove the dental dam clamp. The forceps have two beaks that fit into the holes of the jaws of the clamp. Once the beaks are securely in the holes, pressure is applied to the handle of the forceps and the clamp jaws are opened slightly. A lock (sliding bar) on the handle keeps the clamp in this position until it is placed on the anchor tooth. When the handle is squeezed again and the lock is released, the operator has control over the clamp and can make adjustments to the clamp position. Once the clamp is stable, the beaks of the forceps are removed from the clamp and the forceps are removed from the mouth.

Dental Floss

Dental floss is used for a variety of reasons with dental dam isolation.

1. A piece of dental floss, about eighteen inches long, is tied to the bow of the dental dam clamp before the clamp is placed. If the clamp accidentally slips off the anchor tooth, the floss makes it easy to retrieve.
2. The floss is used to ease the dental dam material through tight contacts.
3. The dental floss assists in **inverting**, or tucking, the dental dam material around the teeth to prevent moisture leakage.

Lubricant

A small amount of lubricant is placed on the back or underside of the dental dam to facilitate slipping to the dam material over the teeth.

Scissors

Scissors are used to cut the **interseptal** dental dam during removal of the dam from the patient's mouth. When cutting the interseptal dam material, direct the scissors away from the tissues to prevent tearing of the dam material and to completely cut the interseptal dam.

Inverting or Tucking Instrument

The dental floss can be used to invert or tuck the dental dam; however, sometimes an instrument is needed to do this. Options include a periodontal probe, spoon excavator, or the flat side of the T-ball burnisher. These instruments are used to turn under the edge of the dental dam that is around the tooth.

Preparation Before Placement of the Dental Dam

Before the dental dam is placed, the procedure should be explained to the patient and the operator should examine the oral cavity to determine the area of isolation.

Determining the Area to Be Isolated

Before the dental dam is punched, the area to be isolated needs to be determined and then examined. Follow these steps:

1. Determine the tooth to be restored and then determine the anchor tooth, which is usually one or two teeth distal to the tooth being restored. When learning, a good rule of thumb is to punch to the canine of the opposite quadrant.
2. The size and the shape of the arch are examined so that they can be duplicated on the dental dam as closely as possible to the patient's arch.
3. The area is examined for missing teeth, teeth that are out of alignment, or fixed prosthetics. The dental dam is punched accordingly.
4. The area is flossed to identify tight contacts and open spacing.

Dividing the Dental Dam

Select the size and weight dental dam that best suits the patient and the procedure.

To begin, fold the dam in half and then crease the fold. This horizontal line is the division between the maxillary and mandibular arches. With the dam folded in half, fold the dam vertically into equal thirds and crease along each fold. The center third is where the dam will be punched. This represents the width of the arches of most patients.

Punching the Dental Dam

After the dental dam is divided, it is ready to be punched for the placement. There are many places to begin punching the dental dam, thus, it is important for the operator to visualize the patient's arch on the dam. Often, the **key hole punch** is punched first. The key punch hole is the largest hole punched in the dental dam. It is the hole that slides over the clamp and onto the anchor tooth. The next holes are punched moving forward, about 3 to 3.5 mm apart. This is the amount of dental dam that slides between the teeth. It is called the **septum**. The punch table is adjusted for the size of the teeth.

Placement and Removal of the Dental Dam

The dental assistant assists the dentist with the dental dam in states where it is not legal for him or her to place the dental dam. In states where the dental assistant can place the dental dam, the assistant punches the dam, selects the clamp, and places and removes the dental dam without the chairside presence of the dentist (Procedure 23–1).

PROCEDURE

23-1 Placing and Removing Dental Dam

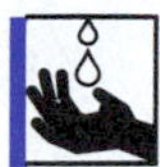
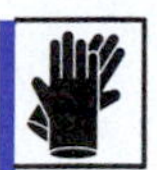
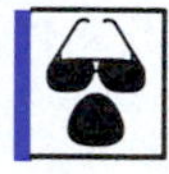
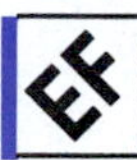

This procedure is performed by the dentist or dental assistant. The patient has been anesthetized before the placement of the dental dam, before the cavity preparation begins. The dental assistant has prepared all equipment and supplies needed for the entire procedure. Only the items needed for the dental dam procedure are listed.

EQUIPMENT AND SUPPLIES

- Dental dam material
- Dental dam napkin
- Dental dam punch
- Assortment of clamps
- Dental dam forceps
- Dental dam frame
- Dental floss
- Lubricant
- Cotton tip applicator
- Tucking instrument (plastic instrument, T-ball burnisher, or spoon excavator)
- Scissors

PROCEDURE STEPS *(Follow aseptic procedures)*

Placement of Dental Dam

1. Inform the patient about the dental dam procedure.
2. Examine the patient's oral cavity to determine the anchor tooth, shape of the arch, tooth alignment, missing teeth, and the presence of crowns and bridges. Also, examine the gingival tissues and check for tight contacts.
3. Prepare the dam material by dividing it into sixths and then punch the dam, aligning the stylus and the holes carefully.
4. Center the punch in the upper or lower middle third of the dental dam. Holes are punched according to size of tooth, the key punch being the largest to accommodate the anchor tooth and the clamp.
5. Holes are punched following the pattern of the patient's arch. Lubricate the dental dam on the tissue side of the dam with a water-soluble lubricant.
6. Select the clamp or several clamps to try on the tooth.
7. Attach a safety line (floss) on all clamps that are to be tried on. When trying on the clamps, keep the end of the safety line in hand.
8. Secure the clamp on the clamp forceps and spread the jaws slightly to lock the forceps.
9. Place the clamp over the anchor tooth. To widen the jaws of the clamp, squeeze the forceps handle slightly to release the locking bar.
10. Fit the lingual jaws of the clamp on the lingual side of the tooth first. Next, spread the clamp and slide the buccal jaws of the clamp over the height of contour of the buccal surface of the tooth. Release the pressure on the clamp forceps slightly against the tooth to evaluate the clamp, but do not release the clamp from the forceps.
11. The jaw points of the clamp should be at the CEJ, adapting to the gingival embrasures on the buccal and lingual. The clamp should be secure on the tooth, not pinching any gingival tissue. The clamp may be adjusted to the

(continued)

PROCEDURE 23-1 *continued*

tooth by moving the wrist to the left and right and by putting more pressure on the distal or mesial of the clamp.

12. When the clamp is in place, confirm with the patient that the clamp position is comfortable.
13. Place the dental dam over the clamp bow by grasping the dam material and placing the index fingers on each side of the key hole punch. Spread the hole wide enough to slip over the clamp. Stretch the hole over the anchor tooth and one side of the clamp, then expose the other clamp jaw so that the entire clamp and anchor tooth are exposed. Pull the safety line through the dam and drape to the side of the patient's mouth.
14. Isolate the most forward tooth, usually the opposite canine. The dam material is secured on the distal of this tooth with a double loop of floss, a corner cut of the dental dam material, or stabilizing cord.
15. Place the dental napkin around the patient's mouth.
16. Place the frame or holder to stretch the dam to cover the oral cavity. The frame can be placed either under or over the dental dam material, depending on the type of frame and the preference of the operator.
17. Isolate the remaining teeth, gently working the dental dam between the contacts with dental floss. When using the floss, catch the edge of the hole with the floss and pull it over the tooth, into and through the contact (Figure 23–3). Using the air syringe to dry the teeth at this time facilitates the placement of the dam material.
18. Invert or tuck the dam material. (The edge of the dam that surrounds the tooth must be inverted or tucked into the sulcus of the gingiva to seal the tooth and prevent leakage. There are several ways to do this. Carefully pull the dental dam material slightly apically, and the dam often inverts when it is released. When using the floss to place the dam interproximally, the dam may be inverted. Or, use a T-ball burnisher, a plastic instrument, or a spoon excavator to tuck the buccal and lingual surfaces. Use the instrument with the air from the air-water syringe to dry the surface and then invert the edge of the dam. Continue until all edges of the dam are sealed.

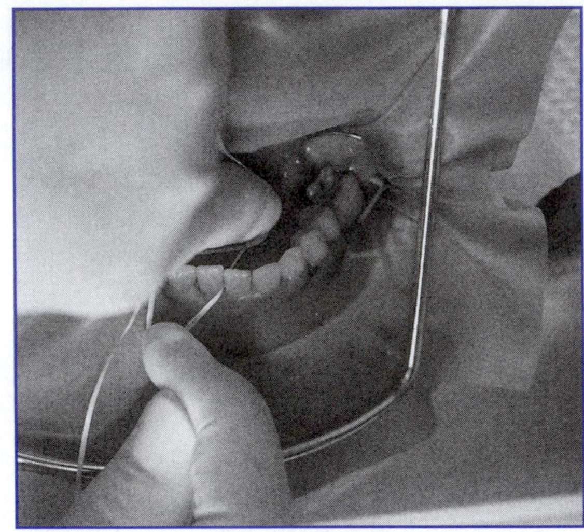

FIGURE 23–3 Dental assistant placing the dam between the contacts with floss.

19. Coat all tooth-colored restorations with lubricant.
20. Place and position a saliva ejector and/or a bite-block under the dam for patient comfort, if needed.
21. Double-check dam placement and patient comfort.

Alternate Technique for Placing Dental Dam

Some operators prefer to carry the clamp, dental dam material, and, in some placements, even the frame to the tooth when applying the clamp. This technique requires practice and confidence when placing the clamp but takes less time. The clamp is selected (usually a winged clamp), and the ligature is secured on the bow of the clamp. The bow of the clamp and the forcep holes on the jaws are exposed through the dental dam material. The clamp forceps are placed in the forcep holes and secured. The operator holds the rest of the dam material up and out of the way while placing the clamp and dam on the anchor tooth. After the clamp is secured on the tooth, the wings of the clamp are exposed and placement is completed following the procedure steps.

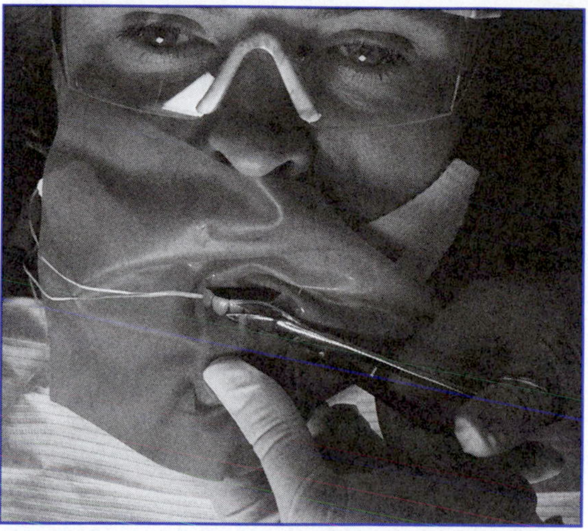

FIGURE 23–4 Pulling the dental dam material toward the facial, the operator cuts the interseptal dam.

Removal of Dental Dam

When the operator is ready to remove the dental dam, the area is rinsed and dried using the evacuator and the three-way syringe.

1. Explain to the patient the procedure to remove the dental dam and caution him or her not to bite down when the dam is removed.
2. Free the interseptal dam with scissors. To protect the patient, slip the index or middle finger underneath the dam material and stretch it facially, away from the tooth. Slant the scissors toward the occlusal surface, and clip each septum with the scissors (Figure 23–4). Pulling the dam material toward the facial, the operator cuts the interseptal dam.
3. Remove the dental dam clamp. Place the forceps in the clamp holes and squeeze the handles to open the clamp jaws. Usually, the clamp can be lifted straight off the tooth; however if this is not possible, rotate the clamp facially so the jaws clear the lingual and then rotate the clamp lingually to clear the buccal.
4. Remove the frame or holder and the dam material.
5. Remove the napkin, wiping the area around the mouth.
6. Examine the dam material by spreading the dental dam material out flat and examining to make certain that all the interseptal material is present. If any pieces are missing, floss between the teeth to dislodge any small segment of remaining dam.
7. Massage the gingiva around the anchor tooth to increase circulation of the area.
8. Rinse the patient's mouth thoroughly.

Preparation of a Tooth for Restoration

During the preparation of a tooth for an amalgam or a composite restoration, one or more axial surfaces are often removed. Once these surfaces are removed, the only way to restore the tooth is to have an artificial wall in place of the missing wall or surface. This wall holds the restorative materials in the preparation during the filling of the cavity. A matrix replaces the surface and acts as the artificial wall.

The **matrix** is a collective term used to refer to the matrix **band** and the **retainer**. The matrix band forms the missing surface or wall and reestablishes the normal contour of the prepared tooth while the tooth is being filled with the restorative material. The matrix band is inserted into the retainer and then placed on the tooth. The retainer is the device that holds the band. It is tightened on the tooth and secures the band in place.

In addition to replacing the missing tooth surface of the cavity preparation, the matrix restores the natural contours of the tooth and the proximal contact with the adjacent tooth. A matrix also contains the restorative material within the walls, thereby preventing any excess material from getting near the gingiva. The matrix must be stable enough to withstand the pressure of the restorative material being placed in the cavity preparation.

Types of Matrices

There are several different matrices available; the type selected depends upon the type of restorative materials being used. For amalgam restorations, the **Tofflemire matrix** or the **Automatrix** is used; for composite material, a **plastic strip matrix** or **shell matrix** is used.

WEDGES

Once the matrix is in place, a wedge (small, triangular piece of wood or plastic) is inserted interproximally against the matrix band or strip near the gingival margin of the preparation. This **wedge** holds the band securely in place and prevents excess filling material from escaping between the tooth and the matrix band.

Placement of Wedges

Wedges are only used when the preparation includes one or two proximal surfaces. For example, if the tooth has a mesiocclusal (MO) cavity, only one wedge would be required and it would be placed on the mesial. Either wooden or plastic wedges can be used on the posterior teeth. On the anterior teeth, where light-cured materials are used, plastic wedges are preferred.

On the posterior teeth, wedges are usually placed from the lingual. Cotton pliers or a hemostat is used to place and remove wedges. When placing the wedge, the smallest of the three sides is placed toward the gingiva.

TOFFLEMIRE MATRIX

The Tofflemire matrix is the most common matrix used for amalgam restorations. It has two parts: the retainer and the band (Figure 23–5).

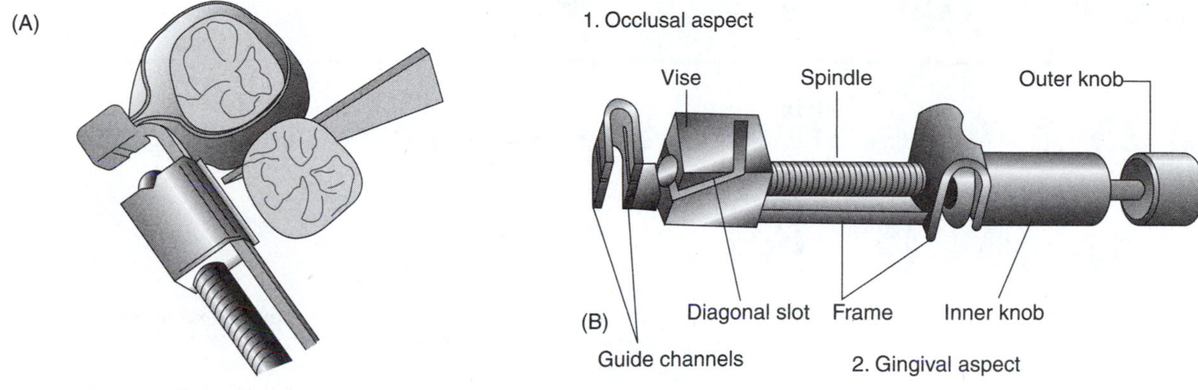

FIGURE 23–5 (A) Matrix and wedge in place. (B) Parts of the straight Tofflemire retainer: Guide channels, vise, diagonal slot, spindle, inner knob, outer knob, and frame. 1. Occlusal view. 2. Gingival view.

Parts of the Tofflemire Matrix Retainer

The Tofflemire matrix retainer has a top (occlusal) side and a bottom (gingival) side. The occlusal side is directed toward the occlusal surface and is the smooth side of the guide channels and the vise. The gingival side is directed toward the gingival tissues and has the diagonal slot on the vise and the open ends of the guide channels.

Matrix Bands

Matrix bands are made of stainless steel and are approximately all the same length. They differ in the shape of one edge and their widths. The size and shape of the cavity prep indicate which band is used (Procedure 23–2, 23–3 and 23–4).

- Hold the retainer with the guide channels and diagonal slot on the vise facing the operator.
- Keep the guide channels and the vise within one-quarter inch of each other.
- The looped matrix band correlates to the shape of the tooth, with the smaller circumference at the gingiva and the larger circumference at the occlusal.

Plastic Strip Matrix

The thin, transparent, strip matrix is used with composite, glass ionomer, or compomer restorative materials on anterior teeth (Procedures 23–5 and 23–6).

PROCEDURE

23-2 Assembly of the Tofflemire Matrix

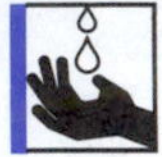 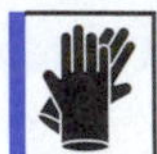 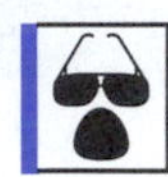 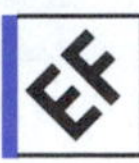

This procedure is performed by the dentist or dental assistant. The assembly is completed before the procedure begins.

EQUIPMENT AND SUPPLIES

- Tofflemire retainer
- Assortment of matrix bands
- Ball burnisher

PROCEDURE STEPS *(Follow aseptic procedures)*

1. Use a ball burnisher to soften the matrix.
2. Hold the retainer so the guide channels and the diagonal slot on the vise are facing the operator.
3. Holding the frame of the retainer, rotate the inner knob (adjustment knob) until the vise is within one-quarter inch of the guide channels.
4. Turn the outer knob (locking knob) until the pointed end of the spindle is clear (below) of the slot in the vise.
5. Prepare the matrix band for placement in the retainer by holding the band to look like a smile, with the gingival edge on the top and the occlusal edge on the bottom.
6. Bring the ends together to form a teardrop-shaped loop. Be careful not to crease the band at any time. The larger circumference of the band, the occlusal, will be on the bottom and the smaller, the gingival, will be on the top.
7. With the gingival edge still on the top, place the occlusal edge of the band in the diagonal slot of the vise. The loop is extended toward the guide channels.
8. Place the matrix band in the appropriate guide channels. The direction of the matrix band depends on the tooth being restored.

Hold the matrix retainer with the guide channel up, facing the operator and the matrix band looped. Then:

- If the matrix is to be applied to the maxillary right or mandibular left quadrant, place the matrix band in the guide channels toward the operator's right.
- If the matrix is to be applied to the maxillary left or mandibular right quadrant, place the matrix band in the guide channels toward the operator's left.

9. Once the band is placed in the vise slot with the guide channels, turn the outer knob until the tip of the spindle is tight against the band in the vise slot.
10. Move the inner knob to increase or decrease the size of the loop to match the diameter of the tooth.
11. If the band becomes creased or bent during the assembly, it can be smoothed out by inserting the handle of the mouth mirror into the loop and running it around the inside of the loop.

PROCEDURE

23-3 Placement of the Tofflemire Matrix

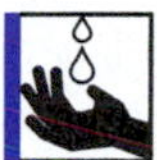
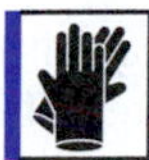
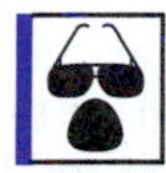
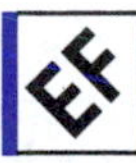

This procedure is performed by the dentist or dental assistant. After the Tofflemire matrix is assembled, it is ready for positioning on the prepared tooth.

EQUIPMENT AND SUPPLIES

- Assembled Tofflemire retainer and matrix band
- Cotton pliers or hemostat
- Ball burnisher
- 2 × 2 gauze sponges
- Assortment of wedges

PROCEDURE STEPS *(Follow aseptic procedures)*

1. Place the matrix band over the prepared tooth with the smaller edge of the band toward the gingiva. The slot on the vise is directed toward the gingiva. Keep the retainer parallel to the buccal surface as the loop is placed around the tooth.
2. Move the loop through the interproximal surface. Place one finger over the loop to stabilize the loop and the retainer.
3. Once the matrix band is around the tooth, adjust the guide channel to center the retainer on the buccal surface of the tooth.
4. Turn the inner knob to tighten the band around the tooth. The band should be securely around the tooth and the retainer should be snug to the tooth. If the band is too tight or too loose, the contour of the restoration may change the contours of the tooth and the proximal contact.
5. Check the margins of the matrix band. The band should extend no more than 1 to 1.5 mm beyond the gingival margin of the cavity preparation on the gingival edge, and the occlusal edge should extend no more than 2 mm above the highest cusp (Figure 23–6).

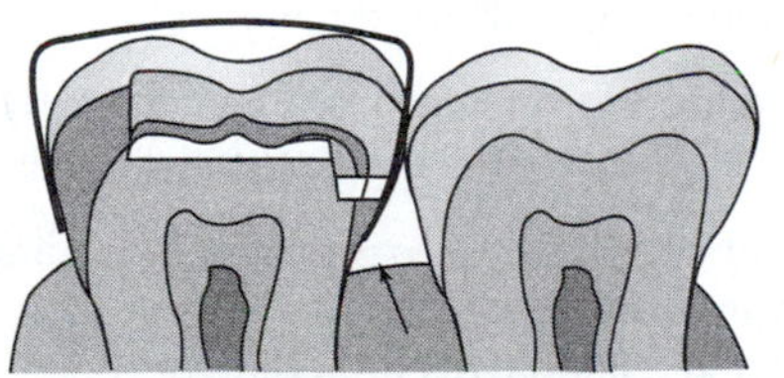
(A) Band should be tight near the gingival margin

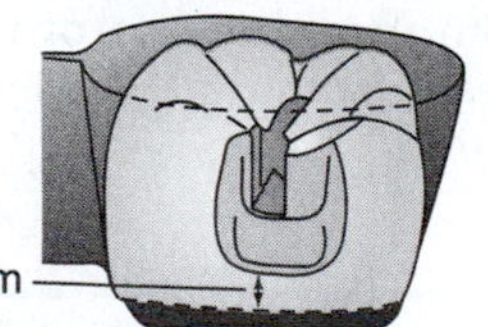

(B) Band should extend 1.0 to 1.5 mm beyond cavity preparation near the gingiva

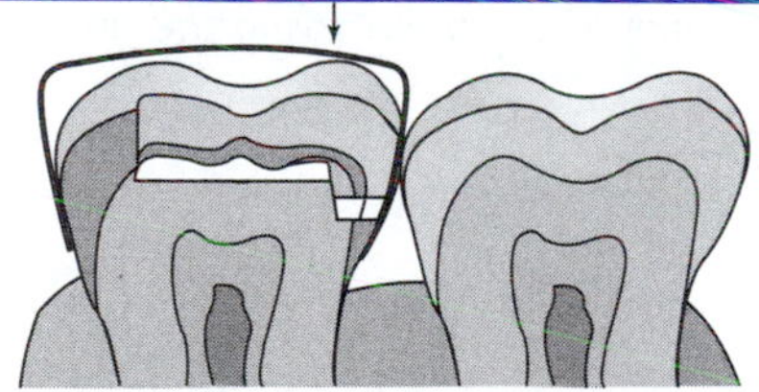
(C) Band should fit the circumference of the tooth near the occlusal surface

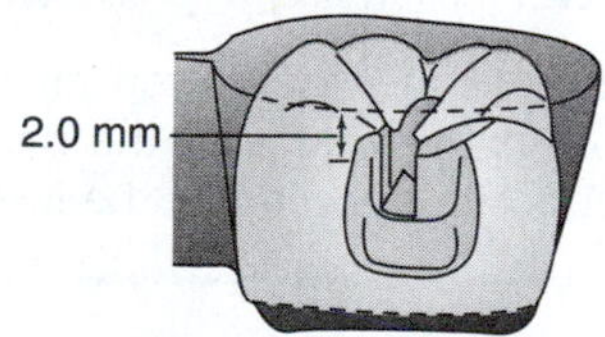

(D) Band should extend no more than 2 mm above the cusp of the tooth and occlusal ridge

FIGURE 23–6 Criteria for correct placement of the matrix band.

(continued)

PROCEDURE 23-1 *continued*

6. To ensure contact with the adjacent teeth, the band needs to be contoured. To accomplish this, use a ball burnisher. Place the burnisher on the inner surface of the band and apply pressure until the band becomes slightly concave at the contact area.
7. Once the matrix band has been placed on the tooth, a wedge(s) is (are) placed to stabilize the band at the gingival margin of the preparation. (Refer to Wedges for placement suggestions.)
8. Check the seal at the gingival margin of the preparation with an explorer. There should be no gap between the band and the preparation.

PROCEDURE

23-4 Removal of the Wedge(s) and Tofflemire Matrix

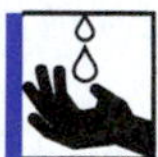
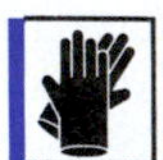
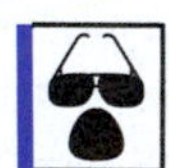
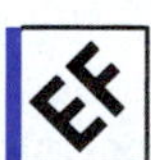

This procedure is performed by the dentist with the assistance of the dental assistant. Once the tooth has been filled with restorative material, the matrix and wedge are removed to finish carving the anatomy of the tooth.

EQUIPMENT AND SUPPLIES

- Cotton pliers or hemostat
- 2 × 2 gauze

PROCEDURE STEPS *(Follow aseptic procedures)*

1. To remove the wedge, use cotton pliers or a hemostat. Grasp the wedge at the base and pull in the opposite direction of the insertion.
2. To remove the retainer, hold the matrix in place with a finger on the occlusal surface, then turn the outer knob of the retainer to loosen the spindle in the vise.
3. Separate the retainer from the band by lifting the retainer toward the occlusal surface.
4. Using cotton pliers, gently free the band from around the tooth, then lift one end of the band in a lingual occlusal direction.
5. Lift the band from the proximal surface and repeat with the other end of the band. The tooth is ready for the final carving.

PROCEDURE

23-5 Placement of the Strip Matrix

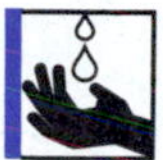 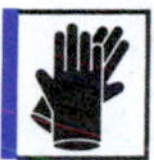 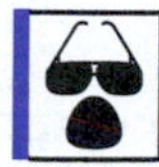 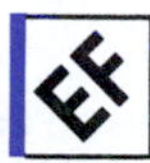

This procedure is performed by the dentist or the dental assistant. After the tooth has been prepared, the strip matrix is placed.

EQUIPMENT AND SUPPLIES

- Strip matrix
- Cotton pliers
- Mouth mirror
- Assortment of clear wedges

PROCEDURE STEPS *(Follow aseptic procedures)*

1. Contour the strip by drawing the strip over the rounded edge of the handle of the mouth mirror. The procedure is the same here as it is with the Tofflemire matrix band.
2. Place the strip matrix between the teeth. Hold the strip tightly and slide toward the gingiva.
3. Adjust the position of the strip so that the entire preparation is covered by the strip.
4. Seat the wedge to secure the strip in place.
5. Restorative materials are placed and the strip matrix is pulled tightly around the tooth to adapt the material to the convex surface of the tooth.
6. The strip matrix is held in place by hand or with a clip retainer until the material has been cured.

PROCEDURE

23-6 Removal of the Strip Matrix

 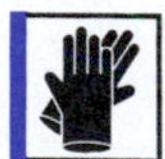 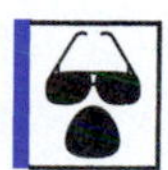 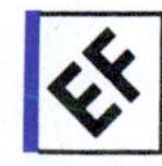

This procedure is performed by the dentist once the restorative material is placed and cured.

EQUIPMENT AND SUPPLIES

- Cotton pliers or hemostat
- 2 × 2 gauze sponges

PROCEDURE STEPS *(Follow aseptic procedures)*

1. Once the material has been cured and is completely hardened, remove the clip retainer, if one was used. Then, remove the wedges with cotton pliers.
2. The strip matrix is gently pulled away from the restorative material.
3. Remove the strip by pulling the matrix strip in a lingual incisal or facial incisal direction.

The strip can be made of nylon, acetate, celluloid, or resin and is approximately three inches long and three-eighths inch wide. The functions of the strip matrix are to:

- Provide anatomical contour and proximal contact relation
- Protect the restorative material from losing or gaining moisture during the setting time
- Allow the polymerizing light to reach the composite restorative material

CHAPTER 24

Gingival Retraction and Temporary Restorations

CDA

OBJECTIVES

The student should strive to meet the following objectives and demonstrate an understanding of the facts and principles presented in this chapter:

1. Explain the function of gingival retraction.
2. Describe the different types of gingival retraction.
3. Explain the steps of placing and removing gingival retraction cord.
4. Demonstrate the knowledge and skills necessary to contour prefabricated temporary crowns and to fabricate and fit temporary restorations.
5. Demonstrate the knowledge and skills necessary to fit aluminum crowns and custom self-cured composite temporary crowns.

KEY TERMS

direct matrix techniques (p. 410)
electrosurgery unit (p. 407)
gingival retraction (p. 404)
indirect matrix technique (p. 410)
ischemia (p. 405)
matrix (p. 410)

INTRODUCTION

After a tooth is prepared for a crown, **gingival retraction** is done to ensure that an impression with clear margins can be obtained. During this process, all hemorrage must be arrested and all the hard and soft tissue the operator wants reproduced must be clean and dry. The margins ideally are supragingival, or above the gingiva, however, many may be subgingival, or below the gingiva. The tissue must be retracted horizontally to allow room for sufficient impression material and displaced vertically to expose the margin completely. Retraction may be done chemically, mechanically, surgically, or in combination.

Retraction cord is available in a variety of sizes, configurations, and chemical treatments. The cord comes in a dispensing package for easy use. It may be twisted, braided, or woven to hold its shape.

TYPES OF GINGIVAL RETRACTION

Mechanical Retraction

Mechanical retraction can be accomplished in a number of ways. Without the use of drugs, tissue shrinkage or hemostasis is not accomplished; however, the tissue can be displaced to allow access to the margin. Retraction cord is placed in the sulcus of healthy and inflamed free gingiva. The cotton cord is left in place for ten to fifteen minutes (instead of the five minutes as it would be with chemical retraction cord).

If the cord is placed too deeply, the crevice opens at the bottom but is narrow at the top (Figure 24–1A). The operator may be able to get the impression material into the crevice after the cord is removed, but the material has a tendency to fracture near the edge of the preparation. If the cord is placed too shallowly in the crevice, the space is inadequate to allow an accurate reproduction of the margin of the preparation (Figure 24–1B). The proper position of the tucked cord is 1 to 3 mm into the V-shaped crevice (Figure 24–1C). The dentist may want two cords placed to retract the gingival tissues. The crevice is V shaped, and this dictates the size of cords to use. The smaller cords are placed at the depth of the crevice, and the larger cord is placed on top (Figure 24–1D).

Chemical Retraction

Chemical retraction (Procedure 24–1) may be done prior to the placement of the cord, or by impregnating the cord and then placing it, or both ways. One of the newer ways is to use a topical hemostatic solution, astringent with dentoinfusion tubes, and a plastic lure lock syringe. The solution is placed using a disposable metal tip bent to the desired area. As the solution is placed, the blood and the solution merge together and are washed away with the air-water

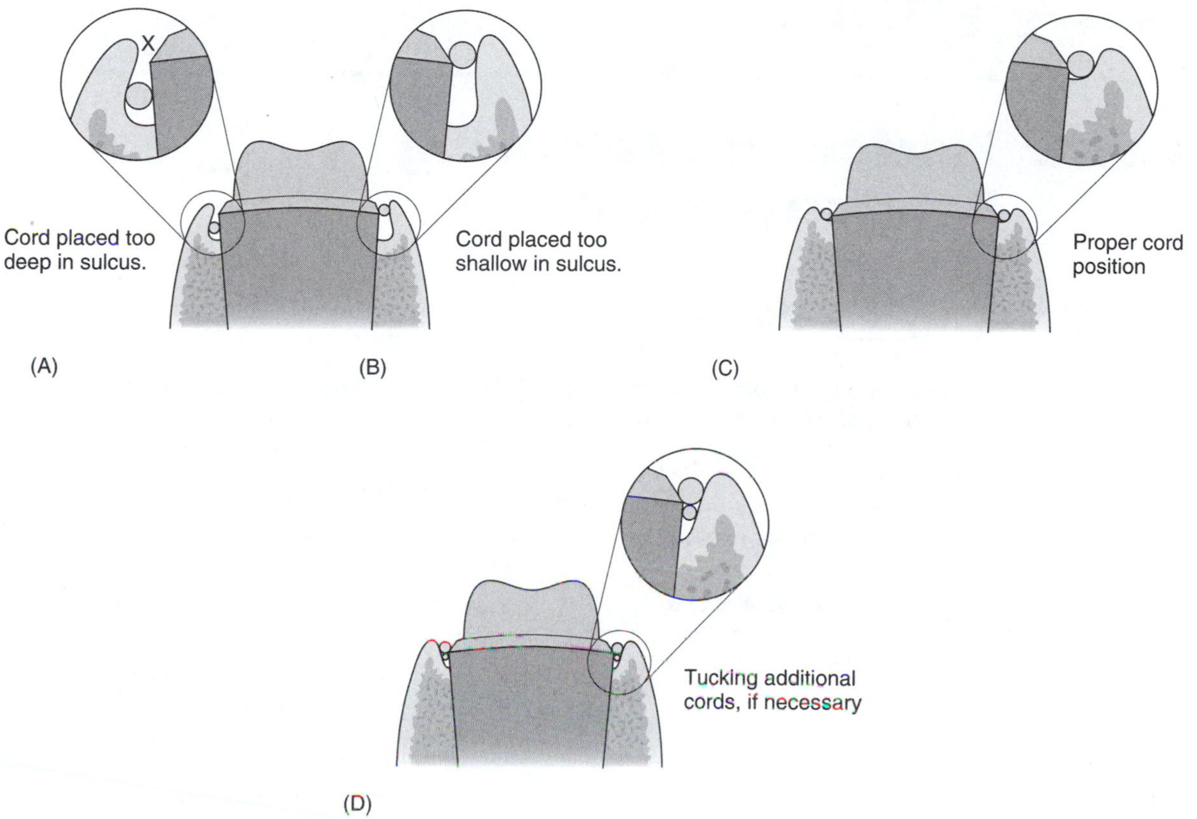

FIGURE 24–1 (A) Retraction cord placed too deeply. (B) Retraction cord placed too shallowly. (C) Retraction cord placed properly. (D) Double retraction cords placed properly.

syringe. What is left in the tissue is a temporary coagulum seal that does not allow any seepage. The tissue may appear slightly darkened, however this technique allows hemorrhage to be arrested. A retraction cord is packed vertically to expose the prepared margin. This packing of the cord allows for horizontal retraction to allow for sufficient bulk of impression material to flow around the margin.

The retraction cord could also be impregnated with aluminum chloride or astringent of aluminum salts for chemical retraction. This technique causes a shrinking of the tissues, or **ischemia**, to obtain clear access to the margin of the preparation. A substance used to obtain this result is epinephrine, which is an astringent and a vasoconstrictor. It provides hemostasis and shrinks the tissues by constricting the blood vessels. Epinephrine brings on an increase in the heart beat, or **tachycardia,** in some patients. The epinephrine is contraindicated for patients with heart disease, diabetes, or hyperthyroidism.

PROCEDURE

24-1 Placing and Removing Retraction Cord

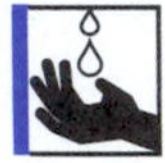
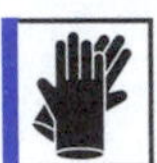
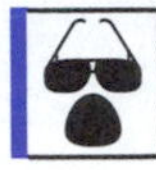
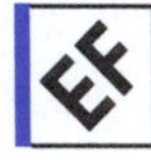

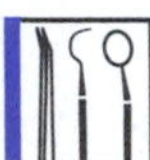

This procedure is performed by the dentist or the expanded-function dental assistant. After the tooth has been prepared, the retraction cord is placed. The equipment and supplies are included as part of the crown/bridge tray setup. The specific items needed to place and remove the retraction cord are listed.

EQUIPMENT AND SUPPLIES

- Basic setup: Mouth mirror, explorer, cotton pliers
- HVE tip and air-water syringe tip
- Scissors
- Hemostat
- Retraction cord(s)
- Retraction cord placement instrument or plastic instrument
- Cotton rolls, 2 × 2 gauze sponges

PROCEDURE STEPS *(Follow aseptic procedures)*

1. The dentist prepares the tooth for the crown.
2. Rinse and dry the area in preparation for placement of the retraction cord.
3. Cotton rolls are placed on the facial surface and, if mandibular, on the lingual surface. The area is carefully dried.
4. The dentist selects the retraction cord(s) to be placed around the tooth.
5. The length of the cord needed is determined by the circumference of the prepared tooth.

NOTE: The desired length is determined by wrapping the cord around the small finger for an anterior tooth and around a larger finger for a molar.

6. The cord is cut to the appropriate length.
7. Twist the cord ends to compress the fibers together.
8. The cord is looped and placed in a hemostat or cotton pliers.
9. The cord is looped around the margin of the prepared tooth and tightened slightly. This facilitates slipping the cord into the sulcus area. Normally, the ends of the cord are toward the buccal surface for easy access.
10. The hemostat or cotton pliers is/are released, leaving the cord in the sulcus.
11. The retraction cord is packed into position with a packing instrument or a plastic instrument.
12. The cord is gently packed around the cervical area, apical to the preparation.
13. The cord is packed around the tooth and overlaps, usually on the facial surface.
14. A tip of the cord is left showing out of the sulcus for easy removal just prior to taking the impression.
15. The retraction cord is left in place for five minutes when chemical retraction cord is used and for ten to fifteen minutes for mechanical retraction.
16. The end of the retraction cord is grasped and removed in a circular motion just prior to the impression material being placed.

NOTE: The dental assistant should watch for patients who exhibit hypertension, knowing that most hyperthyroid and diabetic patients are usually hypertensive. Usually, the dentist prefers to use chemical retraction cord, thus, the patient's medical history should be reviewed carefully.

Surgical Retraction

Instead of retraction, the dentist may choose to remove the tissue around the preparation. This approach is accomplished by using a surgical knife or by performing electrosurgery. With the surgical knife, the dentist excises the tissue and exposes the margin of the preparation. The area where the tissue has been removed may bleed and cause additional treatment to get a good impression of the area.

The dentist may decide to use an **electrosurgery unit**, which cauterizes the tissues as it removes them. After the tissue is removed, the sulcus is cleaned with a hydrogen rinse. Immediately following the procedure, the final impression is taken.

Temporary (Provisional) Restorations

After a tooth has been prepared for a crown and prior to the seating of the crown, a temporary restoration must be adapted and temporarily cemented on the tooth to protect it in the interim. These temporary restorations stabilize and protect the tooth during the time required to make the crown(s) or bridge(s) during the time requested.

Temporary Restoration Criteria

- The temporary restoration is comfortable and esthetically acceptable to the patient.
- The temporary restoration remains stable, with proper mesial and distal contacts and occlusal alignment, until the permanent crown is cemented.
- The temporary restoration is easily removed, without damaging the tooth, when the permanent restoration is ready for placement.
- The temporary restoration fits snugly and accurately along the prepared margin of the tooth. There is less than ½ mm of space between the temporary restoration and the finish line of the margin.
- The temporary restoration is contoured in a similar fashion to the original tooth, therefore protecting the gingiva from irritation and interproximal areas from food impaction.

Types of Temporary Restorations

Temporary restorations, also known as provisional restorations, can be made of a number of materials, both custom and preformed. In many states, the function of fabricating and placing a temporary restoration is delegated to the dental assistant under the supervision of the dentist. Most offices use preformed aluminum and acrylic crowns, along with custom acrylic or composite crowns.

Preformed Aluminum Temporary Crowns

Preformed aluminum temporary crowns are supplied in different sizes and anatomic features. They are used on the posterior teeth because they lack esthetic value. Some are made without any anatomy and resemble thimbles with parallel straight sides and flat occlusal surfaces. More contouring is necessary to adapt this model to the tooth (Procedure 24–2). Both can be filled with acrylic or composite material to obtain a more custom fit prior to setting the temporary restorations in place over the prepared teeth.

PROCEDURE

24-2 Sizing, Adapting, and Seating an Aluminum Temporary Crown

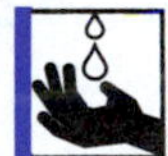
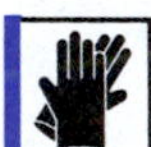
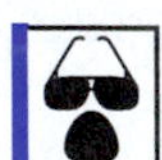
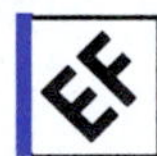
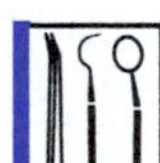

This procedure is performed by the dentist or the dental assistant at the dental unit after a tooth has been prepared for a crown.

EQUIPMENT AND SUPPLIES

- Maxillary and/or mandibular selection of aluminum temporary crowns
- Millimeter ruler
- Basic setup: Mouth mirror, cotton pliers, and explorer
- Crown and collar scissors
- Contouring pliers
- Acrylic or composite temporary material (optional)
- Sandpaper discs, rubber wheel, and mandrel
- Temporary cement, pad, and spatula
- Articulating paper
- Dental floss

PROCEDURE STEPS *(Follow aseptic procedures)*

1. Measure the available space for the temporary crown from the mesial to distal with the millimeter ruler.
2. Determine the correct crown to try in. The aluminum crown is for the correct tooth in the dentition and the size is chosen according to the measurement taken with the millimeter ruler. (Prevent cross-contamination while tak-

ing the crown from the container. Do not use contaminated instruments.) Any crown tried that does not fit must be sterilized before replacing it in the selection tray.

3. Try the selected crown on the prepared tooth and check for mesial and distal width. The crown will be above the occlusal plane at this time.
4. The length of the crown is determined by placing the aluminum crown over the prepared tooth and using an explorer to mark the height. Another way to do this is to scribe the tooth at the occlusal surface where it aligns with the other teeth on the arch and then taking that amount off the gingival area. Either method shows that the margin of the gingival needs to be trimmed to fit.
5. Using a crown and collar scissors (with curved blades), trim the gingival margin. Crowns are never straight across the surface but are longer on the buccal and lingual margins. Use the rounded edges of the scissors to trim.

NOTE: Trimming a small amount at first allows refitting to further check the desired result (Figure 24-2). Taking too much off renders the crown useless. Making several trims to get the desired effect is a better method. Using the scissors in a continuous cutting action gives a much smoother surface. Avoid sharp, uneven edges that cause the patient discomfort around the gingival surface.

6. After the desired length is achieved, use the contouring pliers to invert the gingival edge in an inward manner. This crimping aids in the adaptation of the circumference edge of the aluminum crown to the finish line of the preparation.
7. Smoothing of the rough and jagged edges is done with sandpaper discs and a rubber wheel. Check that all edges are smooth and polished.
8. Place the aluminum crown on the prepared tooth and check the occlusion with the articulating paper and the contacts with dental floss.

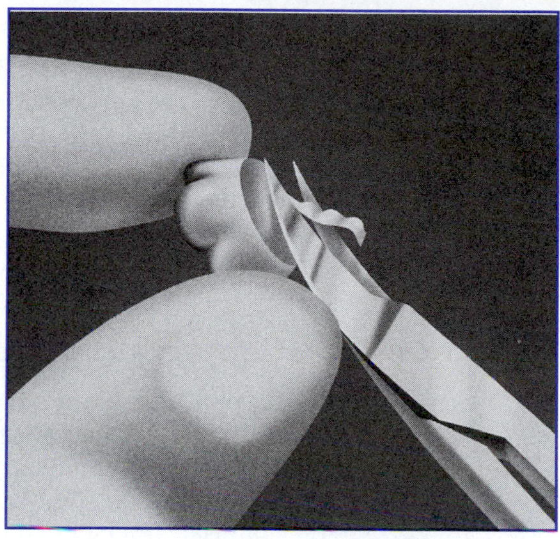

FIGURE 24–2 The aluminum crown is trimmed with crown and collar scissors. (*Courtesy of 3M Dental Products Division*)

NOTE: If the contacts are weak, use a burnisher on the inside to extend the crown outward to get a better contact.

9. If an acrylic or a composite lining is used, the crown is filled with the material and placed on the prepared tooth. The patient is asked to bite into normal occlusion.

NOTE: The tooth may require light lubrication with petroleum jelly to avoid retention of the material.

The material sets according to manufacturer's directions and is then removed. Any excess material is polished away.

NOTE: Some operators prefer to do this step earlier in the procedure.

10. A final check for marginal fit, contour, and occlusion is done before cementation takes place.

Preformed Acrylic Temporary Crown

Preformed acrylic or plastic temporary crowns are available in different sizes, shapes, and shades. The advantage of this type of crown is that it is more esthetically pleasing for anterior use. The plastic temporary crown is a form used to match the appropriate shape and contour of the tooth. It is filled with acrylic material and then removed. The preformed acrylic crowns have tabs on the incisal edge for easy placement. These tabs are removed prior to cementation. The preformed acrylic crowns (Procedure 24–3) are used more easily because they require little adjustment and can be seated immediately.

Custom Acrylic or Composite Temporary Restorations

When making custom acrylic or composite temporary restorations (Procedure 24–4), a matrix is used. The matrix can be direct or indirect. A **matrix** is a form shaped in the pattern of the tooth prior to preparing the tooth. **Direct matrix techniques** (making the matrix directly from the tooth) uses alginate, impression material, freehand (block) technique, wax, thermo-forming beads, or a thermo-plastic button in the matrix. The **indirect matrix technique** (making the matrix on a model or cast) utilizes wax, a vacuum-formed shell, and thermo-forming bead and button matrices.

The alginate and impression materials render more anatomically accurate temporaries. The other materials meet the criteria for a temporary restoration form adequately and may prove to be less costly and more easily made. The utility wax is heated in warm water and then formed over the tooth or model to obtain the shape of the tooth and then cooled. Thermo-forming beads and buttons are heated in hot water and formed on the tooth prior to preparation or on a cast when using the indirect matrix technique. The vacuum-formed shell is made on a vacuum unit using a cast covered with very thin sheets of acrylic resin. After it is heated, this sheet is cut to the desired size for use in making the temporary restoration.

Matrix Used for Direct Technique in Making Temporary Restorations

- Alginate impression
- Impression material
- Freehand (making a block of the material and covering the prepared tooth)
- Wax
- Thermo-forming beads or buttons

Matrix Used for Indirect Technique in Making Temporary Restorations)

- Wax
- Thermo-forming beads or buttons
- Vacuum-formed shell

PROCEDURE

24-3 Sizing, Adapting, and Seating a Preformed Acrylic Crown

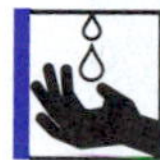
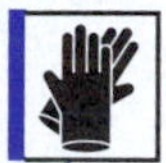
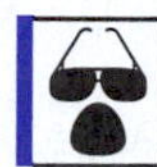

This procedure is performed by the dentist or the dental assistant after the preformed acrylic provisional has been prepared, sized, and contoured to the prepared tooth.

EQUIPMENT AND SUPPLIES

- Maxillary and/or mandibular selection of acrylic temporary crowns
- Mirror, explorer, and cotton pliers
- Acrylic or composite temporary material (optional)
- Acrylic bur
- Temporary cement, pad, and spatula
- Articulating paper
- Dental floss
- Saliva ejector

PROCEDURE STEPS *(Follow aseptic procedures)*

Preparing the Preformed Acrylic Temporary Restoration

1. After the tooth has been prepared for a crown, a preformed acrylic temporary restoration is selected and adapted. Choose a crown that has enough width to contact on the adjacent teeth, is long enough to be in proper occlusion, and is the correct shade.
2. Retrieve this crown without cross-contaminating the other acrylic crowns. The tab at the incisal edge allows the operator to try the crown over the prepared tooth.
3. If necessary, adjustments are made with an acrylic bur. Polish with a rag wheel and pumice.
4. Remove the tag, place the crown, and check the occlusion with articulating paper.
5. Make adjustments, if necessary, and again polish the adjustment areas for a smooth surface for patient comfort.

Cementing the Acrylic Provisional Crown

1. The prepared tooth is rinsed and dried with cotton rolls in place.
2. Temporary cement such as zinc oxide eugenol, is mixed with a spatula and placed in the preformed acrylic crown.
3. The preformed acrylic crown is placed in position over the prepared tooth and the patient is asked to bite in occlusion or the operator holds the crown in place until the cement is set.

NOTE: Some operators like the patient to bite on a cotton roll over the preformed acrylic crown while the cement sets.

4. After the cement is set, remove the excess with an explorer.
5. The contacts are checked with floss and the margins are inspected to determine all the excess cement has been removed and that the crown fits correctly.
6. A final check for occlusion is done with articulating paper.
7. Instructions are given to the patient for care of the temporary preformed acrylic crown.

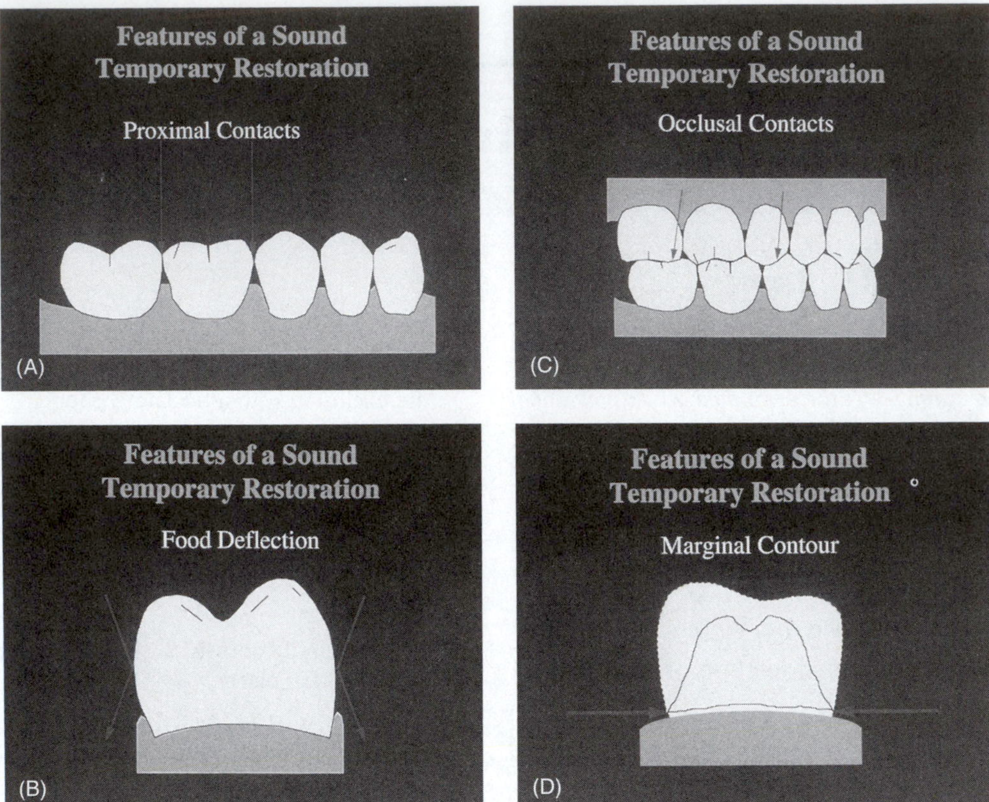

FIGURE 24–3 Criteria for a custom acrylic or composite temporary restoration. (A) Good proximal contacts. (B) Good occlusal contacts. (C) Good food deflection. (D) Good marginal contours. (*Courtesy of 3M Dental Products Division*)

A custom acrylic or composite temporary restoration must have good proximal contacts, good occlusal contacts, good food deflection, and good marginal contours (Figures 24–3A through D).

Self-Cure Methyl Methacrylate. There are several categories of materials that achieve the desired outcome of a custom temporary restoration. One of the older materials that is routinely used is the methyl methacrylates. The advantages of this material are that it has good physical properties, good esthetics, better color stability than the R'methacrylates, and a lower cost. The disadvantages are the strong odor, high shrinkage, and high exothermic heat given off during the self-cure chemical setting.

Self-Cure R'Methacrylate. The R' (resin) methacrylates have one of the active ingredients, such as vinyl, ethyl, or isobutyl, in place of the methyl. In comparison with methyl methacrylates, they exhibit less shrinkage and give off a lower level of exothermic heat during the self-cure chemical setting. They are similar in cost, are the weakest of the methacrylates, have poor color stability, and have the same strong odor as methyl methacrylates.

Both the methyl and the R'methacrylates are supplied in a powder and liquid that are mixed together to form a creamy mass. After mixing, they are allowed to condition for approximately thirty seconds and are then placed in the matrix. A dull surface appears on the top of the material; it is placed in the mouth over the prepared tooth and held in place for the initial set. At this time the material takes on a rubbery appearance. Most manufacturers suggest the material be alternately placed on and removed from the prepared tooth during the four to six minutes, when the degree of exothermic heat is the greatest. The excess can be trimmed off easily using scissors. The final set takes place in six to eight minutes and the material becomes hard plastic. The range of setting time from start to finish is eight to ten minutes. The temporary restorations are removed from the matrix and trimmed with an acrylic bur to the desired shape and size (see Figures 24–3A through D for criteria).

After the temporary has been trimmed, it is polished with pumice and a rag wheel. Some of the materials in this category come with glazes. This glaze is applied after the polishing and allowed to dry for five minutes before the temporary is cemented.

Self-Cure Composite Material. Materials in the category of self-cure composite are double the price of the methacrylates. They are much stronger because they are made as composites and not plastics. They do not have the odor, the shrinkage, or the exothermic reaction during setting, and they have excellent color stability.

Materials in this category are supplied in two pastes, either in two tubes or in a cartridge that fits into extruding guns with auto mixing tips. Both the tubes and the cartridge tips must remain clean and flowing to obtain the correct dispensed amount of the material. If they become clogged, use an explorer to clear the old material out. Dispense a small, pea-shaped amount on the pad before beginning to ensure that everything is working properly.

The material is placed in the matrix and over the prepared tooth for up to two minutes. During the rubber stage (from four to six minutes), it is removed from the mouth to complete curing. The total time from start to finish for this material classification is up to seven minutes. After the material is set, the surface has a greasy layer due to the oxygen in the air, which can be removed with alcohol or any organic solvent. The trimming is done with a diamond bur and no polish is necessary. If additional material is required on the temporary, light-cured composite can be used and trimmed accordingly. After completing the temporary, cement in place with a temporary luting cement (Procedure 24–5).

PROCEDURE

24-4 Adapting, Trimming, and Seating a Matrix and Custom Temporary Restoration

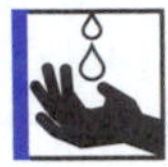
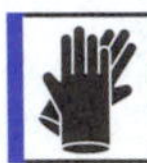
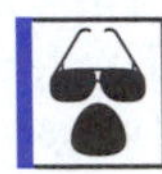
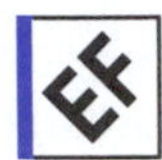
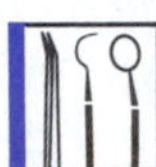

This procedure is performed by the dentist or the dental assistant at the dental unit after the tooth has been prepared for a crown.

EQUIPMENT AND SUPPLIES

- Basic setup: Mouth mirror, explorer, and cotton pliers
- Thermo-plastic buttons/hot water (one possible option for use in making a matrix)
- Composite temporary material
- Diamond bur
- Temporary cement, pad, and spatula
- Articulating paper
- Dental floss

PROCEDURE STEPS *(Follow aseptic procedures)*

Making the Thermo-Forming Matrix Prior to the Tooth Preparation

1. Place the thermo-forming matrix buttons in hot water (one button per prepared tooth).
2. Allow the white or blue color of the button to become clear. When that takes place, the material is pliable and able to be adapted.
3. Adapt the material over the tooth and tightly conform it to the tooth area and slightly below the gingival.
4. When the material cools (air can be used to make this more rapid), the matrix appears milky colored and firm. Remove the matrix from the area and set it aside.

Preparing the Custom Temporary Restoration

1. After the tooth has been prepared for a crown, coat the teeth with a light application of petroleum jelly.
2. If using the composite self-curing temporary material in two tubes, dispense on the paper pad by holding tubes at a 45° angle.
3. Rotate the end-dispensing handle of the base until a click is heard. (The base is the larger of the two tubes. The smaller of the two holds the catalyst and has two dispensing ends.) Rotate the end-dispensing handle of the catalyst. Two small amounts are expelled. Each click of the dispensing handle is enough material for one temporary.
4. If a shade is being used, mix it with the base. If a mottled effect is desired, mix the shade after the base and catalyst are mixed together.
5. Mix the material together to obtain a creamy substance (about thirty seconds).
6. Place the material in the matrix.
7. Place the matrix over the prepared tooth (manipulation time is about one and one-half minutes).
8. Hold it in place in the mouth for two minutes.

9. Remove it from the mouth and set it aside for two minutes.
10. Remove the crown or bridge from the matrix. The additional curing time takes one minute. There are seven minutes total time from start to finish of the set.
11. Remove the greasy layer with alcohol or any other organic solvent.
12. Trim with a diamond or an acrylic bur (Figure 24–4).
13. Check the contacts with dental floss.
14. Check the occlusion by having the patient bite on the articulating paper.
15. Check the margins with the explorer and mirror.

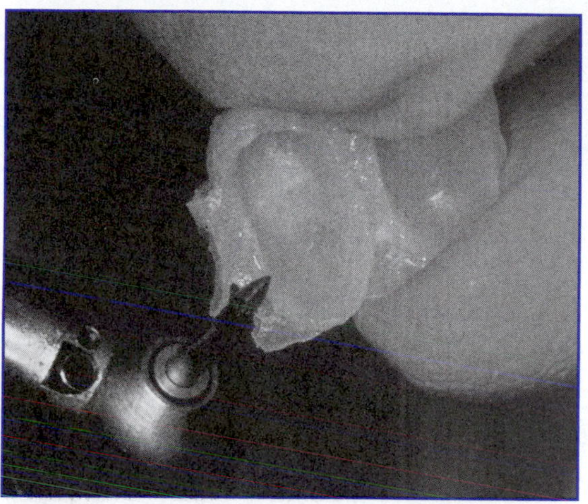

FIGURE 24–4 Trimming the temporary.

Multi-Cured Temporary Materials. Several multi-cured temporary materials are on the market. They have extended working time in the rubbery stage and improved operator control because they can be light cured on demand. They have good strength and are higher in cost. Some of the materials in this group are methacrylates and some are composites having the characteristics of the self-curing materials. The biggest advantage of this group is light-curing control, which allows for a quicker set and unlimited setting time.

PROCEDURE

24-5 Cementing the Custom Self-Curing Composite Temporary Crown

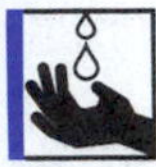 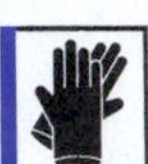 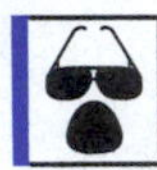 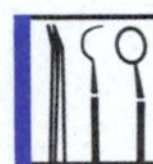

This procedure is performed by the dentist or the dental assistant at the dental unit after the temporary restoration has been prepared and is ready to be cemented in place over the prepared tooth.

EQUIPMENT AND SUPPLIES

- Basic setup: Mouth mirror, explorer, and cotton pliers
- Cotton rolls
- Temporary luting cement
- Paper pad
- Mixing spatula
- Plastic filling instrument
- Dental floss

PROCEDURE STEPS *(Follow aseptic procedures)*

1. The prepared tooth is rinsed and dried with cotton rolls in place.
2. The temporary cement material is mixed with a spatula and placed in the custom composite temporary crown.
3. The temporary crown is placed in position over the prepared tooth and the patient is asked to bite in occlusion or the operator will hold the crown in place until the cement is set.

NOTE: Some operators like the patient to bite on a cotton roll over the preformed acrylic crown while the cement sets.

4. After the cement is set, the excess is removed with an explorer.
5. The contacts are checked with floss and the margins are inspected to determine whether all excess cement has been removed and whether the crown fits correctly.
6. A final check for occlusion is done with articulating paper.
7. Instructions are given to the patient for care of the temporary preformed acrylic crown.

INDEX